Neuroanesthesia:
Handbook
of Clinical and
Physiologic Essentials

Neuroanesthesia: Handbook of Clinical and Physiologic Essentials

SECOND EDITION

Edited by

Philippa Newfield, M.D.

Assistant Clinical Professor of Anesthesia and Neurosurgery, University of California, San Francisco, School of Medicine, San Francisco; Attending Anesthesiologist, Children's Hospital of Los Angeles, Los Angeles

James E. Cottrell, M.D.

Professor and Chairman, Department of Anesthesiology, State University of New York Health Science Center at Brooklyn, College of Medicine, Brooklyn

Foreword by Charles B. Wilson, M.D.

Professor and Chairman, Department of Neurological Surgery, University of California, San Francisco, School of Medicine, San Francisco

Little, Brown and Company
Boston/Toronto/London

Library of Congress Catalog Card No. 91-60326

ISBN 0-316-60471-2

Printed in the United States of America

RRD-VA

To Maurice Albin, M.D.,
whose unfailing adherence to a single standard
of clinical and scientific excellence has been
an inspiration to anesthesiologists and
neurosurgeons the world over

Contents

Foreword

Writing a foreword to the second edition of this book became a pleasant assignment because I could dispense with the qualifications in my foreword to the first edition. Today, one hardly needs to "justify" neuroanesthesia, and anyone with half a wit knows that neurosurgery depends on neuroanesthesia as much as the central nervous system depends on the heart and lungs.

Drs. Cottrell and Newfield have correlated, modified, and updated the first handbook of neuroanesthesia. If you do not have the first edition, you will miss nothing if you acquire this edition. For those of you who did obtain the first edition, this edition is even better. The editors have done a first-rate job in revising, and I was very pleased to be asked for a foreword to it.

Charles B. Wilson, M.D.

Preface

With the second edition of *Neuroanesthesia: Handbook of Clinical and Physiologic Essentials,* the editors are gratified to note two significant developments. First, the original concept of this book—written for both anesthesiologists and neurosurgeons, to provide a convenient, accessible compendium of the many facets of clinical neuroanesthesia and the scientific foundations on which they are based—has been realized. This book has come to enjoy a valued place in the libraries of trainees and practitioners alike because the information regarding perioperative management and the effects on cerebral pathophysiology is presented clearly, concisely, and authoritatively, with current references.

The other source of gratification is the fact that the second edition contains new as well as updated information reflecting the scientific and medical progress that has been made in the neurosciences. Newly detailed in this edition are research on cerebral protection and its application to clinical care, management of anesthesia for the latest neurodiagnostic and interventional neurotherapeutic modalities, treatment of vasospasm after subarachnoid hemorrhage, and recent advances in the treatment of patients with ischemic cerebrovascular disease. The effect of anesthetics on cerebral physiology and electrophysiologic monitoring of the brain and spinal cord are revisited in light of the development of new anesthetic drugs, new equipment, and the evolution of standards for intraoperative monitoring of the central nervous system.

The chapters in the second edition are divided into three areas: General Considerations, Intensive Care, and Anesthetic Management. Discussions of cerebral physiology, blood flow and metabolism, electrophysiologic monitoring, and cerebral protection and resuscitation are included in General Considerations. Intensive Care addresses respiratory and cardiovascular management as well as fluid and electrolyte balance in the neurosurgical patient.

Both neurosurgeons and anesthesiologists contributed to the section on the anesthetic management of neurosurgical problems, such as tumors of the pituitary and posterior fossa, trauma to the head and spinal cord, intracranial aneurysms, ischemic cerebrovascular disease, neurovascular lesions in pregnancy, and neurogenic airway and swallowing disorders. Consideration of pediatric neurosurgery merits a separate chapter because children, despite their smaller size, require care equal to that accorded adults in terms of their monitoring needs and the effects of anesthetics on cerebral pathophysiology. Indeed, adequate monitoring, adequate intravenous access, and prompt restoration of blood volume figure prominently among the hallmarks of pediatric neuroanesthesia. The discussion of anesthesia for the diagnostic and therapeutic procedures performed by neuroradiologists is significant because the same anesthetic judgment and precautions exercised in the operating room must be observed in other locations, as well. The selection of anesthetic drugs for monitored anesthesia care in the neuroradiology suite is based on their effect on intracranial dynamics, just as it is for general anesthesia for the definitive operation in the operating suite.

That neurosurgeons as well as anesthesiologists have contributed to this book reflects a factor of paramount importance: Consultation, collaboration, and communication between the two specialties have improved the perioperative care of patients who have complicated neurosurgical problems. This spirit of mutual cooperation and regard is equally important in the management of secondary neurological injuries and postoperative sequelae.

Sophisticated monitoring for all neurosurgical patients, now an integral part of perioperative management, is essential to the identification of problematic trends at an early stage, the facilitation of rapid intervention, and the prevention of catastrophe. Because of the complexity of many neurosurgical operations, the information generated by direct measurement of arterial, central venous, pulmonary artery, pulmonary capillary wedge, and intracranial pressure has become central to the perioperative decision making. The principles and techniques of monitoring the evoked potentials, electroencephalogram, and cerebral blood flow and metabolism, as described in the book, also provide valuable data that can be used to guide intraoperative care.

None of these advances would have been possible, however, without the intellectual curiosity and uncompromising resolve to deliver the best possible care evinced by the specialists involved in the treatment of neurosurgical patients. We wish to acknowledge the authors who have so generously contributed to this book and all neuroanesthesiologists who have worked to disseminate the principles of the safe and enlightened practice of neuroanesthesia. We would also like to recognize the cooperation and support of the neurosurgeons, neuroradiologists, neuropathologists, and neuroophthalmologists with whom we enjoy a close working relationship. The willingness of the specialists in each of these disciplines to share knowledge, information, and responsibility accounts for the concerned and informed care that neurosurgical patients enjoy.

PN
JEC

Contributing Authors

A. Elisabeth Abramowicz, M.D.
Assistant Professor, Department of Anesthesiology, State University of New York Health Science Center at Brooklyn College of Medicine, Brooklyn

Robert F. Bedford, M.D.
Clinical Professor of Anesthesiology, University of Virginia School of Medicine; Attending Anesthesiologist, Martha Jefferson Hospital, Charlottesville

Audree A. Bendo, M.D.
Assistant Professor and Director of Neuroanesthesia, Department of Anesthesiology, State University of New York Health Science Center at Brooklyn College of Medicine, Brooklyn

Derek A. Bruce, M.B., Ch.B.
Clinical Assistant Professor, University of Texas Southwestern Medical School; Director, Pediatric Neurosurgical Institute, Humana Advanced Surgical Institutes, Dallas

Neal H. Cohen, M.D., M.P.H.
Professor of Clinical Anesthesia and Medicine, and Vice Chairman, Department of Anesthesia, University of California, San Francisco, School of Medicine; Director, Intensive Care Unit, The Medical Center at the University of California, San Francisco

Peter S. Colley, M.D.
Associate Professor of Anesthesiology, University of Washington School of Medicine; Chief of Neurosurgical Anesthesia, University Hospital, Seattle

James E. Cottrell, M.D.
Professor and Chairman, Department of Anesthesiology, State University of New York Health Science Center at Brooklyn College of Medicine, Brooklyn

Khurshed J. Dastur, M.D.
Attending Neuroradiologist, Department of Diagnostic Radiology, Mercy Hospital, Pittsburgh

Judith Donegan, M.D., Ph.D.
Professor of Anesthesiology, Medical College of Wisconsin; Attending Anesthesiologist, Froedtert Memorial Lutheran Hospital, Milwaukee

Elizabeth A. M. Frost, M.B., Ch.B.
Professor of Anesthesiology, Albert Einstein College of Medicine of Yeshiva University; Attending Anesthesiologist, Bronx Municipal Hospital Center, New York

Joseph P. Giffin, M.D.
Assistant Professor of Anesthesia, State University of New York Health Science Center at Brooklyn College of Medicine; Clinical Director of Anesthesia, Kings County Hospital Center, Brooklyn

Betty L. Grundy, M.D.
Professor of Anesthesiology, University of Florida College of Medicine; Chief, Anesthesiology Service, Veterans Administration Medical Center, Gainesville

Kenneth Grush, M.D.

John Hartung, Ph.D.
Research Associate Professor, Department of Anesthesiology, State University of New York Health Science Center at Brooklyn College of Medicine, Brooklyn

William D. Hetrick, M.D.
Clinical Assistant Professor of Anesthesiology, University of Pittsburgh School of Medicine; Staff Anesthesiologist, Mercy Hospital, Pittsburgh

Andrew Karlin, M.D.
Assistant Professor of Anesthesiology, State University of New York Health Science Center at Brooklyn College of Medicine; Clinical Director, Department of Anesthesiology, Kings County Hospital Center, Brooklyn

Ira Kass, Ph.D.
Associate Professor, Department of Anesthesiology, State University of New York Health Science Center at Brooklyn College of Medicine, Brooklyn

Jane Matjasko, M.D.
Professor and Chairman, Department of Anesthesiology, University of Maryland School of Medicine; Chief of Anesthesiology Services, University Hospital, Baltimore

Robert D. McKay, M.D.
Clinical Associate Professor of Surgery, East Tennessee State University Quillen-Dishner College of Medicine; Staff Anesthesiologist, Bristol Memorial Hospital, Johnson City, Tennessee

Frederick G. Mihm, M.D.
Associate Professor of Clinical Anesthesia, Stanford University School of Medicine; Associate Director, Intensive Care Units, Stanford University Hospital, Stanford

Philippa Newfield, M.D.
Assistant Clinical Professor of Anesthesia and Neurosurgery, University of
California, San Francisco, School of Medicine, San Francisco; Attending
Anesthesiologist, Children's Hospital of Los Angeles, Los Angeles

Mark F. Newman, M.D.
Chief, Cardiothoracic Anesthesia, and Director of Anesthesia Research,
Department of Anesthesiology, Wilford Hall USAF Medical Center, San
Antonio

S. J. Peerless, M.D., F.R.C.S. (C.)
Professor of Neurosurgery, University of Miami School of Medicine;
Attending Surgeon and Director, Institute of Cerebrovascular Disease,
Jackson Memorial Hospital, Miami

Kalmon D. Post, M.D.
Associate Professor and Vice-Chairman, Department of Neurological
Surgery, Columbia University College of Physicians and Surgeons;
Attending Neurosurgeon, Neurological Institute, Columbia-Presbyterian
Medical Center, New York

Donald S. Prough, M.D.
Associate Professor of Anesthesia and Neurology, Bowman Gray School of
Medicine of Wake Forest University; Associate Chief of Professional
Services, North Carolina Baptist Hospital, Winston-Salem

J. G. Reves, M.D.
Attending Anesthetist, Duke University Hospital, Durham

Mark A. Rockoff, M.D.
Associate Professor of Anesthesiology (Pediatrics), Harvard Medical School;
Clinical Director and Vice Chairman, Department of Anesthesiology, The
Children's Hospital, Boston

Mark A. Rosen, M.D.
Associate Professor of Anesthesia, Obstetrics, Gynecology, and Reproductive
Sciences, University of California, San Francisco, School of Medicine;
Attending Anesthesiologist, Moffitt-Long Hospital, San Francisco

Diane R. Rosner, M.D.
Assistant Professor of Anesthesiology, Medical College of Wisconsin;
Clinical Director of Anesthesia, Director of Pediatric Neuroanesthesia,
Children's Hospital of Wisconsin, Milwaukee

Lee D. Rowe, M.D.
Assistant Clinical Professor of Otolaryngology, The University of
Pennsylvania School of Medicine; Attending Surgeon, Pennsylvania and
Northeastern Hospitals, Philadelphia

Bernard Wolfson, M.B., Ch.B., F.F.A.R.C.S.
Clinical Professor of Anesthesiology, University of Pittsburgh School of Medicine; Staff Anesthesiologist, Department of Anesthesiology, Mercy Hospital, Pittsburgh

Neurosurgeons and Anesthesia:
A Historical View

ADRIAN W. GELB

Although trephining of the skull has been practiced for thousands of years, neurosurgery as we know it—the manipulation and excision of brain tissue—had to wait for three major advancements during the second half of the nineteenth century to come of age. The most important of these advances was the accumulation of knowledge about the functional anatomy of the central nervous system. This knowledge not only enabled surgeons to locate the site of neurologic disease, but also gave them the ability to remove parts of the brain without leaving the patient neurologically devastated. The second major development was the increase in the understanding of the role of microorganisms in postoperative mortality. In 1867, Joseph Lister published his article on antisepsis, which resulted in a dramatic reduction in the incidence of postoperative infections. Nineteen years later, Ernst von Bergmann, one of the first advocates of antisepsis in the management of craniocerebral wounds, introduced steam sterilization of surgical instruments, which further reduced the incidence of postoperative infection. The third major advance occurred in 1846 with the first public demonstration of anesthesia. Anesthesia allowed surgery to be performed painlessly, so that the speed of surgery became less important than the care and accuracy with which it was done.

The management of the airway during neurosurgical procedures was a great challenge to the early anesthesiologist. Not only were he and his anesthetic apparatus frequently in the surgeon's way, but the patients were often in unusual operative positions, such as sitting or prone, which required the anesthesiologist to be a contortionist to ensure both an adequate airway and satisfactory operating conditions. Before the introduction of the pharyngeal airway in 1908, one method of keeping the airway clear was for the anesthesiologist to secure the tongue in a forward position with a large clip or suture. A suitable alternative, endotracheal intubation, was suggested by Sir William Macewen in 1880 but did not become widely used until 30 years later.

Macewen, regarded by Harvey Cushing as "the chief pioneer in craniocerebral surgery," was a Scot who studied with Lister and later followed him as Professor of Surgery at the University of Glasgow. He was one of the first to use the methods of neurologic diagnosis in the localization of a surgical lesion. Although Rickman Godlee, a British surgeon and Lister's nephew, is often credited with having initiated the modern period of neurosurgery by successfully removing a glioma from a patient [10], Macewen had removed a meningioma and a subdural hematoma five years earlier. In 1880, Macewen published

xvii

an article entitled "Clinical Observations on the Introduction of Tracheal Tubes by the Mouth Instead of Performing Tracheostomy or Laryngotomy," in which he described four cases, two of glottic edema and two of upper airway surgery, in which oral intubations were used successfully. The first patient had a tumor removed from the pharynx and the base of the tongue, and the principles followed in that operation are still used today: the trachea was intubated while the patient was awake, the anesthetic was administered through the tube, a throat pack was placed around the tube, and the trachea was extubated when the patient regained consciousness. Despite the final statement in Macewen's 1880 paper, "such tubes may be introduced. . .for the purpose of administering the anesthetic," this technique did not come into use until the development of intratracheal insufflation anesthesia in 1909.

Macewen was profoundly concerned with the anesthetic education of his medical students. He was fully cognizant of the risks of anesthesia and went to some lengths to impress upon his students both the benefits and the dangers of anesthesia—"to have been privileged to hear Macewen unfolding the mysteries of the subject, and describing the successive changes produced by chloroform up to the stage of pupillary dilatation, was sufficient to implant in the student's mind a fitting sense of his responsibility."[1] Students were given a full week of systematic lectures on anesthesia and each one was required to administer at least 12 anesthetics under Macewen's personal supervision.

In 1890 there was much public debate about the safety of anesthesia. This was prompted by the increasing number of untoward incidents being reported. Many influential individuals demanded that it be a legal requirement to have two physicians supervise the administration of anesthesia. Macewen crusaded against this suggestion. He pointed out the obvious impracticality of such a requirement in country districts and suggested instead that more attention be paid to the adequate training of physicians. He maintained that if the lowly accomplishment of vaccination required a certificate of proficiency, then so too did the more important and dangerous function of the anesthesiologist.

One of the major transatlantic debates during the latter half of the nineteenth century was whether ether or chloroform should be the preferred agent for intracranial operations. Despite chloroform's poor safety record (it was associated with an intraoperative death three months after its introduction and continued to be a factor in intraoperative mortality thereafter), the British preferred it to ether because it produced a slight decrease in blood pressure and thus less bleeding to obscure the operative field. In addition, it was less likely than ether to cause excitement, bronchorrhea, or postoperative headache. Ether, however, was the drug of choice in the United States because it was thought to be safer, and the mild hypertension it produced was not viewed as a disadvantage. It is difficult to determine to what extent geographic chauvinism was a factor in the predilection of each country for "its" agent. Some anesthesiologists believe that the relative safety of ether made surgeons quite content to have nurses administer the drug, and that this is in part responsible for the development of the subspecialty of nurse-anesthesia in the United States today. The greater risks associated with chloroform necessitated the presence of a physician at all times, hence the absence of this nursing specialty in Britain and the Commonwealth countries.

Sir Victor Horsley, one of the founders of neurosurgery as a separate specialty in Britain, was a great proponent of chloroform, despite the associated mortality. He based his support for chloroform not only on his clinical impressions and the animal experiments he performed, but also on his personal response to being anesthetized with nitrous oxide, ether, and chloroform.

Indeed, Horsley the scientist was not satisfied with a single observation even when he himself was the subject. He was, for example, anesthetized at least fifteen times with nitrous oxide in order to verify its effects[5]. His description of this experience makes rather startling reading. ". . .after the usual symptoms tending the commencement of the administration of the pure gas were fully marked, absolute unconsciousness followed in 90 to 120 seconds. The anesthesia was pushed until rigidity and sometimes cyanosis resulted. The recovery of consciousness was very frequently attended with considerable muscular spasm and semi-coordinated convulsive struggles and excitement."

Over the years, vaporizers were developed to dispense chloroform more safely, but most did not gain popular acceptance because anesthesiologists regarded their practice as a subtle art that should not be encumbered by scientific apparatus. In 1901, at the suggestion of A. D. Waller, a British physiologist who had demonstrated the neurotoxicity of chloroform, Horsley was instrumental in establishing the British Medical Association Special Chloroform Committee. The committee concluded that 2% was the maximum safe dose, and Vernon Harcourt, a physical chemist on the committee, designed a vaporizer to fulfill this requirement, which enjoyed widespread acceptance. This was due, in part, to the quality of the vaporizer, but probably more importantly, to the growing realization that if lives were to be saved, there would have to be a dramatic change in the way in which chloroform was used.

Horsley insisted on the use of this vaporizer during his cases, and he had strong views on what percentage was needed for each stage of the operation: 2% for skin, 1% for bone, 1.5% for dura, and 0.5% or less thereafter [6]. Although the surgeon was well satisfied with his anesthetic protocol, Zebulon Mennell, the anesthetist with whom Horsley worked for many years, wrote that "it was customary at the National Hospital for a male nurse to be allotted for restraining the patient's movements, not only when the sensitive skin was being dealt with at the beginning and end of the operation, but often throughout its whole duration, and it was common for the patients to complain of 'dreams' after the operation" [9]. Surgeons and anesthesiologists always seem to have differed on what constitutes good anesthesia.

Although Horsley and others may have charted the amount of anesthetic administered and the patient's response to it, the anesthetic chart as we know it today was developed by Harvey Cushing. Cushing stands out as one of the giants of neurosurgery. Not only was he the first physician to devote his time exclusively to neurosurgery, but he also contributed greatly to the development of surgical technique and apparatus (including the Bovie cautery), the classification and pathologic description of tumors, and the elucidation of neurophysiology. While a student at Harvard Medical School, Cushing, like most of his colleagues, received no formal instruction in anesthesia but often administered ether for operations. On one such occasion, the patient died during the procedure. The distraught Cushing and his friend and fellow student Amory Codman began to look for ways of safeguarding the patient. At the suggestion of F. B. Harrington, one of their teachers, they developed an anesthetic chart that was first used in 1894. The following year, Cushing modified the chart to emphasize the importance of monitoring the pulse, respiration, and temperature. These charts were the first formal anesthetic records.

In 1901, Cushing visited Italy, where he was presented with one of Dr. Scipione Riva-Rocci's sphygmomanometers. Cushing introduced the use of this device at the Johns Hopkins Hospital and insisted on the routine monitoring and recording of blood pressure throughout his operations. In addition to using a precordial stethoscope for continuous heart monitoring, he thought that intraoperative pulse and blood pressure should always be related to the patient's normal values as obtained under normal ward conditions. In keeping with his concerns about patient safety, he believed that an apparatus for artificial respiration should be immediately available during surgery. On the subject of anesthesia for neurosurgery, Cushing wrote, "Regardless of the drug to be employed, it is essential that it be administered by an expert—preferably by one who makes this his specialty" [2].

Despite Cushing's use of a tourniquet around the head to reduce scalp bleeding and Horsley's development of bone wax, obscuring of the surgical field by bleeding remained a problem. Surgeons had long noted that when a patient had partially exsanguinated, the operation became easier because the field was not hidden. James Gardner, an American neurosurgeon, attempted to take therapeutic advantage of this phenomenon by purposely inducing hypotension. In 1946, he published data on the successful use of arteriotomy for the preoperative removal, and then postoperative retransfusion, of a patient's own blood for excision of a meningioma [3]. Griffiths and Gillies, anesthetists in Edinburgh, preferred a pharmacologic approach and used spinal anesthesia to induce hypotension [4]. These two papers introduced the use of deliberate and controlled hypotension in surgery. They also further illustrate the useful interchange that can occur between surgeons and anesthesiologists.

References

1. Bowman, A. K. *The Life and Teaching of Sir William Macewen.* London: William Hodge, 1942.
2. Cushing, H. Technical methods of performing certain cranial operations. *Surg. Gynecol. Obstet.* 6:227, 1908.
3 Gardner, W. J. The control of bleeding during operation by induced hypotension. *J.A.M.A.* 132:572, 1946.
4. Griffiths, H. W. C., and Gillies, M. D. Thoraco-lumbar sympathectomy anaesthetic procedure. *Anaesthesia* 3:134, 1948.
5. Horsley, V. Note on the patellar knee-jerk. *Brain* 6:369, 1883.
6. Horsley, V. On the technique of operations on the central nervous system. *Br. Med. J.* 2:411, 1906.
7. Keys, T. E. *The History of Surgical Anesthesia.* New York: Dover, 1963.
8. Macewen, W. Clinical observations on the introduction of tracheal tubes by the mouth instead of performing tracheostomy or laryngotomy. *Br. Med. J.* 2:122, 1880.
9. Mennell, Z. Anesthesia in intracranial surgery. *Am. J. Surg.* 38:44, 1924.
10. Pearce, J. M. S. The First Attempts at Removal of Brain Tumors. In F. C. Rose and W. F. Bynum (eds.), *Historical Aspects of the Neurosciences.* New York: Raven, 1982.
11. Thomas, K. B. *The Development of Anaesthetic Apparatus.* Oxford: Blackwell, 1975.
12. Walker, A. E. *A History of Neurological Surgery.* New York: Hafner, 1967.

I

General Considerations

1

Physiology and Metabolism
of the Brain and Spinal Cord

JUDITH DONEGAN

I. Blood flow
A. Normal values
1. Cerebral blood flow [13]
a. Adults. Total cerebral blood flow (CBF) in adults is about 50 ml/100 gm/min. However, flow is nonuniform; it varies both with histologic tissue type (gray or white matter) and with anatomic area. Of the two tissue types, gray matter has the higher flow at about 80 ml/100 gm/min. For white matter, the value is closer to 20 ml/100 gm/min. Overall flow normally decreases with age, the major change being in the gray matter. CBF in the various anatomic regions of the brain differs widely. An important determinant of regional CBF (rCBF) is regional metabolic activity; thus, rCBF may vary from minute to minute.

b. Infants and children. The CBF of the newborn infant (40 ml/100 gm/min) [2] is lower than that of the adult, while the CBF in young children (90–100 ml/100 gm/min) [9] is higher.

2. Spinal cord blood flow.
The flow in the white matter of the cord, similar to that of the cerebral white matter, is 15 to 20 ml/100 gm/min. Gray matter flow in the spinal cord is about 60 ml/100 gm/min in adults.

B. Methods of measurement
Some methods of measuring CBF and spinal cord blood flow are applicable only to animal studies because they require extensive surgical manipulation or tissue sampling. These techniques include the use of radioactive microspheres, classic autoradiography, and venous outflow. The following methods are available for use in awake and anesthetized humans.

1. Inhalation of inert gas.
This method, as originally developed by Kety and Schmidt in 1945 [10], used nitrous oxide (N_2O) as the tracer gas. It determines the mean transit time for N_2O molecules through the brain by measurement of the gas in arterial and jugular venous blood samples collected during a 10- to 15-minute period of gas inhalation. Other inert gases that have been used include argon, krypton-85 ([85]Kr), and xenon-133 (^{133}Xe), the most commonly used today. Nonradioactive xenon can also be employed when combined with computed tomographic (CT) scanning.

Regional as well as total flows can be obtained with the use of multiple collimated scintillation detectors placed in various positions over the skull. These detect photons (ionizing radiation), and the rate of photons received by a detector is directly related to the concentration of the photon-emitting radionuclide (^{133}Xe) in the volume of tissue seen by the detector.

2. Intra-arterial injection of inert gas. This method, described by Lassen and Ingvar in 1961 [14], also measures the mean transit time of a freely diffusible tracer molecule. Although ^{85}Kr was originally used as the tracer, ^{133}Xe is now most commonly employed. The gas is dissolved in saline solution and injected as a bolus into the internal carotid or the vertebral artery. Scintillation detectors are used to measure the radionuclide, as in the inhalation method. Neither of the inert gas methods is useful for obtaining spinal cord blood flow owing to the difficulty of selective recording from the cord.

3. Positron emission tomography (PET) uses radionuclides that emit positrons (^{11}C, ^{15}O, ^{13}N, ^{18}F) [1]. The radionuclide is administered by inhalation or intravenous injection. PET has proven useful for determining CBF and metabolism. A cyclotron is required to generate the positron-emitting radionuclides.

4. Nuclear magnetic resonance. Methods are being developed whereby CBF can be measured using nuclear magnetic resonance. The methods essentially employ the Kety-Schmidt principle but are not sufficiently developed for routine clinical use as yet.

5. Venous occlusion plethysmography has been used to estimate intracranial blood flow in newborns [2].

C. Regulation of cerebral and spinal cord blood flow

1. The spinal cord blood flow is regulated by the same factors as is the CBF [7].

2. Autoregulation. In the normal individual, CBF remains almost constant despite wide variations in the cerebral perfusion pressure (CPP) [26] (Fig. 1-1). This phenomenon, termed *pressure autoregulation,* occurs not only in the vasculature of the central nervous system, but also in the vessels of many other organs, including the heart and the kidneys. The CPP of the brain is determined by the difference between the mean arterial systemic blood pressure (MAP) and the intracranial pressure (ICP): CPP = MAP − ICP. The normal value for CPP is about 100 mmHg. A decrease of perfusion pressure to 50 mmHg is associated with slowing of the electroencephalogram (EEG). At pressures of 25 to 40 mmHg, the EEG becomes flat; and when CPP falls below 20 mmHg, irreversible tissue damage takes place if body temperature is normal. Since, in the normal person, the ICP does not vary markedly, MAP is the major factor affecting CPP.

Autoregulation is an active vascular response. During increases in MAP, the cerebral vessels constrict (i.e., cerebrovascular resistance increases), and during decreases in arterial pressure, the cerebral

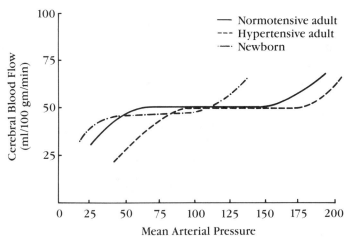

Fig. 1-1. Autoregulatory curve of the cerebral vasculature in the normotensive adult, the hypertensive adult, and the newborn.

vessels dilate (i.e., cerebrovascular resistance decreases). The lower limit of autoregulation is about 50 to 60 mmHg and the upper limit is about 150 mmHg. When MAP falls below 50 to 60 mmHg, CBF decreases. When MAP exceeds 150 mmHg, "autoregulatory breakthrough" occurs. This breakthrough is associated with an increase in CBF, disruption of the blood-brain barrier at many sites, and formation of cerebral edema.

a. The time required for autoregulation to compensate for abrupt changes in systemic arterial blood pressure is 30 to 120 seconds.

b. The mechanism of cerebrovascular autoregulation is not completely understood. The two major theories involve myogenic and metabolic control.

   (1) Myogenic. This hypothesis states that autoregulation is an intrinsic response of the smooth muscle of the arterial wall. When the smooth muscle is stretched by increasing pressure, it contracts, producing vasoconstriction. The response of the smooth muscle to a reduction in systemic arterial tension is relaxation, thus producing vasodilatation.

   (2) Metabolic. According to the metabolic hypothesis, blood flow is regulated by the metabolic activity of the tissue. Therefore, anything that interferes with oxygen delivery to the tissue (e.g., hypotension) results in the liberation of acid metabolites, which then produce local vasodilatation and increased blood flow.

c. Causes of loss of autoregulation include

   (1) Hypoxia

   (2) Ischemia

   (3) Hypercapnia

(4) Trauma

(5) Some anesthetic agents

d. In persons who are hypertensive, the autoregulatory curve is of normal shape but is shifted to the right [24]. Thus, the lower and upper limits of autoregulation are higher than in normotensive patients (Fig. 1-1).

e. Blood flow in the spinal cord is autoregulated over the same range of blood pressures as is CBF [7,15].

f. CBF autoregulation has been demonstrated in newborn animals. Consistent with the lower systemic blood pressure in newborns, the autoregulatory curve is shifted to the left so that both the upper and lower limits of autoregulation are lower than they are in the adult animal [5] (Fig. 1-1).

3. Arterial blood gases and pH

   a. Arterial blood carbon dioxide tension ($PaCO_2$). Variations in $PaCO_2$ profoundly affect CBF. CBF varies linearly with $PaCO_2$ from 20 to 80 mmHg in normocapnic persons (Fig. 1-2).

   (1) The time course of the response is approximately 30 seconds.

   (2) The exact mechanism by which CO_2 exerts its effect on cerebral vessels is not completely understood. The prevailing theory is that changes in CO_2 produce alterations in the pH of the cerebrospinal fluid (CSF) surrounding the vessels and in the walls of the arterioles [23], although this is still controversial [17]. This alteration occurs because CO_2 crosses the blood-brain barrier freely, whereas bicarbonate crosses more

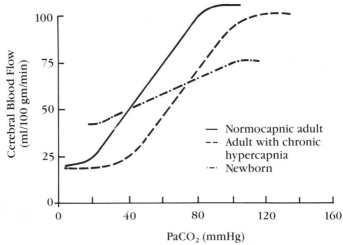

Fig. 1-2. Relationship between cerebral blood flow (CBF) and arterial carbon dioxide tension ($PaCO_2$) in the normocapnic adult, the hypercapnic adult, and the newborn.

slowly. Thus, increases in $PaCO_2$ decrease pH in the CSF and arteriolar walls. Because bicarbonate ions do cross the blood-brain barrier, changes in CSF pH and CBF resulting from alterations in $PaCO_2$ last only a few hours. After this time, CBF returns to normal despite continuing hypocapnia or hypercapnia [21,27].

(3) Spinal cord blood flow reacts to CO_2 in a manner similar to CBF [15].

(4) The cerebral vasculature of young animals responds to changes in $PaCO_2$, but not to the same extent as do adults of the same species [19] (Fig. 1-2).

b. Arterial blood oxygen tension (PaO_2)

(1) Measurable increases in CBF do not occur until the PaO_2 is reduced below 50 mmHg (Fig. 1-3). If CBF as a function of arterial oxygen content (CaO_2) rather than PaO_2 is examined (Fig. 1-4), the resultant curve does not demonstrate a threshold [8]. The reason that some studies have failed to demonstrate an increase in CBF at PaO_2 above 50 mmHg may be that in most species substantial reductions in CaO_2 do not occur until PaO_2 falls below 50 mmHg.

(2) The mechanism for the increase in flow with hypoxia is not completely understood.

(3) Hyperoxia, produced by the inhalation of 80 to 100% oxygen in the normal individual, is associated with a 10 to 12% decrease in CBF.

(4) Spinal cord blood flow reacts to oxygen (O_2) in a manner similar to CBF [11].

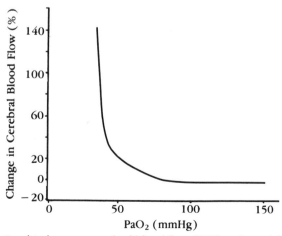

Fig. 1-3. Relationship between cerebral blood flow (CBF) and arterial oxygen tension (PaO_2).

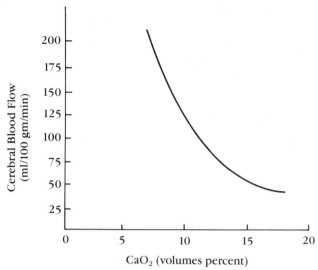

Fig. 1-4. Relationship between cerebral blood flow (CBF) and arterial oxygen content (CaO_2).

(5) The response of the cerebral vasculature of the newborn to changes in CaO_2 appears to be similar to that of the adult [3].

c. pH. Changes in pH from respiratory variation have been discussed in section **3.a.(2)**. Metabolic alterations also affect CBF, although not as profoundly as do changes in $PaCO_2$. Acidemia causes a slight increase in CBF, whereas alkalemia reduces CBF.

4. Cerebral metabolism

a. Total CBF and regional CBF (rCBF). Total CBF generally parallels overall cerebral metabolism [18]. Metabolism, and consequently CBF, are closely correlated with brain activity. When the level of activity is lowest, as in coma, metabolism and CBF are lowest. When overall brain activity is high, as in a grand mal seizure, metabolism and CBF are high (Fig. 1-5). The same is true of activity, metabolism, and CBF at the regional level. For example, when stereognostic test objects are placed in a subject's hand, there is an increase in rCBF of the hand area of the contralateral postcentral gyrus.

b. Sleep. Changes in CBF occurring during sleep and unrelated to variations in either $PaCO_2$ or MAP appear to reflect alterations in cerebral metabolism. CBF is reduced approximately 10% during slow-wave sleep and is increased about 10% during rapid eye movement (REM) sleep.

5. Neurogenic factors. The physiologic importance of the sympathetic and parasympathetic innervation of the cerebral vasculature has been extensively debated and is still a matter of some controversy [4]. Although neurogenic influences appear to be less im-

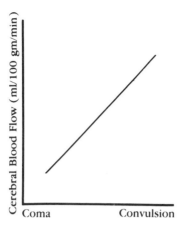

Fig. 1-5. Relationship between cerebral blood flow (CBF) and cerebral metabolism.

portant for overall cerebrovascular regulation than the factors just discussed, they may be operative at the upper and lower limits of autoregulation.

6. **Hematocrit.** The hematocrit affects CBF primarily by altering blood viscosity. A rise in hematocrit increases viscosity and thus reduces CBF. Decreased hematocrit has the opposite effect. Measureable changes in CBF are not seen with hematocrits between 30 and 50%.

7. **Body temperature.** A decrease in body temperature lowers cerebral metabolism, resulting in a decrease in CBF. The depression in metabolism is about 5% per degree centigrade reduction in body temperature. Similarly, raising body temperature increases CBF and cerebral metabolism.

II. Cerebral metabolism
A. Cerebral metabolic rate for oxygen (CMRO$_2$)
1. **Normal values.** About 20% of resting oxygen uptake is consumed by the brain, which uses oxygen at a rate of 1.3 to 1.6 μmol/gm/min (3.0–3.5 ml/100 gm/min) [22]. As is true for CBF, CMRO$_2$ is higher in children than in adults [9], but lower in the fetus and newborn than in the adult [6].

2. **Regional differences.** Regional differences in CMRO$_2$ exist. The metabolic rate of the cerebral cortex is the highest in most species studied.

3. **Processes that require oxygen**
   a. The most important oxygen-consuming process in the brain is the **reduction of molecular oxygen** by the electron transport system. This process produces high-energy phosphate compounds and water.
   b. **The mixed function oxidase systems** and the **oxygen transferase systems,** two other processes that require oxygen, are

involved in synthesis and detoxification. These systems contribute little to the overall oxygen consumption of the brain.

4. **Oxygen stores.** Oxygen stores in the brain are almost nonexistent. Consciousness is lost when PaO_2 declines to approximately 30 mmHg. If delivery of oxygen to the brain ceases, loss of consciousness occurs within 5 to 11 seconds [20].

B. **Cerebral metabolic rate for glucose (CMRgl)**

1. **Normal values.** Glucose is consumed by the brain at a rate of about 0.27 μmol/gm/min (5 mg/100 gm/min) [22]. More than 90% of glucose consumption is aerobic. A small amount of "anaerobic" metabolism occurs normally, producing lactic acid. The anaerobic metabolism does not signify a lack of oxygen, since the normal oxygen tensions in the brain do not limit cellular respiration. The production of lactic acid has to do, rather, with lactate concentration gradients, since if lactate levels in the brain rise, lactate production stops and, in fact, the brain can take up and metabolize lactate.

2. **Relationship between $CMRO_2$ and CMRgl.** Because most of the glucose metabolism requires oxygen, under normal steady-state conditions there is a fixed relationship between $CMRO_2$ and CMRgl. The general equation for the reaction is

Glucose + 6 $O_2 \rightarrow$ 6 CO_2 + 6 H_2O

Thus, the ratio of oxygen to glucose is normally six. Under certain conditions, including hypoxia (which activates glycolysis), hypercapnia (which inhibits glycolysis), and hypoglycemia (when ketone bodies are produced), the relationship does not hold. In these instances, CMRgl is not synonymous with cerebral metabolic rate.

3. **Metabolism of alternative substrates.** During starvation, the brain can metabolize acetoacetate and beta-hydroxybutyrate. These compounds appear to be the only substrates that can support cerebral energy production in the absence of glucose. Amino acids are not important in the absence of glucose, and fatty acids are not used by the brain.

C. **Production of high-energy phosphate compounds.** The aerobic metabolism of glucose produces adenosine triphosphate (ATP) according to the following equation:

Glucose + 6 O_2 + 38 ADP + 38 $P_i \rightarrow$ 6 CO_2 + 44 H_2O + 38 ATP

The hydrolysis of ATP into adenosine diphosphate (ADP) and inorganic phosphate (P_i) is accompanied by a release of energy. Thus, the oxidation of glucose provides energy for the various synthetic and transport processes of the brain. The level of ATP is not an accurate indicator of the energy level of the brain, however, as the storage form of ATP is phosphocreatine (PCr). In addition, ATP can be produced from ADP by the adenylate kinase reaction.

$$ADP + ADP \leftrightharpoons ATP + AMP$$

Phosphocreatine can provide ATP according to the equation

$$PCr + ADP + H^+ \leftrightharpoons ATP + Cr$$

During periods of hypoxia, ATP levels are preserved at the expense of PCr and ADP, until the hypoxic stress becomes severe.

III. Cerebrospinal fluid (CSF)
A. Secretion and circulation of CSF
1. **Normal values.** CSF normally is formed at a rate of about 0.35 ml/min. The total amount of CSF circulating in the cerebrospinal subarachnoid space is 130 to 150 ml.
2. **Sites of formation.** Most CSF is formed in the choroid plexus and the ependymal lining of the cerebral ventricles. Some CSF is formed extrachoroidally by the cerebral capillary endothelium, and some may be derived from the water of oxidative metabolism.
3. **Composition.** CSF is not an ultrafiltrate of plasma, but is actively secreted by the choroid plexus and other sites. The sodium concentration of CSF is approximately 7% higher than the sodium concentration of plasma. Potassium, calcium, bicarbonate, and glucose levels are lower in CSF than in plasma, whereas chloride and magnesium levels are higher. Protein concentration in the CSF is extremely low. The pH of CSF, 7.3, is more acidic than that of plasma, and PCO_2 is higher in CSF (51 mmHg). CSF is isotonic to plasma.
4. **Factors affecting secretion**
   a. **Physiologic parameters.** The following factors reduce the rate of CSF secretion.
   (1) Decreased choroidal blood flow and choroidal capillary hydrostatic pressure
   (2) Decreased body temperature
   (3) Increased serum osmolality
   (4) Increased intraventricular hydrostatic pressure
   b. **Drugs.** Drugs that have been shown to inhibit CSF formation in mammals include acetazolamide, ouabain, corticosteroids, spironolactone, furosemide, and vasopressin. Ouabain and corticosteroids produce their effect by inhibiting Na^+, K^+-ATPase. The mechanism of action of the other drugs is less clear; it may be related to their effects on sodium transport, or, in the case of acetazolamide, the effect on bicarbonate formation.

5. Circulation of CSF. CSF flows from its sources within the ventricles through the medial (foramen of Magendie) and lateral (foramina of Luschka) foramina of the fourth ventricle into the cerebellomedullary cistern (cisterna magna). From the cisterna magna, the fluid circulates in the subarachnoid spaces surrounding the brain and spinal cord. The flow in the spinal subarachnoid space is extremely sluggish compared to the flow in the cranial subarachnoid space.

B. Absorption of CSF

1. Sites of absorption. The major sites of absorption of CSF are the arachnoid villi that protrude into the cerebral venous sinuses. Ten to fifteen percent of the absorption occurs in the spinal subarachnoid space, while the ependyma and meningeal lymphatics take up small amounts of CSF as well. From these sites, CSF is returned to the venous system.

2. The mechanism of absorption. The mechanism of CSF absorption is not completely understood. At one time it was thought that the arachnoid villi had valves that prevented backflow of CSF from the cerebral sinuses to the subarachnoid space. Another theory was that the arachnoid villi consisted of a number of tubes that provided direct communication between the subarachnoid space and the venous sinuses and permitted CSF to move into the sinuses by bulk flow. There is no histologic evidence, however, for either valves or open channels in the arachnoid villi.

More recently, giant vacuoles in the lining cells of the arachnoid villi have been described. These appear to develop from invaginations of the basal cell surface and open onto the apical cell surface, thus forming in essence a dynamic system of channels through the cells. These channels allow bulk flow of CSF to occur through the cells of the arachnoid villi.

3. Factors affecting absorption. The absorption of CSF is governed by a hydrostatic force. The pressure in the cerebral ventricles and the subarachnoid space is normally higher than the pressure in the venous sinuses, and the process of formation of transcellular channels is hydrostatic pressure-sensitive. Thus, factors that alter the hydrostatic pressure gradient between CSF and sinuses affect absorption. Increases in CSF pressure, such as the increases that occur with meningitis and subarachnoid hemorrhage, cause linear increases in CSF absorption. Increases in venous pressure, such as may result from coughing, straining, positive end-expiratory pressure, and congestive heart failure, decrease the rate of absorption. Dural sinus thrombosis also inhibits absorption because it obstructs the venous outflow tract.

IV. Intracranial pressure
A. General principles

1. The term **intracranial pressure (ICP)** as currently used means *supratentorial CSF pressure;* that is, the pressure in a lateral ventricle or in the subarachnoid space over the convexity of the cerebral cortex. This definition is a simplification of the concept of CSF pressure, as this pressure may be markedly different in different areas of the cranium, and as CSF pressure in the cranial subarachnoid space may differ from pressure in the spinal subarachnoid space. In a normal person in the recumbent position, the CSF pressure measured at the lumbar cistern accurately reflects ICP. However, many factors, including the assumption of the upright position, can alter the relationship between cranial and spinal CSF pressure. In addition, in the presence of intracranial mass lesions, infratentorial CSF pressure (as measured in the cisterna magna or lumbar cistern) often falls while supratentorial pressure rises. Therefore, the measurement of supratentorial CSF pressure is a useful clinical concept.

2. **Volume of cranial contents.** Because the cranial vault is a rigid structure, ICP is affected by the volume of the various components found within the cranium.
   a. **Brain volume.**
   b. **Blood volume.** The intracranial blood volume occupies approximately 4% of the total intracranial volume.
   c. **CSF volume.** The CSF occupies 10% of the total intracranial volume.

3. The **normal value** for intracranial pressure is about 10 mmHg in children as well as in adults.

B. Intracranial compliance

1. **Pressure-volume curve** (Fig. 1-6). Intracranial compliance can be illustrated diagrammatically by the pressure-volume curve obtained in rhesus monkeys by Langfitt and colleagues [12]. They plotted supratentorial CSF pressure as a function of the volume of an expanding epidural balloon.
   a. Sullivan and coworkers [25] showed that the concept of a single pressure-volume curve is invalid, since equal volume changes in different intracranial compartments produce different effects on ICP. In addition, the shape of the curve varies from person to person and is dependent on factors such as blood pressure and $PaCO_2$. Nevertheless, the analysis of the phases of an idealized curve can be used as an aid to understanding intracranial compliance.
   b. The various phases of the pressure-volume curve may be described as a flat horizontal portion (representing high com-

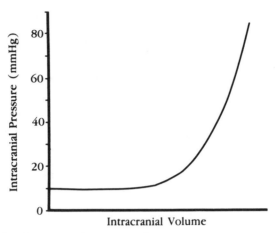

Fig. 1-6. Idealized intracranial pressure-volume curve.

pliance), a steep terminal portion (representing low compliance), and an intermediate portion (representing a transition stage). During the phase of high compliance, a considerable increase in total intracranial volume may take place before ICP increases. This initial stability occurs because there is a certain degree of elasticity in the craniospinal system; in addition, an increase in the volume of one of the intracranial contents can be partially compensated for by a decrease in the volume of the remaining contents. For example, during development of a mass lesion or of edema of the brain, some compensation is achieved by displacement of cranial CSF into the spinal subarachnoid space, by an increase in the rate of CSF absorption, by a decrease in the rate of CSF production, and by a decrease in cerebral blood volume that occurs as a result of venous compression by the mass.

2. **Testing intracranial compliance.** A patient may have normal or nearly normal ICP and yet be at the limit of compensatory mechanisms. Further perturbations, such as those that can occur during the induction of anesthesia, may therefore be associated with large increases in ICP and a worsening of neurologic status. A method for determining which patients are in this category was devised by Miller and colleagues [16], who designed a method for testing intracranial compliance in patients whose ICP is being monitored by an intraventricular catheter. The ICP response to the injection of 1 ml of fluid through the catheter is assessed. An increase of greater than 4 mmHg is almost always associated with a significant mass lesion and is an indication of poor compliance.

References

1. Baran, J. C., Steinling, M., Tanaka, E., et al. Quantitative measurement of CBF, oxygen extraction fraction (OEF) and $CMRO_2$ with the ^{15}O continuous inhalation technique and positron emission tomography (PET): Experimental evidence and normal values in man. *J. Cereb. Blood Flow Metab.* 1:(Suppl):S5, 1981.
2. Cross, K. W., Dear, P. R. F., Hathorn, M. K. S., et al. An estimation of intracranial blood flow in the new-born infant. *J. Physiol.* 289:329, 1979.
3. Donegan, J. H., Traystman, R. J., Koehler, R. C., et al. Cerebrovascular hypoxic and autoregulatory responses during reduced brain metabolism. *Am. J. Physiol.* 249:H421, 1985.
4. Gross, P. M., Heistad, D. D., Strait, M. R., et al. Cerebral vascular responses to physiological stimulation of sympathetic pathways in cats. *Circ. Res.* 44:288, 1979.
5. Hernandez, M. J., Brennan, R. W., and Bowman, G. S. Autoregulation of cerebral blood flow in the newborn dog. *Brain Res.* 184:199, 1980.
6. Hernandez, M. J., Brennan, R. W., Vannucci, R. C., and Bowman, G. S. Cerebral blood flow and oxygen consumption in the newborn dog. *Am. J. Physiol.* 234:R209, 1978.
7. Hickey, R., Albin, M. S., Bunegin, L., and Gelineau, J. Autoregulation of spinal cord blood flow: Is the cord a microcosm of the brain? *Stroke* 17:1183, 1986.
8. Jones, M. D., Jr., Traystman, R. J., Simmons, M. A., and Molteni, R. A. Effects of changes in arterial O_2 content on cerebral blood flow in the lamb. *Am. J. Physiol.* 240 (Heart Circ. Physiol. 9):H209, 1981.
9. Kennedy, C., and Sokoloff, L. An adaptation of the nitrous oxide method to the study of the cerebral circulation in children; normal values for cerebral blood flow and cerebral metabolic rate in childhood. *J. Clin. Invest.* 36:1130, 1957.
10. Kety, S. S., and Schmidt, C. F. The determination of cerebral blood flow in man by the use of nitrous oxide in low concentrations. *Am. J. Physiol.* 143:53, 1945.
11. Kobrine, A. I., Evans, D. E., and Rizzoli, H. V. Effects of progressive hypoxia on long tract neural conduction in the spinal cord. *Neurosurgery* 7:369, 1980.
12. Langfitt, T. W., Weinstein, J. D., and Kassell, N. F. Cerebral vasomotor paralysis produced by intracranial hypertension. *Neurology* 15:622, 1965.
13. Lassen, N. A., and Christensen, M. S. Physiology of cerebral blood flow. *Br. J. Anaesth.* 48:719, 1976.
14. Lassen, N. A., and Ingvar, D. H. The blood flow of the cerebral cortex determined by radioactive Krypton-85. *Experientia* 17:42, 1961.
15. Marcus, M. L., Heistad, D. D., Ehrhardt, J. C., and Abboud, F. M. Regulation of total and regional spinal cord blood flow. *Circ. Res.* 41:128, 1977.
16. Miller, J. D., Garibi, J., and Pickard, J. D. Induced changes of cerebrospinal fluid volume. Effects during continuous monitoring of ventricular fluid pressure. *Arch. Neurol.* 28:265, 1973.
17. Nilsson, B., and Siesjo, B. K. Evidence Against H^+ as a Regulator of Cerebral Blood Flow. In C. Owman and L. Edvinsson (Eds.), *Neurogenic Control of the Brain Circulation.* Elmsford, N.Y.: Pergammon Press, 1977. Pp. 295–300.
18. Raichle, M. E., Grubb, R. L., Jr., Gado, M. H., et al. Correlation between regional cerebral blood flow and oxidative metabolism. In vivo studies in man. *Arch. Neurol.* 33:523, 1976.
19. Reivich, M., Brann, A. W., Jr., Shapiro, H., et al. Reactivity of cerebral vessels to CO_2 in the newborn rhesus monkey. *Europ. Neurol.* 6:132, 1971/72.
20. Rossen, R., Kabat, H., and Anderson, J. P. Acute arrest of cerebral circulation in man. *Arch. Neurol. Psychiatr.* 50:510, 1943.
21. Severinghaus, J. W. Role of cerebrospinal fluid pH in normalization of cerebral blood flow in chronic hypocapnia. *Acta Neurol. Scand.* 14:116, 1965.

22. Siesjo, B. K. *Brain Energy Metabolism.* Chichester, N.Y.: Wiley, 1978.
23. Skinhoj, E. Regulation of cerebral blood flow as a single function of the interstitial pH in the brain. *Acta Neurol. Scand.* 42:604, 1966.
24. Strandgaard, S., Olesen, J., Skinhoj, E., and Lassen, N. A. Autoregulation of brain circulation in severe arterial hypertension. *Br. Med. J.* 1:507, 1973.
25. Sullivan, H. G., Miller, J. D., Griffith, R. L., III, and Becker, D. P. CSF pressure transients in response to epidural and ventricular volume loading. *Am. J. Physiol.* 234:R167, 1978.
26. Wagner, E. M., and Traystman, R. J. Hydrostatic determinants of cerebral perfusion. *Crit. Care Med.* 14:484, 1986.
27. Warner, D. S., Turner, D. M., and Kassell, N. F. Time-dependent effects of prolonged hypercapnia on cerebrovascular parameters in dogs: Acid-base chemistry. *Stroke* 18:142, 1987.

2

Effect of Anesthesia on Cerebral Physiology and Metabolism

JUDITH DONEGAN

I. Inhalation anesthetics
A. Nitrous oxide (N_2O)
1. **Effect on cerebral blood flow (CBF) and cerebral oxygen consumption ($CMRO_2$).** The somewhat variable results of N_2O on CBF and $CMRO_2$ that have been reported in the literature probably reflect differences in species, methodology, and the effects of other drugs administered with N_2O. The weight of the evidence appears to support the theory that N_2O is a cerebral vasodilator.
   a. **Dog.** An increase in both $CMRO_2$ and CBF associated with the administration of 60 to 70% N_2O to dogs has been reported [55,67]. Archer and colleagues used positron emission tomography to examine the effects of 50% N_2O and 2% isoflurane, superimposed on a background anesthetic of fentanyl, on regional cerebral blood volume (rCBV) during normocapnia and hypocapnia [4]. During normocapnia, the addition of 50% N_2O was associated with an 11% increase in rCBV; 2% isoflurane without nitrous oxide caused rCBV to increase by 36%. During hypocapnia (arterial carbon dioxide tension [$PaCO_2$] = 25 mmHg), rCBV was reduced 17%, and the addition of 50% N_2O to the background fentanyl anesthetic did not alter rCBV; however, rCBV increased 15% when isoflurane was introduced.
   b. **Rabbits.** Seventy percent N_2O added to 0.5 minimal alveolar concentration (MAC) of halothane or isoflurane during normocapnia caused CBF to increase (halothane, 40%; isoflurane, 20%), and when N_2O was added to a background anesthetic of 1 MAC of either of the two agents an even greater increase in CBF was produced [17]. When 0.5 MAC halothane or isoflurane was supplemented with morphine, the effect of N_2O on CBF was not different from the effect with 0.5 MAC alone. In another study in which 70% N_2O was added to 1 MAC halothane during conditions of normocapnia and hypocapnia, the presence of hypocapnia did not blunt the cerebrovascular response to N_2O [68].
   c. **Other species.** In swine and goats, N_2O has been associated with increases in CBF and $CMRO_2$ [35, 50].
   d. **Human beings.** The results of a study in humans in which 60% N_2O was added to 0.8% halothane showed that, during N_2O inhala-

17

tion, the CBF equivalent (CBF/CMRO$_2$) increased by 67% [56]. The authors theorized that decreases in CMRO$_2$ during N$_2$O should not be large enough to explain the findings completely. They felt the evidence was strongly suggestive of an increase in CBF resulting from N$_2$O. Other groups of investigators obtained no change in CBF and a 15 to 20% decrease in CMRO$_2$ with 70% N$_2$O [62,72]. Thus, it appears that the inhalation of 60 to 70% N$_2$O in humans is associated with at least a relative cerebral hyperemia.

2. **Effect on intracranial pressure (ICP).** Nitrous oxide raises ICP, the effect being most pronounced in patients who have intracranial disorders [26]. The rise in pressure is thought to result from cerebral vasodilatation that leads to increases in CBF and cerebral blood volume (CBV). Increases may be attenuated or prevented by prior administration of thiopental or diazepam, but not by hyperventilation before the introduction of N$_2$O [51, 68].

3. **Effect on autoregulation and carbon dioxide response.** Autoregulation is well preserved during anesthesia with 70% N$_2$O in response to both hypotension and hypertension [62]. In addition, the response of the cerebral vasculature to CO$_2$ is not altered by 70% N$_2$O [72].

B. **Volatile anesthetics.** In general, the volatile anesthetics produce dose-dependent increases in CBF, thus increasing cerebral blood volume and ICP. Other dose-related effects of volatile anesthetics include a decrease in cerebral metabolic rate and abolition of autoregulation (Fig. 2-1).

1. **Halothane**

   a. **Effect on CBF and CMRO$_2$.** Halothane in clinical doses increases CBF and decreases CMRO$_2$, thus uncoupling the normal relationship between metabolism and flow and increasing the CBF equivalent [63]. The effect on CBF is a result of vasodilatation, presumably secondary to a direct effect of halothane on the cerebral vasculature. The decrease in cerebrovascular resistance is dose-dependent as halothane concentration is increased from 0.5 to 4.0% [36]. Nikki and colleagues have demonstrated that the vascular dilatation is not mediated by β-adrenergic receptors [47]. A study in goats examined the temporal relationship between the onset of anesthesia and the alterations in flow and metabolism [2]. Two percent halothane produced an increase in CBF of 100%; this increase occurred before there was a significant change in CMRO$_2$ or any evidence of anesthesia. During prolonged anesthesia with halothane, the CBF returns toward normal, although the time course of this adaptation remains controversial [1,47,71].

   That CBF may actually be decreased by low inspired concentrations of halothane was demonstrated by a study done on monkeys [45]. During the inhalation of 0.5% halothane, CBF decreased by 17% and CMRO$_2$ by 30%. In contrast, at 1 and 2% halothane, CBF increased by 26 and 97% respectively, although CMRO$_2$ continued

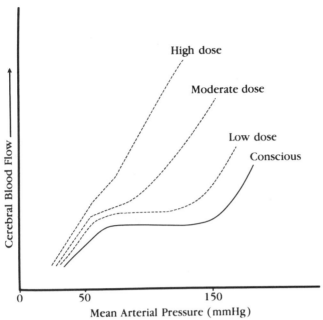

Fig. 2-1. Dose-dependent effect of the volume anesthetics on cerebrovascular autoregulation.

to fall. The authors suggested that at low concentrations the decrease in CBF might result from the marked reduction in $CMRO_2$, which the vasodilatory effect of halothane is unable to overcome. At higher concentrations, there is little further reduction in $CMRO_2$ (40% at 1% halothane, 50% at 2% halothane), and the direct dilator effects of halothane predominate. The cerebral metabolic rate for glucose (CMRgl) is decreased by halothane in proportion to the reduction in $CMRO_2$ [61]. Regional differences in the reduction of glucose metabolism have been demonstrated; the greatest change occurs in the occipital lobes.

b. Effect on ICP. Halothane increases ICP primarily as a result of cerebral vasodilatation and increased CBV [5]. The rate of cerebrospinal fluid (CSF) production is reduced by halothane [6], but the resistance to its reabsorption is increased [7]. The administration of thiopental or the establishment of hypocapnia prior to the introduction of halothane may ameliorate the increase in ICP. Halothane has been shown to produce more brain surface protrusion during craniotomy than either enflurane or isoflurane [19].

c. Effect on autoregulation and CO_2 response. Impairment of autoregulation by halothane is dose-dependent. At 0.5%, it is partially intact, and at 1 to 2%, there is complete loss of autoregulation [43,45]. Carbon dioxide responsiveness is retained [18,43].

2. Enflurane (Ethrane)

a. Effect on CBF and CMRO$_2$. Increases in CBF with enflurane are not quantitatively as great as increases with halothane. The maximum rise is approximately 12 to 20%. Enflurane is a potent depressor of CMRO$_2$ and CMRgl. At 1 MAC, cerebral metabolism is reduced by about 35%. In a canine study, this was found to be the maximal change [40], but in a study in humans, metabolism was depressed 50% when 3% enflurane was inhaled [73]. In both studies, the appearance of a seizure pattern in the electroencephalogram (EEG), which may occur spontaneously during moderately deep levels of enflurane anesthesia, was associated with a reversal of the metabolic depression. A 48% increase in CMRO$_2$ was seen in the canine study when such an EEG pattern appeared.

b. Effect on ICP. Enflurane, like halothane, raises ICP, especially in patients who are at the limit of their compensatory ability. In addition, since hypocapnia increases the likelihood of seizure activity on the EEG during enflurane anesthesia, the use of hyperventilation in an attempt to attenuate the ICP response is not feasible. Enflurane produces an increase in CSF production [10] and an increase in resistance to reabsorption [9].

c. Effect on autoregulation and CO$_2$ response. The autoregulatory response of the cerebral vasculature is at least partially effective at 0.5 MAC enflurane, whereas at 1 MAC it is abolished [43]. Responsiveness to CO$_2$ is maintained during enflurane anesthesia [43].

3. Isoflurane (Forane)

a. Effect on CBF and CMRO$_2$. In dogs, isoflurane produced an increase in CBF (33% at 1 MAC) and a decrease in CMRO$_2$ (23% at 1 MAC) [16], while a study comparing the cerebrovascular and metabolic effects of halothane and isoflurane in the cat demonstrated significant increases in CBF with halothane but not with isoflurane [69]. Isoflurane, however, was associated with greater decreases in CMRO$_2$ than was halothane at an equipotent dose. This study measured CBF using intra-arterial xenon-133 (^{133}Xe) with the collimated scintillation counter placed over the right posterior parietal area of the skull, and thus measured flow in a supratentorial region of the brain. In another study that compared the cerebrovascular effects of halothane and isoflurane in dogs, in which microspheres were used to measure CBF, isoflurane was associated with less flow increase in the cerebral hemispheres than was halothane, but isoflurane produced a greater increase in brainstem blood flow [12]. In patients with small supratentorial tumors, CBF and metabolism were measured during anesthesia with isoflurane at an inspired concentration of 0.75% with 67% nitrous oxide and again when the inspired isoflurane concentration was 1.5% [34]. Doubling the inspired concentration of isoflurane produced no change in CBF (measured with intravenous ^{133}Xe), but $CMRO_2$ decreased from 2.4 to 1.9 ml $O_2/100$ gm/min. As is true for other potent inhalation agents, the effects of isoflurane on cerebral glucose utilization vary regionally [49]. Decreases are produced in cortical areas and sensory relay nuclei while increases may be seen in the limbic system. In a study that compared brain energy metabolites in rats given 1 MAC of either halothane, enflurane, or isoflurane, the major difference noted was that those animals that received isoflurane had higher levels of glucose in both plasma and brain than did animals that received halothane or enflurane [31].

b. Effect on ICP. Isoflurane and halothane at 1 MAC both produced significant increases in ICP when administered to rabbits following cryogenic brain injury [59]. Patients with supratentorial brain tumors and a significant midline shift on the preoperative computed tomographic (CT) scan were found to have increases in ICP (8.0 ± 1.9 mmHg) associated with the inhalation of 1% isoflurane even during hypocapnia ($PaCO_2 = 29$ mmHg) [25]. Increases in anterior fontanel pressures in preterm neonates were similar (9–11%) with 0.75% isoflurane, 0.5% halothane, 20 μg/kg fentanyl, and 2 mg/kg ketamine [22]. Isoflurane produces no change in CSF production [8] and decreases the resistance to reabsorption [9].

c. Effect on autoregulation and CO_2 response. As is true for the other potent volatile anesthetic agents, isoflurane produces a dose-dependent reduction in cerebral autoregulation. Responsiveness to $PaCO_2$ is well preserved at 1 MAC [18].

II. Intravenous anesthetics
A. Barbiturates

1. **Effect on CBF and $CMRO_2$.** Barbiturates, in doses large enough to produce unconsciousness, constrict cerebral vessels and increase cerebrovascular resistance, thereby decreasing CBF and CBV. The reduction in flow parallels a reduction in $CMRO_2$ and CMRgl, and the alteration in flow has been attributed entirely to metabolic changes [39]. The cerebral effects of barbiturates are dose dependent; neither CBF nor metabolism is markedly altered by sedative doses. The onset of anesthesia with barbiturates, as defined by loss of response to pain in one study and by EEG changes in another, occurs when CBF and $CMRO_2$ have declined 25 to 30% [2,64]. With increasing doses of barbiturates, CBF and $CMRO_2$ are further decreased to the point at which the EEG becomes isoelectric. At this point, both flow and metabolism are approximately 50% of normal, and additional doses of drug have little effect on either (Fig. 2-2).

a. Analysis of tissue concentrations of phosphocreatine (PCr), adenosine triphosphate (ATP), and adenosine monophosphate during

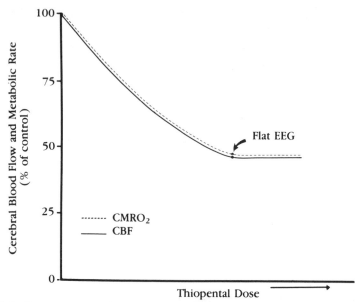

Fig. 2-2. Decrease in cerebral blood flow (CBF) and cerebral metabolic rate for oxygen ($CMRO_2$) produced by barbiturates. The change is dose dependent until the EEG becomes isoelectric.

    barbiturate anesthesia has demonstrated that the cerebral energy state is unchanged.

  b. Acute tolerance to the anesthetic effects and the cerebral hemodynamic effects of barbiturates occurs. The plasma concentration of barbiturate at the time of awakening is dependent on the dose of the drug administered. The larger the dose, the higher the plasma concentration on awakening, suggesting that the central nervous system (CNS) develops a resistance to the effects of the drug after a single administration. Acute tolerance to the reduction of CBF and $CMRO_2$ by thiopental has been demonstrated in dogs [3]. In animals that received a single dose two hours before the start of an infusion of the drug, flow and metabolism did not decrease to the same extent as in animals that received only the infusion (17 vs. 40%).

2. Effect on ICP. Barbiturates, because they reduce CBF and CBV, can lower ICP significantly. This property has been used as a therapeutic measure in patients who have increased ICP secondary to head injury and encephalitis [53]. Barbiturates may successfully lower pressure when other methods (e.g., hyperventilation, osmotic agents, or steroids) fail. The barbiturates are also valuable as induction agents in patients who have raised ICP who require anesthesia and surgery. The intravenous administration of barbiturates not only lowers ICP but may protect against the increases in ICP that often accompany laryngoscopy, intubation, suctioning, and head positioning.

3. **Effect on autoregulation, CO_2, and O_2 responses.** Barbiturates administered in sedative or anesthetic doses do not alter autoregulation or CO_2 responsiveness of the cerebral vasculature. The cerebrovascular response to hypoxia has not been studied in humans but has been demonstrated to remain intact in monkeys anesthetized with barbiturates.

B. **Narcotics.** Analgesic and premedicant doses of narcotics have little effect on either CBF or ICP unless $PaCO_2$ increases secondary to respiratory depression.

1. **Morphine and meperidine (Demerol)**
   a. **Effect on CBF and $CMRO_2$.** In dogs, morphine was found to cause parallel, dose-related decreases both in $CMRO_2$ and in CBF [65]. The maximum decrease occurred at 1.2 mg/kg, which reduced $CMRO_2$ by 15% and CBF by 55%. In control dogs, CBF decreased 35% during the course of the experiment. Thus, the vasoconstrictor effect of morphine accounted for about 20% of the reduction in flow. The effect of meperidine on the $CMRO_2$ in dogs is similar to the effect of morphine [38]. In contrast, CBF, $CMRO_2$, and CMRgl were essentially unchanged in human volunteers by the administration of a total of 3 mg/kg morphine combined with 70% N_2O and 30% O_2 [29].
   b. **Effect on ICP.** In normocapnic, normotensive individuals, morphine and meperidine in anesthetic doses do not affect ICP significantly. Since CO_2 responsiveness is maintained, an increase in $PaCO_2$ will be associated with a rise in ICP, whereas hyperventilation will decrease ICP.
   c. **Effect on autoregulation and CO_2 response.** Under normocapnic conditions, autoregulation remains intact during anesthesia with morphine (2 mg/kg) and N_2O [28]. Cerebrovascular response to CO_2 is maintained with the narcotics.

2. **Fentanyl (Sublimaze)**
   a. **Effect on CBF and $CMRO_2$.** Fentanyl, in a dose of 0.006 mg/kg, decreased CBF by 47% and $CMRO_2$ by 18% in dogs, with both effects lasting approximately 30 minutes [41]. The reduction of CBF was primarily due to an increase in cerebrovascular resistance. In humans, fentanyl 10 μg/kg combined with diazepam and nitrous oxide produced a 34% decrease in CBF and $CMRO_2$ [70]. However, fentanyl 5 μg/kg in combination with droperidol 0.25 mg/kg was not associated with changes in either CBF or $CMRO_2$ [57]. A study in rats demonstrated maximal reductions in CBF (50%) and $CMRO_2$ (35%) at fentanyl doses of 100 μg/kg [13]. Larger doses of 200 or 400 μg/kg did not produce further reduction in flow or metabolism but were associated with seizure activity in 25% of the animals.
   b. **Effect on ICP.** Fentanyl has little or no effect on ICP under conditions of normocapnia or hypocapnia [44,46]. It does not

change the rate of CSF production [6], and it decreases the resistance to reabsorption of CSF [7].

    c. Effect on autoregulation and CO_2 response. Cerebral responses to changes in arterial oxygen tension (PaO_2), $PaCO_2$, and arterial blood pressure remain intact when fentanyl, in doses of up to 100 μg/kg, is administered to dogs [37].

3. Sufentanil. Sufentanil administered to rats in doses of 5 to 160 μg/kg produced maximal decreases of CBF (53%) and $CMRO_2$ (43%) at a dose of 80 μg/kg [30]. In the same animal model, sufentanil reduced glucose utilization in cortical structures but produced increases in some limbic structures [74].

C. Other agents

1. Droperidol and fentanyl citrate (Innovar)

    a. Effect on CBF and $CMRO_2$. When administered to dogs in a dose of 0.3 mg/kg, droperidol decreased CBF approximately 40% without altering $CMRO_2$ significantly [41]. The reduction in CBF was due to cerebral vasoconstriction and a marked increase in cerebrovascular resistance. Innovar reduced CBF by 50 to 60% and $CMRO_2$ by 23%. Thirty minutes after injection, the effects on CBF and metabolism resembled the effects of droperidol alone. Thus, droperidol acted as a potent, long-lasting cerebral vasoconstrictor, and the effects of droperidol and fentanyl on CBF and $CMRO_2$ appeared to be additive in the first 30 minutes following injection but not thereafter. In a study performed on healthy patients, the administration of the combination drug (Innovar) was not associated with significant changes in either CBF or $CMRO_2$ [57]. Similar results were obtained in humans in a study of regional hemispheric flow using droperidol and phenoperidine [11]. Thus, while species differences exist, the neuroleptics appear to have little effect on CBF and metabolism in humans.

    b. Effect on ICP. The combination of droperidol, 5 mg, and fentanyl, 0.1 mg, has been shown to reduce ICP both in patients who have normal CSF pathways and in patients who have intracranial space-occupying lesions [20]. In a study in which droperidol was given in large doses (7.5–12.5 mg), ICP was not reduced in normocapnic patients who had space-occupying lesions, but MAP was depressed and cerebral perfusion pressure (CPP) was decreased significantly [44]. This blood pressure response is most likely related to the alpha-adrenergic blocking effect of droperidol. The addition of fentanyl, 0.2 to 0.3 mg, did not affect ICP but produced a further decrease in MAP and CPP. Hyperventilation reduced ICP, causing CPP to rise. Neuroleptanesthesia may be used safely in patients who have increased ICP, provided that hyperventilation is used concurrently and hypotension is avoided.

c. Effect on autoregulation and CO_2 response. The combination of droperidol and fentanyl produces marked cerebral vasoconstriction in dogs, and hypocapnia ($PaCO_2 = 20$ mmHg) has no further effect [41]. The vessels, however, respond to hypercapnia. Therefore, CO_2 responsiveness is not lost, but the vessels are maximally constricted by Innovar and unable to respond further when hypocapnia is induced. The cerebral autoregulatory response during Innovar anesthesia has not been examined.

2. Ketamine

a. Effect on CBF and $CMRO_2$. Ketamine is a potent dilator of the cerebral vasculature. Total increases in CBF of 60% with little change in $CMRO_2$ and CMRgl have been reported in humans [66]. Marked regional differences in the increases in CBF have been found [27]. The effects of ketamine on local cerebral glucose utilization vary in different regions of the brain [15]. Increases occur in the limbic system, extrapyramidal motor system, and corpus callosum, while reductions occur in the somatosensory and auditory systems.

b. Effect on ICP. Ketamine produces a marked rise in ICP both in patients who have normal CSF pressures and in patients whose ICP is elevated [23]. This effect is presumably secondary to an increase in CBF and can be minimized, but not completely prevented, by concurrent hyperventilation [58]. For this reason, it is best to avoid ketamine altogether in patients who have intracranial disorders.

c. Effect on autoregulation and CO_2 response. There is presumptive evidence to indicate that autoregulation remains intact during ketamine anesthesia. Cerebrovascular CO_2 responsiveness appears to be maintained, since hypocapnia lowers ICP during ketamine anesthesia, suggesting that it decreases CBF.

3. Benzodiazepines. Diazepam has been shown to decrease CBF and $CMRO_2$ to the same extent ($\sim25\%$) in head-injured patients [14]. In normal dogs the reduction in CBF and metabolism was approximately 15% [33]. Lorazepam produced a similar result in monkeys [54]. CBF was reduced by 26%, $CMRO_2$ by 21 to 30%, and CMRgl by 42%. Midazolam 0.15 mg/kg decreased CBF by 35% in human volunteers [21]. Reductions in CBF and $CMRO_2$ have been demonstrated in dogs [48]. In a group of patients with brain tumors but without significantly elevated ICP, anesthetic induction with midazolam 0.32 mg/kg was not associated with a change in ICP [24], although midazolam has been reported to reduce ICP in patients with elevated ICP [32].

4. Etomidate. Etomidate has been shown to decrease both CBF and $CMRO_2$ in humans [52] and in dogs [42] and to reduce ICP when administered in a dose of 0.3 mg/kg to patients with severe cerebral injury [60].

References

1. Albrecht, R. F., Miletich, D. J., and Madala, L. R. Normalization of cerebral blood flow during prolonged halothane anesthesia. *Anesthesiology* 58:26, 1983.
2. Albrecht, R. F., Miletich, D. J., Rosenberg, R., and Zahed, B. Cerebral blood flow and metabolic changes from induction to onset of anesthesia with halothane or pentobarbital. *Anesthesiology* 47:252, 1977.
3. Altenburg, B. M., Michenfelder, J. D., and Theye, R. A. Acute tolerance to thiopental in canine cerebral oxygen consumption studies. *Anesthesiology* 31:443, 1969.
4. Archer, D. P., Labrecque, P., Tyler, J. L., et al. Cerebral blood volume is increased in dogs during administration of nitrous oxide or isoflurane. *Anesthesiology* 67:642, 1987.
5. Artru, A. A. Relationship between cerebral blood volume and CSF pressure during anesthesia with halothane or enflurane in dogs. *Anesthesiology* 58:533, 1983.
6. Artru, A. A. Effects of halothane and fentanyl on the rate of CSF production in dogs. *Anesth. Analg.* 62:581, 1983.
7. Artru, A. A. Effects of halothane and fentanyl anesthesia on resistance to reabsorption of CSF. *J. Neurosurg.* 60:252, 1984.
8. Artru, A. A. Isoflurane does not increase the rate of CSF production in the dog. *Anesthesiology* 60:193, 1984.
9. Artru, A. A. Effects of enflurane and isoflurane on resistance to reabsorption of cerebrospinal fluid in dogs. *Anesthesiology* 61:529, 1984.
10. Artru, A. A., Nugent, M., and Michenfelder, J. D. Enflurane causes a prolonged and reversible increase in the rate of CSF production in the dog. *Anesthesiology* 57:255, 1982.
11. Barker, J., Harper, A. M., McDowall, D. G., et al. Cerebral blood flow, cerebrospinal fluid pressure and e.e.g. activity during neuroleptanalgesia induced with dehydrobenzperidol and phenoperidine. *Br. J. Anaesth.* 40:143, 1968.
12. Boarini, D. J., Kassell, N. F., Coester, H. C., et al. Comparison of systemic and cerebrovascular effects of isoflurane and halothane. *Neurosurgery* 15:400, 1984.
13. Carlsson, C., Smith, D. S., Keykhah, M. M., et al. The effects of high-dose fentanyl on cerebral circulation and metabolism in rats. *Anesthesiology* 57:375, 1982.
14. Cotev, S., and Shalit, M. N. Effects of diazepam on cerebral blood flow and oxygen uptake after head injury. *Anesthesiology* 43:117, 1975.
15. Crosby, G., Crane, A. M., and Sokoloff, L. Local changes in cerebral glucose utilization during ketamine anesthesia. *Anesthesiology* 56:437, 1982.
16. Cucchiara, R. F., Theye, R. A., and Michenfelder, J. D. The effects of isoflurane on canine cerebral metabolism and blood flow. *Anesthesiology* 40:571, 1974.
17. Drummond, J. C., Scheller, M. S., and Todd, M. M. The effect of nitrous oxide on cortical cerebral blood flow during anesthesia with halothane and isoflurane, with and without morphine, in the rabbit. *Anesth. Analg.* 66:1083, 1987.
18. Drummond, J. C., and Todd, M. M. The response of the feline cerebral circulation to $PaCO_2$ during anesthesia with isoflurane and halothane and during sedation with nitrous oxide. *Anesthesiology* 62:268, 1985.
19. Drummond, J. C., Todd, M. M., Toutant, S. M., and Shapiro, H. M. Brain surface protrusion during enflurane, halothane, and isoflurane anesthesia in cats. *Anesthesiology* 59:288, 1983.
20. Fitch, W., Barker, J., Jennett, J. B., and McDowall, D. G. The influence of neuroleptanalgesic drugs on cerebrospinal fluid pressure. *Br. J. Anaesth.* 41:800, 1969.
21. Forster, A., Juge, O., and Morel, D. Effects of midazolam on cerebral blood flow in human volunteers. *Anesthesiology* 56:453, 1982.
22. Friesen, R. H., Thieme, R. E., Honda, A. T., and Morrison, J. E., Jr. Changes in anterior fontanel pressure in preterm neonates receiving isoflurane, halothane, fentanyl, or ketamine. *Anesth. Analg.* 66:431, 1987.

23. Gardner, A. E., Dannemiller, F. J., and Dean, D. Intracranial cerebrospinal fluid pressure in man during ketamine anesthesia. *Anesth. Analg.* 51:741, 1972.
24. Giffin, J. P., Cottrell, J. E., Shwiry, B., et al. Intracranial pressure, mean arterial pressure, and heart rate following midazolam or thiopental in humans with brain tumors. *Anesthesiology* 60:491, 1984.
25. Grosslight, K., Foster, R., Colohan, A. R., and Bedford, R. F. Isoflurane for neuro-anesthesia: Risk factors for increases in intracranial pressure. *Anesthesiology* 63:533, 1985.
26. Henriksen, H. T., and Jorgensen, P. B. The effect of nitrous oxide on intracranial pressure in patients with intracranial disorders. *Br. J. Anaesth.* 45:486, 1973.
27. Hougaard, K., Hansen, A., and Brodersen, P. The effect of ketamine on regional cerebral blood flow in man. *Anesthesiology* 41:562, 1974.
28. Jobes, D. J., Kennell, E. M., Bitner, R., et al. Effects of morphine-nitrous oxide anesthesia on cerebral autoregulation. *Anesthesiology* 42:30, 1975.
29. Jobes, D. J., Kennell, E. M., Bush, G. L., et al. Cerebral blood flow and metabolism during morphine-nitrous oxide anesthesia in man. *Anesthesiology* 47:16, 1977.
30. Keykhah, M. M., Smith, D. S., Carlsson, C., et al. Influence of sufentanil on cerebral metabolism and circulation in the rat. *Anesthesiology* 63:274, 1985.
31. Kofke, W. A., Hawkins, R. A., Davis, D. W., and Biebuyck, J. F. Comparison of the effects of volatile anesthetics on brain glucose metabolism in rats. *Anesthesiology* 66:810, 1987.
32. Larsen, R., Hilfiker, O., Radke, J., and Sonntag, H. Midazolam: Wirkung auf allgemeine Hamodynamik, Hirndurchblutung und cerebralen Sauerstoffverbrauch bei neurochirurgischen Patienten. *Anaesthetist* 30:18, 1981.
33. Maekawa, T., Sakabe, T., and Takeshita, H. Diazepam blocks cerebral metabolic and circulatory responses to local anesthetic-induced seizures. *Anesthesiology* 41:389, 1974.
34. Madsen, J. B., Cold, G. E., Hansen, E. S., and Bardrum, B. The effect of isoflurane on cerebral blood flow and metabolism in humans during craniotomy for small supratentorial cerebral tumors. *Anesthesiology* 66:332, 1987.
35. Manohar, M., and Parks, C. Regional distribution of brain and myocardial perfusion in swine while awake and during 1.0 and 1.5 MAC isoflurane anaesthesia produced without or with 50% nitrous oxide. *Cardiovasc. Res.* 18:344, 1984.
36. McDowall, D. G. The effects of clinical concentrations of halothane on the blood flow and oxygen uptake of the cerebral cortex. *Br. J. Anaesth.* 39:186, 1967.
37. McPherson, R. W., and Traystman, R. J. Fentanyl and cerebral vascular responsivity in dogs. *Anesthesiology* 60:180, 1984.
38. Messick, J. M., Jr., and Theye, R. A. Effects of pentobarbital and meperidine on canine cerebral and total oxygen consumption rates. *Can. Anaesth. Soc. J.* 16:321, 1969.
39. Michenfelder, J. D. The interdependency of cerebral functional and metabolic effects following massive doses of thiopental in the dog. *Anesthesiology* 41:231, 1974.
40. Michenfelder, J. D., and Cucchiara, R. F. Canine cerebral oxygen consumption during enflurane anesthesia and its modification during induced seizures. *Anesthesiology* 40:575, 1974.
41. Michenfelder, J. D., and Theye, R. A. Effects of fentanyl, droperidol and Innovar on canine cerebral metabolism and blood flow. *Br. J. Anaesth.* 43:630, 1971.
42. Milde, L. N., Milde, J. H., and Michenfelder, J. D. Cerebral functional, metabolic and hemodynamic effects of etomidate in dogs. *Anesthesiology* 63:371, 1985.
43. Miletich, D. J., Ivankovich, A. D., Albrecht, R. F., et al. Absence of autoregulation of cerebral blood flow during halothane and enflurane anesthesia. *Anesth. Analg. (Cleveland)* 55:100, 1976.

44. Misfeldt, B. B., Jorgensen, P. B., Spotoft, H., and Ronde, F. The effects of droperidol and fentanyl on intracranial pressure and cerebral perfusion pressure in neurosurgical patients. *Br. J. Anaesth.* 48:963, 1976.

45. Morita, H., Nemoto, E. M., Bleyaert, A. L., and Stezoski, S. W. Brain blood flow autoregulation and metabolism during halothane anesthesia in monkeys. *Am. J. Physiol.* 233:H670, 1977.

46. Moss, E., Powell, D., Gibson, R. M., and McDowall, D. G. Effects of fentanyl on intracranial pressure and cerebral perfusion pressure during hypocapnia. *Br. J. Anaesth.* 50:779, 1978.

47. Nikki, P. H., Nemoto, E. M., Bleyaert, A. L., et al. Absence of B-adrenergic receptor involvement in cerebrovascular dilation by halothane in monkeys. *Anesth. Analg.* 66:39, 1987.

48. Nugent, M., Artru, A. A., and Michenfelder, J. D. Cerebral metabolic, vascular and protective effects of midazolam maleate. *Anesthesiology* 56:172, 1982.

49. Ori, C., Dam, M., Pizzolato, G., et al. Effects of isoflurane on local cerebral glucose utilization in the rat. *Anesthesiology* 65:152, 1986.

50. Pelligrino, D. A., Miletich, D. J., Hoffman, W. E., and Albrecht, R. F. Nitrous oxide markedly increases cerebral cortical metabolic rate and blood flow in the goat. *Anesthesiology* 60:405, 1984.

51. Phirman, J. R., and Shapiro, H. M. Modification of nitrous oxide–induced intracranial hypertension by prior induction of anesthesia. *Anesthesiology* 46:150, 1977.

52. Renou, A. M., Vernhiet, J., Macrez, P., et al. Cerebral blood flow and metabolism during etomidate anaesthesia in man. *Br. J. Anaesth.* 50:1047, 1978.

53. Rockoff, M. A., Marshall, L. F., and Shapiro, H. M. High dose barbiturate therapy in humans: A clinical review of 60 patients. *Ann. Neurol.* 6:194, 1979.

54. Rockoff, M. A., Naughton, K. V. H., Shapiro, H. M., et al. Cerebral circulatory and metabolic responses to intravenously administered lorazepam. *Anesthesiology* 53:215, 1980.

55. Sakabe, T., Kuramoto, T., Inoue, S., and Takeshita, H. Cerebral effects of nitrous oxide in the dog. *Anesthesiology* 48:195, 1978.

56. Sakabe, T., Kuramoto, T., Kumagae, T., and Takeshita, H. Cerebral responses to the addition of nitrous oxide to halothane in man. *Br. J. Anaesth.* 48:957, 1976.

57. Sari, A., Okuda, Y., and Takeshita, H. The effects of thalamonal on cerebral circulation and oxygen consumption in man. *Br. J. Anaesth.* 44:330, 1972.

58. Sari, A., Okuda, Y., and Takeshita, H. The effect of ketamine on cerebrospinal fluid pressure. *Anesth. Analg.* 51:560, 1972.

59. Scheller, M. S., Todd, M. M., Drummond, J. C., and Zornow, M. H. The intracranial pressure effects of isoflurane and halothane administered following cryogenic brain injury in rabbits. *Anesthesiology* 67:507, 1987.

60. Schulte, J., Thiemig, I., and Entzian, W. Wirkungen von etomidate und thiopental auf den stickoxydulbedingten intrakraniellen druckansteig. *Anaesthetist* 29:525, 1980.

61. Shapiro, H. M., Greenberg, J. H., Reivich, M., et al. Local cerebral glucose uptake in awake and halothane anesthetized primates. *Anesthesiology* 48:97, 1978.

62. Smith, A. L., Neigh, J. L., Hoffman, J. C., and Wollman, H. Effects of general anesthesia on autoregulation of cerebral blood flow in man. *J. Appl. Physiol.* 29:665, 1970.

63. Smith, A. L., and Wollman, H. Cerebral blood flow and metabolism: Effects of anesthetic drugs and techniques. *Anesthesiology* 36:378, 1972.

64. Stulken, E. H., Jr., Milde, J. H., Michenfelder, J. D., and Tinker, J. H. The nonlinear responses of cerebral metabolism to low concentrations of halothane, enflurane, isoflurane and thiopental. *Anesthesiology* 46:28, 1977.

65. Takeshita, H., Michenfelder, J. D., and Theye, R. A. The effects of morphine and N-allylnormorphine on canine cerebral metabolism and circulation. *Anesthesiology* 37:605, 1972.

66. Takeshita, H., Okuda, Y., and Sari, A. The effects of ketamine on cerebral circulation and metabolism in man. *Anesthesiology* 36:69, 1972.
67. Theye, R. A., and Michenfelder, J. D. The effect of nitrous oxide on canine cerebral metabolism. *Anesthesiology* 29:1119, 1968.
68. Todd, M. M. The effects of $PaCO_2$ on the cerebrovascular response to nitrous oxide in the halothane-anesthetized rabbit. *Anesth. Analg.* 66:1090, 1987.
69. Todd, M. M., and Drummond, J. C. A comparison of the cerebrovascular and metabolic effects of halothane and isoflurane in the cat. *Anesthesiology* 60:276, 1984.
70. Vernhiet, J., Renou, A. M., Orgogozo, J. M., et al. Effects of a diazepam-fentanyl mixture on cerebral blood flow and oxygen consumption in man. *Br. J. Anaesth.* 50:165, 1978.
71. Warner, D. S., Boarini, N. F., and Kassell, N. F. Cerebrovascular adaptation to prolonged halothane anesthesia is not related to cerebrospinal fluid pH. *Anesthesiology* 63:243, 1985.
72. Wollman, H., Alexander, S. C., Cohen, P. J., et al. Cerebral circulation during general anesthesia and hyperventilation in man. *Anesthesiology* 26:329, 1965.
73. Wollman, H., Smith, A. L., and Hoffman, J. C. Cerebral blood flow and oxygen consumption during electroencephalographic seizure patterns induced by anesthesia with Ethrane. *Fed. Proc.* 28:356, 1969.
74. Young, M. L., Smith, D. S., Greenberg, J., et al. Effects of sufentanil on regional cerebral glucose utilization in rats. *Anesthesiology* 61:564, 1984.

3

Electrophysiologic Monitoring: Electroencephalography and Evoked Potentials

BETTY L. GRUNDY

Electrophysiologic monitoring can help minimize neurologic damage during neurosurgical operations [10,11,23]. When the function of neural elements at risk is measured intraoperatively, surgical manipulations can be altered or treatment can be instituted to reduce the chance of injury. In some cases, electrophysiologic mapping of functional or diseased areas may be critical. Because electroencephalographic (EEG) and evoked potential monitoring provide information otherwise obtainable only by clinical examination of awake patients, these methods may, in some cases, obviate the need to do major procedures under regional anesthesia or to waken patients intraoperatively for the assessment of neurologic function.

The past decade has seen important progress in automated aids to electrophysiologic monitoring of the nervous system, but many questions are still unanswered [7]. Machines can only execute with literal faithfulness the instructions we give them, and our knowledge is still too limited for us to give perfect instructions. At present, EEG and evoked potential monitoring in clinical neuroanesthesia is limited less by hardware (the machines themselves) than by software (programming, or instructions for the machines), and less by software than by our clinical knowledge about what measurements are useful and what values are alarming. Perhaps the most serious problem in relatively inexperienced hands is quality control in signal acquisition.

I. **Applications in clinical neuroanesthesia.** Electrophysiologic monitoring of the nervous system is useful when some part of the nervous system amenable to monitoring is at risk or requires identification, when equipment and personnel are available to obtain technically satisfactory recordings and interpret them accurately, and when prompt responses to monitoring data with an appropriate treatment are possible [10].

Both the convexity of the cerebral cortex and specific sensory pathways can be monitored noninvasively using surface electrodes. EEG monitoring is useful when cerebral perfusion or oxygenation may be compromised, as during carotid endarterectomy, cardiopulmonary bypass, or induced hypotension. Evoked potentials are useful when the surgical

This work was supported in part by Grant Number GM 27942 from the National Institute of General Medical Sciences and by Merit Review Research funds from the Department of Veterans Affairs.

30

procedure might compromise a sensory pathway amenable to monitoring. For example, we monitor somatosensory evoked potentials during the resection of spinal cord lesions, brainstem auditory evoked potentials during operations in the posterior fossa, and visual evoked potentials during the resection of large pituitary tumors. Direct monitoring of motor pathways with electrical or magnetic stimulation of the motor cortex or cervical spinal cord is still largely experimental.

A. **Technical considerations.** Though Gibbs, Gibbs, and Lennox [8] advocated EEG monitoring during surgery in 1937, and Dawson [3] described sensory evoked potentials only ten years later, these methods are just now beginning to find widespread clinical use in the operating room. Barriers to effective application are rapidly giving way to advances both in technology and in the clinical neurosciences. More and more anesthesiologists are conducting or cooperating with electrophysiologic monitoring of the brain and spinal cord in everyday clinical practice. Progress has been made in the following areas.

1. **Signal acquisition.** Meticulous recording technique may be somewhat more difficult to achieve in the operating room than in the laboratory, but it is no less essential. Currently available technology allows efficient and clinically useful recording of electrophysiologic signals during anesthesia and surgery [2,26].

   a. **Recording montage (electrode placement).** Measurements must be made where events of interest are occurring. Single-channel EEG displays reflect only global insults or drug effects and have limitations even in these applications. Nevertheless, they can provide useful information during profound hypotension, cardiopulmonary bypass, or drug-induced coma. For single-channel EEG monitoring, biparietal or fronto-occipital electrode placements are popular. Other electrode positions may be indicated to avoid impinging on the surgical field.

   Use of two or four recording channels greatly increases the value of EEG monitoring. For example, electrical asymmetry is often the first indication of compromised cerebral function [18], and asymmetry can never be detected with single-channel recording. Sixteen or more channels unquestionably provide even more information than two or four channels, but both machines and personnel may be overloaded with data unless either a fully trained EEG technologist or an electroencephalographer is available to observe the record continuously.

   Electrodes should be placed according to the International Ten Twenty System [19]. Scalp locations over particular cortical areas are estimated from measurements of head circumference, distance between the nasion and inion, and distance between the ears (Fig. 3-1). It is helpful to have an experienced EEG technolo-

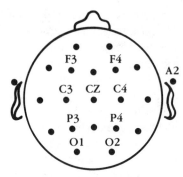

Fig. 3-1. Electrode positions designated by the International Ten Twenty System. The locations not labeled in this drawing also have standard letter and number designations. Note that all even numbers are to the right of the midline, all odd numbers to the left.

gist measure the head and place the electrodes. Symmetrical placement is particularly important when signals are processed by computer. Signal amplitude varies with the distance between scalp electrodes; because voltage asymmetries are of diagnostic interest, unevenly spaced electrodes hinder accurate interpretation of signals and displays.

For EEG monitoring during carotid endarterectomy, we use a full set of electrodes and a 16-channel strip-chart EEG monitored by an experienced EEG technologist when these are available. Otherwise, we use a two-channel device developed for use in the operating room or critical care unit, the Neurotrac (Interspec, Conshohocken, Pennsylvania). This monitor, as well as several other two- or four-channel machines, can be easily used by a single anesthesiologist with no technical assistance. Electrodes can be placed on the forehead and earlobe or mastoid (FP1–A1, FP2–A2) more easily than in hair-bearing areas of the scalp. For single-channel EEG monitoring during hypotension or drug-induced coma, we suggest P3–P4 (Fig. 3-1). More complex "brain-mapping" devices require a trained operator.

Montages for evoked potential monitoring vary according to sensory modality; they are discussed in section **III.**

b. **Application of electrodes.** We use 10-mm silver–silver chloride cup electrodes attached with collodion, filled with salt gel, and sealed with collodion and gauze. Gold or tin disk electrodes may also be used. The hair is parted but not cut. We twist the electrode wires together at about two turns per inch and position them to avoid mechanical disturbance. Fetal scalp electrodes twist into the subdermal tissue. They are more secure than straight subdermal needles, but perhaps less comfortable.

Electrodes can also be attached using conductive pastes. The application is simpler than with collodion, but electrodes are less secure and may be dislodged intraoperatively.

In areas without hair, a stick-on electrode with a saline gel pellet covering a silver–silver chloride disk is convenient (Cleartrace 1700-030, Medtronic, Haverhill, Massachusetts).

Sterile electrodes can be placed within the surgical field. We use platinum needle electrodes in subcutaneous tissue, ligament, or muscle. Wick electrodes, specially constructed metal electrodes, or electrode sets embedded in Silastic* sheets can be applied directly to the cerebral cortex or other neural structures.

Electrode impedances must be low and matched. Skin preparation with an abrasive gel minimizes the need for light skin abrasion with a blunt-tipped needle. Impedance should be measured at a frequency within the recording bandwidth, usually 20 or 30 Hz. We record electrode impedances before and after monitoring and at frequent intervals during the procedure, keeping them below 3000 ohm. With our methods of electrode application, impedances remain stable for many hours.

The commercially available Electro-Cap† may facilitate electrode placement when electrodes can be placed anywhere on the head and only standard electrode placements are required. Tin disk electrodes in ceramic holders are mounted in stretchable nylon caps of various sizes. Application is quick and easy but positioning is less secure than with other methods, and movement of an electrode away from the prepared area of the scalp interrupts recording from that electrode. This is a more serious limitation in the operating room than in the diagnostic laboratory because access to the head is often restricted, and, therefore, corrective adjustments may be impossible.

c. **Electrical interference.** Electrical impulses generated by the nervous system are small. The usual calibration mark on a clinical EEG tracing is 50 μV, compared to the 1 mV standardization mark on an electrocardiogram. Some evoked potentials are less than 1 μV in amplitude. To see these small signals in an electrically hostile recording environment, such as the operating room or intensive care unit, special precautions are necessary.

(1) **Leakage currents from other electrical devices** attached to the patient present little difficulty if standard safety requirements for electrically sensitive patients are met: leakage current from each device to the patient should be less than 10 μamp, the electrical system should provide balanced

---

* Dow Corning, Inc., Midland, Michigan.
† Electro-Cap, Dallas, Texas.

voltage for all line-powered devices attached to a patient, and provision should be made for dissipating static electricity.

(2) **Ground-loop interference** picked up by cables between patient and machine can be minimized by initial signal amplification near the recording electrodes and eliminated by radiotelemetry or by fiberoptic transmission. Even without these special devices, adequate recording is usually possible if cables are electrically shielded and are kept away from other electrical cords and devices.

(3) **Interference from the electrosurgical machine** remains an unsolved problem. Recording must be interrupted, either manually or automatically, during electrocoagulation. Eventually, it may be possible to analyze the activity produced by the electrosurgical machine and subtract this activity from the total signal acquired, obviating the need to suspend monitoring.

2. **Signal processing and display.** Machines serve many functions in electrophysiologic monitoring of the nervous system. Small electrical signals are filtered and amplified. Responses to sensory stimulation are made apparent by summation, averaging, or other techniques. Data are compressed to make trends stand out, or are stored for complex off-line analyses. Information of interest to the neuroanesthesiologist can be extracted and displayed in a useful format once the measurements required and the appropriate formats for presentation are developed. When quantitative measurements of interest and safe limits are defined, alarms can be generated.

Filter and amplifier settings vary according to the mode of recording. Excessive filtering can provide beautiful but erroneous wave forms. Heavily filtered artifacts may resemble physiologic signals, but they bear no relationship to the neurophysiologic state of the patient. When electrophysiologic signals are processed before display, the unprocessed wave form should be monitored to ensure adequate quality of the acquired data. Automatic artifact rejection is helpful but can, like excessive filtering, give misleading results.

II. Electroencephalogram

A. **Generators.** The EEG is generated by the pyramidal cells in the granular layer of the cerebral cortex. These cells, with their long dendritic trees oriented perpendicularly to the cortical surface, act in concert to generate dipole fields measurable at the scalp. Voltage fluctuations result not primarily from neuronal action potentials but rather from graded summations of excitatory and inhibitory postsynaptic potentials. A single surface electrode detects the simultaneous electrical activity of many cells; signal strength falls as the distance from the generator increases so that voltage is about 1/20 of its actual value at a distance of 2.5 cm.

B. Traditional EEG recording. The traditional EEG is a strip-chart plot of voltage against time (Fig. 3-2). Sixteen channels are usually recorded, but 8 or 32 channels may be used. Most often, 30 mm horizontally on the strip chart represents 1 second, and 7 mm vertically represents 50 μV, but these parameters vary and must be described. Records normally begin and end with calibration marks of known voltage (usually 50 μV) and "biocalibration," in which EEG activity from a single pair of electrodes is displayed on all channels simultaneously. Comments written on the strip chart by a well-trained technologist are an important part of the EEG record and are critical to interpretation.

1. Normal EEG patterns

    a. Wave forms. Wave forms seen on traditional EEG records are described in terms of frequency, amplitude, distribution, regularity, and specific patterns. Delta waves (1–4 Hz) are normally seen in deep sleep (slow-wave sleep) or deep anesthesia; but during wakefulness or light anesthesia, delta waves suggest compromised neuronal function (Fig. 3-2A). Theta rhythms (4–8 Hz), normally seen during drowsiness, are common during general anesthesia. Alpha rhythm (8–13 Hz) is the characteristically dominant rhythm of the occipital EEG during alert wakefulness with eyes closed (Fig. 3-2B). This rhythm may be seen over the entire scalp while the patient is under anesthesia. Frequencies in the beta range (13–30 Hz) are common in alert patients with eyes open and during light anesthesia. Beta activity is increased by barbiturates and benzodiazepines in doses given to ambulatory patients; characteristic patterns may persist as long as two weeks after withdrawal of chronic therapy.

    b. Pattern variations. EEG patterns vary from person to person, with physiologic changes, and with anesthetic agents and other drugs. Effective EEG monitoring during anesthesia and surgery depends not only on recognition of specific EEG patterns, but also on detection of pattern changes during critical surgical or anesthetic manipulations. Anesthesia should be managed to provide a relatively constant electrophysiologic state so that acute EEG changes caused by surgical intervention or physiologic insult will be apparent.

2. Abnormal EEG patterns

    a. Cortical malfunction. EEG signals can reflect impaired cortical function before irreversible tissue damage occurs. With sudden massive insult, such as cardiac arrest, the EEG becomes flat within seconds. Progressive ischemia produces slowing,

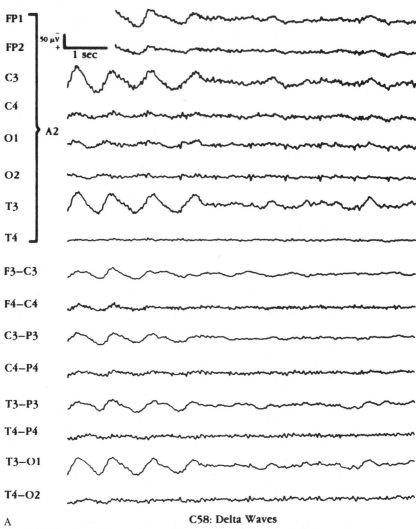

A   **C58: Delta Waves**

Fig. 3-2. Traditional strip-chart EEG recording, 16 channels, 10 seconds per page.
A. Delta waves and loss of amplitude during test occlusion of the left carotid artery.
Because of these EEG changes, a carotid artery shunt was inserted. *B.* Normal EEG
after successful carotid endarterectomy. Note alpha spindles in occipital leads.

then loss of amplitude. In 1145 cases of carotid endarterectomy
with EEG monitoring, 321 patients had EEG changes when the
carotid artery was clamped [30]. In 319 of these, the changes re-
verted to baseline with insertion of a shunt. All patients who had
a regional cerebral blood flow (rCBF) of less than 10 ml/100 gm
brain/min had rapid and severe EEG changes; flows of less than
15 ml/100 gm brain/min were usually associated with EEG alterations. Hypoxia, hypoglycemia, hypothermia, and extreme hypotension can also produce EEG slowing and loss of amplitude.

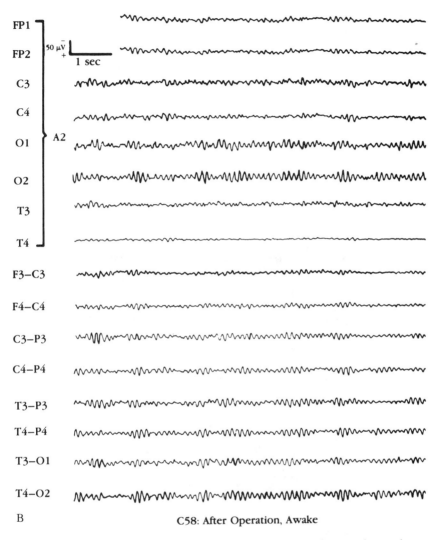

B   C58: After Operation, Awake

These patterns are not specific to the type of injury, but indicate cortical malfunction from any of several causes.

   b. Anesthesia. EEG patterns produced by different anesthetics are more specific; to some extent, they characterize particular drugs. Injury patterns, however, are recognizable during light general anesthesia with virtually all agents. With isoflurane, burst suppression occurs earlier than with most agents, and electrical silence is seen at approximately twice the minimum alveolar concentration (MAC) that produces immobility on skin incision in 50% of patients. In contrast, high-voltage delta waves persist to four times MAC during halothane anesthesia. When EEG monitoring is required at deep levels of anesthesia, isoflurane should be avoided.

C. **Signal processing and display.** Traditional EEG interpretation depends on visual recognition of patterns in plots of voltage against time. This method is tedious and time-consuming. It is inherently limited by the sensitivity and precision of pattern recognition, and it depends on the personal experience, judgment, and attention level of the observer. The amount of data in a lengthy, multichannel EEG record can be overwhelming. Several attempts have been made to overcome these problems by using machines to process signals automatically and generate useful displays [4,25]. We will confine this discussion to methods of EEG analysis and display performed by commercially available devices that have been used for monitoring neurosurgical patients in the operating room.

1. **Power spectral analysis.** Power spectral analysis converts EEG information from the time domain (strip-chart plot of voltage against time) to the frequency domain (plot of power against frequency for a given segment of EEG, usually 4–32 sec). Stockard and Bickford [29] popularized the compressed spectral array (CSA), which is a display of serial power spectra plotted one above the other (with or without hidden-line suppression) to give a time-compressed "mountain and valley" representation of EEG patterns (Fig. 3-3).

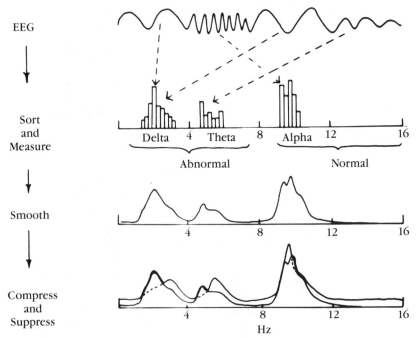

Fig. 3-3. Signal processing for the compressed spectral array (CSA), as popularized by Bickford. From R. G. Bickford, Computer analysis of background activity, EEG Informatics: A Didactic Review of Methods and Applications of Data Processing. A. Remond (Ed.). Amsterdam: Elsevier, 1977.

The numerical data used to generate the CSA are available for further manipulation or for the generation of other displays such as the "pie chart" display used by CNS (Eden Prairie, Minnesota). Digital computers using the Fast Fourier Transform (FFT) can plot power spectra and/or print digital values for several EEG channels on-line (Fig. 3-4). Although moment-to-moment changes in wave shape may be lost in transformation, there is little loss of data unless frequency components are averaged. The length of the EEG segment analyzed and the sampling rate of the analog-to-digital converter determine the frequency resolution possible. Often, more subtle changes become apparent in the CSA only after the lines representing power spectra for several epochs of EEG have been plotted; numerical values are more likely to show changes immediately. The CSA display is available on devices manufactured by Bio-logic Systems (Mundelein, Illinois), Nicolet Biomedical (Madison, Wisconsin), Cadwell Laboratories (Kennewick, Washington), Interspec (Conshohocken, Pennsylvania), and others.

The density modulated spectral array (DSA) also depends on analysis of the EEG power spectrum. This display differs from the CSA in that power in a given frequency band is depicted by different shades of gray or different colors (Fig. 3-5). DSA displays are used on monitors manufactured by Tracor Northern (Middleton, Wisconsin) and others.

3. **Aperiodic analysis.** The Lifescan Monitor by Diatek* is a dual-channel device for displaying processed EEG signals. Each wave in the analog EEG is recognized and plotted as a vertical line of height proportional to the wave's amplitude. Frequency is indicated by the position of this line on the horizontal axis of a three-dimensional display, and frequency bands are color coded (Fig. 3-6). The display moves up a television screen with time, and 4 to 32 minutes of EEG pattern can be seen at once. Aperiodic analysis gives a potentially more complete representation of information in the analog EEG than does power spectral analysis, but a large proportion of the vertical lines representing individual waves are suppressed to simplify the display. Time compression is less than with CSA or DSA and this limits the observation of trends.

4. **Other methods of EEG analysis.** Several methods for processing EEG signals have been reported in the literature. The methods that allow automated pattern recognition and alarm generation appear very promising for use in the operating room, and it seems likely that several such devices will be marketed during the next few years. Inevitably, large, complex devices that require constant attention will become smaller, more rugged, and easier to use, and there will be less need to sacrifice information in facilitating display.

* Diatek, Inc., San Diego, California.

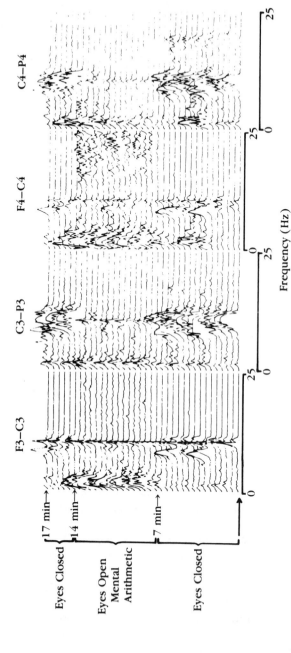

Fig. 3-4. Compressed spectral array (CSA), four channels. Activity in the alpha range, apparent when eyes are closed, diminishes markedly when subject opens eyes and does mental arithmetic.

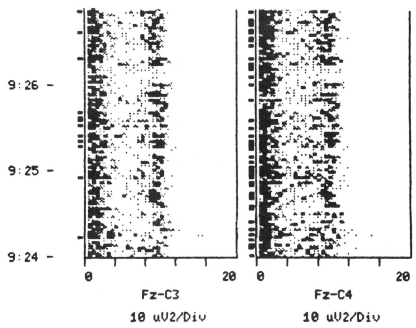

Fig. 3-5. Example of density modulated spectral array recorded in two channels.

Adequate quality control in signal acquisition will continue to be critically important for successful exploitation of improved technology.

III. Evoked potentials

A. General principles. The neuroanesthesiologist who undertakes evoked potential monitoring in the operating room needs to understand not only the basic concepts of evoked potential monitoring but also the technical, pharmacologic, and physiologic factors that must be taken into account if monitoring is to be effective.

1. The concept of evoked potential monitoring. Sensory evoked potentials are the electrical responses of the nervous system to sensory stimulation. If a stimulus (e.g., a small electric pulse) is applied to one part of the nervous system (e.g., the posterior tibial nerve), and if the expected electrophysiologic response can be reproducibly recorded from another part of the nervous system (e.g., the corresponding somatosensory area of the cerebral cortex), then we can assume that the sensory pathways between the site of stimulation and the site of recording (e.g., posterior columns of the spinal cord) are functioning properly. When some part of the sensory pathway is at risk during a neurosurgical operation (e.g., resection of a spinal cord tumor), evoked potentials can be used to monitor neurologic function intraoperatively, guiding the surgeon in manipulation of neural structures (e.g., the spinal cord) and the

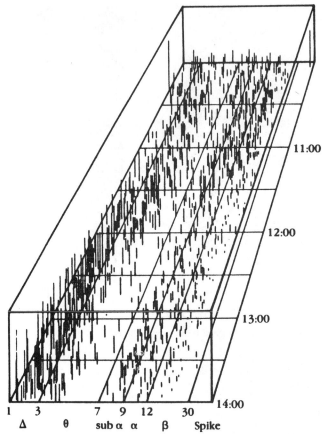

Fig. 3-6. EEG as displayed by Lifescan Monitor by Diatek during enflurane anesthesia, light to deep. Two channels can be displayed side by side.

anesthesiologist in management of physiologic parameters (e.g., arterial blood pressure).

2. **Signal processing.** Cortical evoked potentials can sometimes be seen in traditional EEG recordings, but special techniques are required to make these responses reliably apparent. Although methods such as special filtering of single responses and nonlinear analysis have been applied, most clinical evoked potential recording currently depends on summation or averaging of responses to repeated stimulation. Averaging increases the signal-to-noise ratio so that we can distinguish the signal (the evoked potential) from noise or, for potentials recorded from the scalp, from spontaneous EEG activity. Averaging works because evoked electrophysiologic signals are time-locked to the stimulus while the EEG is to some extent random. Several devices for recording averaged evoked potentials are commercially available.

3. **Categorization of sensory evoked potentials.** The averaged sensory evoked potentials considered here can be categorized according to the distance separating electrodes from neural generators (near-field, far-field), according to poststimulus latency (short, intermediate, long), and according to sensory modality (auditory, visual, somatosensory).

   a. **Distance.** Near-field potentials recorded from the scalp originate primarily in the same pyramidal cells that generate spontaneous EEG signals. These cortical potentials have either intermediate or long latency. Their amplitudes at the scalp are greater than the amplitudes of far-field potentials (those arising at sites farther away from the recording electrode), so that fewer individual responses must be averaged to separate the evoked potential from the on-going EEG.

   Electrophysiologic potentials generated at considerable distance from scalp electrodes can be recorded by averaging large numbers of individual responses. Potentials originating in the brainstem or in a peripheral nerve are transmitted to the scalp by volume conduction. These far-field potentials have shorter poststimulus latencies than do near-field cortical potentials.

   b. **Poststimulus latency.** In general, short-latency potentials are less altered by drugs and reversible changes in physiologic state than are potentials of intermediate or long latency. Long-latency potentials change even with subanesthetic concentrations of anesthetic agents; they are of little use in the operating room. Short- and intermediate-latency potentials are useful for monitoring auditory, visual, and somatosensory function in neurosurgical patients. Intermediate-latency sensory evoked potentials arise from the primary sensory cortex of the sensory modality being tested.

   c. **Sensory modality.** For a discussion of sensory modalities, see sections **B, C,** and **D,** below.

4. **Applications in the operating room.** Inviting applications of intraoperative evoked potential monitoring are summarized in Table 3-1. Of the applications now in clinical use, greatest experience has been gained with somatosensory evoked potential monitoring during surgical procedures on the spine and spinal cord. As experiments in animals and studies of human pathophysiology progressively clarify anatomic correlates of evoked potentials, the operating team can be increasingly confident that stable wave forms indicate intact neural function.

   Technical difficulties, anesthetic agents, and physiologic changes can all interfere with evoked potential monitoring. If electrophysiologic measurements are to influence decision-making in the operating room, definitive answers are essential: Is the change

Table 3-1. Applications of intraoperative sensory evoked potential recording

Auditory evoked potentials
   Resection of acoustic neurinoma
   Posterior fossa procedures
   Resection of temporoparietal lesions
   Epilepsy surgery
   Localization of specific auditory cortex

Somatosensory evoked potentials
   Resection of peripheral nerve lesions
   Resection of spinal cord lesions
   Operative treatment of scoliosis or other spinal deformity
   Posterior fossa procedures
   Stereotactic thalamic procedures
   Identification of rolandic fissure
   Epilepsy surgery
   Resection of parietal lesions

Visual evoked potentials
   Hypophysectomy
   Resection of retro-orbital lesions
   Resection of suprasellar lesions
   Neurovascular procedures involving blood supply to occipital cortex
   Epilepsy surgery

Peripheral nerve potentials and evoked muscle potentials
   Resection of acoustic neurinoma or other posterior fossa lesions impinging on the facial nerve
   Resection of lesions involving peripheral motor nerves
   Resection of central lesions involving motor nerves

produced by a loose electrode, by the anesthesiologist, or by the surgeon? Successful evoked potential monitoring requires meticulous recording technique, appropriate anesthetic management, and identification and constraint of variables other than surgical trespass on neural structures that might alter evoked potentials.

5. Technical factors. Each team must develop standard recording methods with built-in checks for quality control and must demonstrate reliability of evoked potential recording in the particular operating room environment in which monitoring is required. Whenever possible, standard electrode placement should be based on measurement rather than estimation. During supratentorial craniotomy, modified placements are usually necessary. Spontaneous EEG activity should be monitored continuously during averaging on either a strip chart or an oscilloscope. Artifact-reject options available on many machines are helpful; if the proportion of single responses rejected is excessive however (e.g., greater than 25%), the averaged wave form is suspect. Whenever possible, baseline evoked potentials should be recorded in the operating room suite before anesthesia is induced to confirm adequate technical function of the recording system and to provide preanesthetic baseline records for comparison with wave forms recorded intraoperatively. Numerous adequate systems for recording sensory evoked potentials are commercially available.

6. **Pharmacologic factors.** Rosner and Clark [1,27] reviewed early descriptions of the effects of anesthesia on evoked potentials in 1973. Numerous important reports have subsequently helped clarify the effects of several agents and combinations of agents on evoked potentials, but some points remain controversial. Virtually all anesthetics have some effect on evoked potentials, as do many drugs used as adjuncts to anesthesia. In general, short-latency potentials are more robust in the face of pharmacologic onslaughts than are later potentials.

The anesthesiologist should use drugs that only minimally modify the evoked potentials to be monitored. A relatively constant pharmacologic state must be maintained during the critical stages of the operative procedure so that changes in the wave form can be reliably attributed to surgical manipulation rather than to drug effects. New anesthetics and drugs that are not part of a group's established protocol should be avoided until their effects on evoked potentials have been defined.

Particular considerations apply to the following groups of drugs.

a. **Volatile anesthetics.** The volatile agents affect short-latency evoked potentials relatively little. Brainstem auditory evoked potentials, short-latency or "far-field" somatosensory evoked potentials, and evoked muscle potentials elicited by motor nerve stimulation can be reliably recorded during halothane, isoflurane, or enflurane anesthesia. Sensory evoked potentials of intermediate latency can be recorded if very low concentrations of these agents are administered, but at MAC and higher concentrations, these cortical potentials may be severely altered or abolished [24].

b. **Anesthetic gases.** Explosive agents are unacceptable; evoked potential monitoring equipment that is safe for use in the presence of flammable gases is not available. We therefore need consider only nitrous oxide (N_2O). This gas alters evoked potentials less than equipotent concentrations of the volatile inhaled anesthetics. Amplitudes of cortical potentials are somewhat diminished by N_2O, but poststimulus latencies are quite stable. Clinically useful concentrations do affect long-latency evoked responses, but short- and intermediate-latency potentials can be recorded reliably.

N_2O can enlarge closed air spaces, diffusing into these spaces more rapidly than nitrogen can be removed. In the infrequent case of tension pneumocephalus, N_2O would be expected to enlarge the closed air space, further separating the cortex from the recording electrodes (and perhaps further injuring the brain). If the middle ear air space were to be enlarged, auditory evoked potentials might be delayed. The clinical importance of this problem is not clear, but any resulting latency changes should affect all peaks equally. Possible confusion could be avoided by measuring interpeak, as well as absolute, latencies.

   c. **Intravenous anesthetics.** Short- and intermediate-latency potentials can be recorded after moderate doses of barbiturates, narcotics, or diazepam have been administered, but long-latency potentials are altered or abolished. Low doses of barbiturates and narcotics may enhance intermediate-latency somatosensory evoked potentials. Etomidate remarkably increases the amplitude of cortical potentials while slightly increasing latencies [28]. Diazepam in low doses alters but does not abolish these responses. Droperidol is erratic in its effects and should be avoided intraoperatively when potentials of intermediate or long latency are to be recorded. The effects of other intravenous agents have yet to be established.

   d. **Muscle relaxants.** Neuromuscular blocking agents have little if any effect on sensory evoked potentials. That part of an evoked potential arising from the sensory impulses generated by motor activity is lost during the period of neuromuscular blockade. Neuromuscular blockade must, of course, be allowed to dissipate when evoked muscle activity is to be monitored.

7. **Physiologic factors.** Variations in body temperature, arterial blood pressure, intracranial pressure (ICP), tissue perfusion, arterial tensions of oxygen [13] and carbon dioxide, and body chemistry can alter evoked potentials. In general, potentials of longer latency (those further removed in time from stimulation) are more sensitive to such factors than are short-latency potentials, but all may be affected by physiologic changes commonly observed during anesthesia and surgery. For example, even short-latency potentials are delayed by modest hypothermia. Physiologic changes interact with drug effects to alter evoked potentials in complex ways that are not yet fully defined. The neuroanesthesiologist must monitor physiologic variables that can alter evoked potentials and keep them as constant as possible, particularly during critical phases of the surgical procedure.

B. **Auditory evoked potentials**

1. **Generators.** Generators of specific waves in the brainstem auditory evoked potential complex (Fig. 3-7) have been tentatively described on the basis of studies in animals and clinical-pathologic correlations in patients (Table 3-2). Although the identity of these

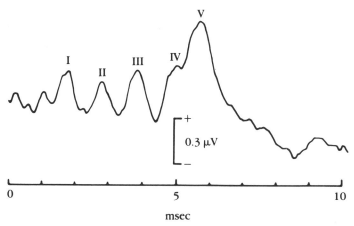

Fig. 3-7. Normal brainstem auditory evoked potential. Stimulation and recording parameters are shown in Table 3-3.

Table 3-2. Purported generators of brainstem auditory evoked potential waves

Wave	Purported generator
I	Extracranial auditory nerve
II	Intracranial auditory nerve and/or cochlear nucleus
III	Superior olive
IV	Lateral lemniscus
V	Inferior colliculus
VI	Thalamus
VII	Thalamocortical radiation

generators has not been definitely established, the concepts are clinically useful. Each wave actually represents not isolated activity from a single source, but a composite of simultaneous activity at multiple sites. Both ascending volleys in axons and action potentials in brainstem nuclei are thought to contribute to the observed wave forms. The cortical components of intermediate- and long-latency auditory evoked potentials, just as the spontaneous EEG recorded at the scalp, probably represent the graded summation of inhibitory and excitatory postsynaptic potentials in pyramidal cells.

   2. Methods. The stimulation and recording parameters used for intraoperative monitoring of brainstem auditory evoked potentials at the University of Florida are shown in Table 3-3. For cortical auditory evoked potentials, we use the same stimulus and the same electrode montage; rates of stimulation and sampling, sweep times, and numbers of repetitions are set to record intermediate-latency evoked potentials (see Table 3-6).

Table 3-3. Stimulation and recording
parameters for brainstem auditory evoked potentials

Stimulation
    Ear insert transducer
    Clicks: alternating rarefaction/condensation
    Volume: 60 decibels above patient's sensation level
    Duration:100 μsec
    Rate: 11.1–31.1 Hz
    Masking contralateral ear: white noise, 30 decibels below stimulus intensity
Recording
    Channel 1: CZ–A1
    Channel 2: CZ–A2
    Ground: FpZ
    Filters: 30–3000 Hz to 100–1000 Hz
    Sensitivity: ± 25 μV full scale
    Sweep time: 15 msec
    Sampling rate for digitization: 10,000–50,000 Hz
    Repetitions: 2000

The large shielded earphones used for auditory stimulation in the evoked potential laboratory are not appropriate for use during craniotomy because they would limit access to the surgical field. A variety of ear-insert transducers are provided with commercially available EP recording systems. With clicks of alternating polarity (rarefaction and condensation), stimulus artifact is minimal. Recording electrodes on the anterior surface of the earlobe are well away from the surgical field.

3. **Applications.** Auditory evoked potentials of both short and intermediate latency are used to assess eighth nerve and brainstem function during neurosurgical operations in the posterior fossa [14]. The patient who has an acoustic neurinoma and intact function of the affected eighth nerve is a prime candidate for intraoperative monitoring. Auditory evoked potentials can also be used to monitor the effects of retractor pressure on the eighth nerve or brainstem, so that the appropriate adjustments can be made before irreversible damage occurs [15]. Moreover, auditory evoked potential alterations may prove to be sensitive indicators of impending transtentorial brainstem herniation. Because they are less affected by anesthetic agents, brainstem auditory evoked potentials (Fig. 3-7) are preferable to intermediate-latency potentials for intraoperative monitoring of eighth nerve and brainstem function. These short-latency potentials are not useful for monitoring cortical function; however, potentials of intermediate latency may be helpful during extracranial-intracranial bypass or resection of temporoparietal lesions when cortical function is at risk.

C. Visual evoked potentials

1. **Generators.** Intermediate-latency visual evoked potentials (VEP) arise in the occipital poles of the cerebral cortex (Fig. 3-8). Whole-field stimulation of either eye normally produces potentials in both the right and left occipital cortex. Satisfactory methods for hemifield stimulation during anesthesia and operation have not been developed. Far-field visual evoked potentials have received little attention.

2. **Methods.** Visual stimulation during anesthesia can be accomplished using light-emitting diodes embedded either in contact lenses or in opaque goggles for use over closed eyes. Only the latter are commercially available. Although pattern-reversal stimulation is usually preferable to flash stimulation in the diagnostic laboratory, in the operating room we are limited to flash stimulation; patterns would not be apparent through closed eyelids. Representative stimulation and recording parameters are shown in Table 3-4.

3. **Applications.** Intraoperative monitoring of visual evoked potentials is most frequently used during operations on the pituitary gland, but monitoring can also be helpful during operations on retrobulbar lesions, lesions of the sphenoid wing, or other lesions impinging on the optic nerves or tracts. In addition, visual evoked potentials may prove useful during neurovascular operations that could jeopardize the blood supply to the occipital poles of the cortex. Ophthalmologists record electroretinograms (ERG) to evaluate retinal disorders, but we have not employed ERG monitoring in neurosurgical patients except to confirm signal input for VEP monitoring.

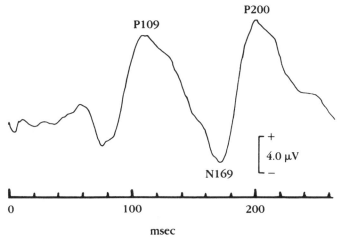

Fig. 3-8. Normal visual (flash) evoked potential. Stimulation and recording parameters are shown in Table 3-4. Peaks are labeled *P* for positive and *N* for negative, with numbers indicating poststimulus latency.

Table 3-4. Stimulation and recording parameters for flash evoked potentials

Stimulation
  Flash: light-emitting diode array on opaque goggles over closed eyelids or mounted
    on scleral contact lens
  Duration: 5 msec
  Rate: 0.9 Hz, pseudorandom interstimulus intervals
Recording
  Channel 1: 01–A2
  Channel 2: 02–A1
  Ground: FpZ
  Filters: 1–250 Hz
  Sensitivity: ± 50–100 μV full scale
  Sweeptime: 250–500 msec
  Sampling rate: 1000 Hz
  Repetitions: 100–200

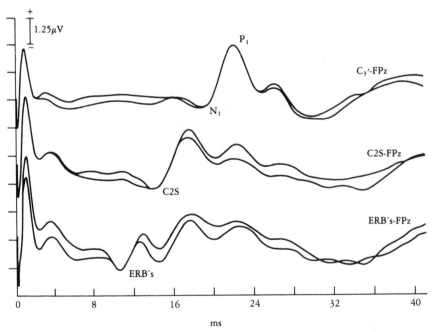

Fig. 3-9. Short-latency median nerve somatosensory evoked potentials. The
smooth waveforms are heavily filtered. From D. O. Peterson, J. C. Drummond, and
M. M. Todd, Effects of halothane, enflurane, isoflurane, and nitrous oxide on
somatosensory evoked potentials in humans. *Anesthesiology* 65:35–40, 1986.

D. Somatosensory evoked potentials

1. Generators. Intermediate-latency somatosensory evoked potentials originate from pyramidal cells in the specific somatosensory
areas of the postcentral gyrus (Figs. 3-9, 3-10), with later components arising in the association areas of the cortex. Purported

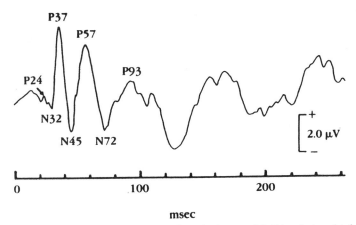

Fig. 3-10. Normal somatosensory cortical evoked potential. Stimulation (right posterior tibial nerve) and recording parameters are shown in Table 3-7. Peaks are labeled to show polarity and poststimulus latency.

Table 3-5. Purported generators of short-latency somatosensory evoked potentials to median nerve stimulation

Peak	Purported generator
N9	Brachial plexus
N11	Spinal roots or dorsal columns
N13, 14	Spinal cord gray matter or dorsal columns
N14, 15	Brainstem and/or thalamus
N20	Primary somatosensory cortex

N = negative.

       generators of short-latency somatosensory evoked potentials are outlined in Table 3-5.

  2. Methods. We use subdermal platinum or surface electrodes to stimulate peripheral nerves with brief electrical pulses. Our stimulation and recording parameters for somatosensory evoked potentials are shown in Tables 3-6 and 3-7.

  3. Applications. Because the somatosensory system has many available sites for stimulation and because this system traverses such a large proportion of the nervous system, somatosensory evoked potential monitoring finds many applications in neurosurgical patients. Spinal cord function has been monitored most frequently [12,16,17,20], but somatosensory function from peripheral nerve to cerebral cortex can be monitored as well. If a sensory pathway is at risk during surgery, it can be monitored by stimulating distally and recording proximally.

  E. Multimodality evoked potentials. Many of the devices now available require that potentials produced by stimulation in each sensory modality be recorded separately. This makes the time needed to

Table 3-6. Stimulation and recording parameters for median nerve somatosensory evoked potentials

Stimulation
    Median nerve at wrist
    Surface or subdermal electrodes
    Constant current square wave pulses slightly above motor threshold (usually 5–15 mamp)
    Duration: 250 μsec
    Rate: 0.9–6.1 Hz
Recording

	Channel 1	Channel 2	Channel 3	Ground
For right median nerve	EPr–FZ	C2S–FZ	C3′–FZ	Right antecubital fossa or either shoulder
For left median nerve	EP$_L$–FZ	C2S–FZ	C4′–FZ	Left antecubital fossa or either shoulder

Filters: 1–1500 Hz to 5–750 Hz
Sensitivity: ± 50 μV full scale
Sweep time: 40–100 msec
Sampling rate: 4000 Hz
Repetitions: 128

Note: C3′ = 2 cm behind C3; C4′ = 2 cm behind C4; EPr = Erb's point right; EP$_L$ = Erb's point left; C2S = spine of second cervical vertebra.

obtain full sets of multimodality evoked potential records excessive for intraoperative monitoring. Greenberg [9] has described the use of multimodality evoked potentials in the critical care unit. Multimodality evoked potential monitoring is valuable during some neurosurgical operations and can be efficiently performed by interweaving dual-stimulus modalities.

IV. Corticography and stereotactic recording. Corticography is important primarily for identifying epileptic foci that are to be resected. Somatosensory evoked potentials recorded directly from the cerebral cortex are used for cortical mapping. Wick electrodes or Silastic sheets with embedded electrodes are placed directly on the exposed cortex, and the responses evoked by somatosensory stimulation are used to identify the sensorimotor strip for the surgeon.

    Spontaneous EEG and evoked potential recordings are important for identifying structures in the depths of the brain during stereotactic operations when these operations are performed without the benefit of intraoperative computerized tomography. Radiographic control of stereotactic operations has largely replaced control by EEG and evoked potential recording, but advances in stereotactic neurosurgery are likely to offer important new opportunities for electrophysiologic monitoring.

Table 3-7. Stimulation and recording parameters for somatosensory evoked potentials (for right posterior tibial nerve stimulation)

Stimulation
  Right posterior tibial nerve at ankle
  Surface or subdermal electrodes
  Constant current square wave pulses slightly above motor threshold, usually 5–15 mamp
  Duration: 250 μsec
  Rate: 0.9–5.1 Hz
Recording
  Channel 1: PFi–FZ
  Channel 2: L3S–iliac crest
  Channel 3: C2S–FZ
  Channel 4: PZ′–FZ
Back
  Filters: 1–1500 Hz to 30–750 Hz
  Sensitivity: ± 50 μV full scale
  Sweep time: 90–250 msec
  Repetitions: 128–500

Note: PFi = ipsilateral popliteal fossa; L3S = spine of third lumbar vertebra; C2S = spine of second cervical vertebra; PZ′ = 2 cm behind PZ.

V. Motor evoked potentials. Peripheral motor nerves have long been functionally monitored during anesthesia by observing the muscle twitch or electromyogram elicited by an electrical current. Until recent years, evaluation of central motor pathways required the cooperation of an awake patient (e.g., the "wake-up" test of spinal cord function during spinal fusion for scoliosis or craniotomy with local anesthesia). Fortunately, somatosensory function in the spinal cord proved to be an excellent indicator of acute insult to motor function as well as to function of the posterior columns, where somatosensory sensation is largely transmitted [16,17]. Examination of the published reports of so-called false-negative somatosensory evoked potential monitoring shows that in all well-documented cases, marked transient changes in somatosensory evoked potentials occurred [6]. In other cases, there were errors in recording or interpretation. For example, obvious technical problems, recording above or below (but not across) the level of injury, failure to monitor continuously, or monitoring only with simultaneous stimulation of both lower extremities during hemicord injury explained many apparently spurious results. Nonetheless, a direct monitor of motor pathway function is of interest. Preliminary observations suggest that this might be even more valuable for intracranial operations than for operations on the spinal cord. During operations on large or complicated intracranial vascular lesions, postoperative motor deficits can sometimes be seen even when somatosensory evoked potentials are continuously monitored and are stable [7].

Transcranial stimulation of the motor cortex with electrical current or with magnetic transients has now been performed in both animals and humans [21,22]. Problems include lack of precise localization of the stimulus with resulting contraction of large paraspinous muscle groups that disrupt the surgical field. This has been managed by using a constant infusion of atracurium or vecuronium to produce subtotal neuromuscular blockade. Stimulation can also be done over the cervical spinal cord, but if only peripheral nerve action potentials are recorded (and not muscle activity), antidromically transmitted sensory impulses in a mixed nerve might be mistaken for motor potentials and lead to erroneous conclusions. Anesthetic management during transcortical stimulation is often complicated by hypertension and tachycardia. These cardiovascular responses to stimulation may lessen if the rate of transcortical stimulation is slowed. With magnetic stimulation, there must be some concern about the possible propulsion of ferromagnetic objects that might lie within the field of the magnet as it discharged. Studies to document the safety of prolonged repetitive stimulation of the cerebral cortex are still incomplete. Intraoperative monitoring of central motor evoked potentials is still largely experimental.

Interestingly, N_2O abolishes the motor evoked potential in rats while the somatosensory evoked potential is well preserved [31]. Effects of other anesthetics on motor evoked potentials have not been defined, but effects of some sedatives have been preliminarily described [5].

VI. Guidelines for anesthetic care. It is essential that surgeons, anesthesiologists, and neurophysiologists fully understand the requirements and constraints under which they mutually work. Reliably functional protocols should be developed for electrophysiologic monitoring in specific situations, and necessary deviations from the protocol should be communicated to team members immediately.

   A. Preoperative assessment. The neuroanesthesiologist and neurosurgeon must jointly determine needs for intraoperative electrophysiologic recording.

   1. Is EEG or evoked potential monitoring likely to provide information that can be acted on intraoperatively to improve the outcome of anesthesia and surgery?

   2. Which electrophysiologic measurements would be altered most readily by the particular neurologic injury for which a patient may be at risk?

   3. What sites for stimulation and recording will be accessible during this procedure?

   4. What physiologic manipulations might facilitate the surgical procedure, minimizing trauma to neural tissue, and how would these physiologic manipulations affect the contemplated EEG or evoked potential monitoring?

B. Pharmacologic management

1. **Monitoring requirements.** The anesthesiologist must select drugs that provide for the patient's safety and comfort, that maximally facilitate the operative procedure, and that minimally alter the EEG or the evoked potentials to be monitored. Once monitoring requirements are defined, the choice of anesthetic technique may be altered accordingly. For example, when intermediate-latency sensory evoked potentials are to be monitored, high concentrations of halogenated agents will not be used. If muscle activity evoked by motor nerve stimulation must be monitored, however, halogenated agents may be specifically chosen to ensure immobility of the patient in the absence of neuromuscular blockade. There are few situations in which individual patients require anesthetic regimens that interfere with intraoperative evoked potential monitoring.

   A relatively constant anesthetic state is needed to facilitate electrophysiologic monitoring, and patients should awaken rapidly at the conclusion of surgery to facilitate clinical neurologic assessment. Balanced anesthesia with nitrous oxide, thiopental, fentanyl, and muscle relaxants is usually suitable. Halothane or isoflurane can be added when neuromuscular blockade must be allowed to dissipate. These volatile agents do not interfere with monitoring of EEG or short-latency evoked potentials. Because early postoperative assessment is important in patients at risk for intraoperative neurologic injury, we avoid drugs with a long duration of action. Ketamine, scopolamine, and large doses of droperidol are particularly undesirable because of their prolonged and erratic effects on mental status in the postoperative period.

2. **Typical anesthetic regimen.** When indicated, we premedicate patients with hydroxyzine, adding meperidine when patients are in pain or when additional sedation is indicated. Induction of anesthesia is with thiopental (2–7 mg/kg) in divided doses and N_2O (50–70%) in oxygen. Vecuronium (0.1 mg/kg) provides muscle relaxation. Sufentanil (0.5 μg/kg or less) is given in divided doses before the skin incision. At the time of incision, thiopental (1 mg/kg) is given as a bolus, and a constant infusion of thiopental is begun at 1 to 3 mg/kg/hr. Incremental doses of vecuronium are administered as necessary. Sufentanil is infused at 0.1 μg/kg/hr. The infusion of thiopental is terminated when wound closure begins or earlier if clinically indicated. Reversal of neuromuscular blockade and withdrawal of N_2O at the conclusion of the procedure produce prompt awakening of the patient. Variations of this technique include replacement of N_2O and thiopental infusion with either low concentrations of isoflurane, or, for total intravenous anesthesia, with propofol.

C. Physiologic management. A primary goal of anesthetic care is maintenance of physiologic stability. However, specific physiologic manipulations are often used to facilitate neurosurgical operations or to minimize neurologic damage. The anesthesiologist can make evoked potential monitoring more effective by maintaining a relatively constant physiologic state during critical monitoring periods. With each change of state (e.g., hypothermia, hypotension, hemodilution), new "baseline" evoked potentials should be recorded for comparison with wave forms recorded during subsequent operative manipulation.

To induce hypotension we use a combination of beta-adrenergic blockade and labetolol, nitroprusside, or trimethaphan. Vasopressors such as phenylephrine or dopamine are used as needed to raise arterial blood pressure. Volume loading to minimize vasospasm is accomplished using albumin and a balanced salt solution. Packed red cells and whole blood are given to maintain an arterial hematocrit of 30 to 35%. Unintentional hypothermia is a common problem. To maintain normothermia, we use heated humidification of inspired gases, radiant and blanket heaters, and cotton webbing wraps for extremities. Elevation of room temperature is rarely necessary.

D. Monitoring. Arterial blood pressure, temperature, blood gas tensions, and hematocrit must be measured; changes in these parameters can alter evoked potentials. In addition, we routinely monitor the electrocardiogram, central venous pressure, urine output, inspired oxygen concentration, neuromuscular blockade, and serum electrolytes, glucose, and osmolality.

VII. Perspective. Intraoperative EEG and evoked potential monitoring are now practical, but some problems remain. Technical difficulties include cost, the lack of standardization in equipment and recording techniques, the need for a high level of operator training, the requirement for excessive operator-machine interaction with some devices, and the inability to record during use of the electrosurgical machine. Totally satisfactory methods of signal analysis have yet to be developed.

All of these problems are amenable to solution using currently available technology. Collaboration among neurophysiologists, clinicians, and manufacturers will facilitate standardization of equipment and recording methods. The levels of operator training and operator-machine interaction now required will be reduced by increasing automation. New developments in signal analysis and pattern recognition will facilitate EEG interpretation and characterization of evoked potential wave forms. Studies of the condition of patients after operative procedures are needed to define intraoperative EEG and evoked potential changes that are predictive of untoward neurologic sequelae.

The present state of EEG and evoked potential monitoring in the operating room resembles, in many respects, the state of electrocardiographic monitoring a generation ago. We know that loss of the signal is ominous, but quantitative description of subtle wave form alterations that may have predictive value is lacking. As technical problems and problems of interpretation are solved, EEG and evoked potential monitoring, like electrocardiographic monitoring, enjoys increasingly widespread use. Cost-effective application of these new methods is now clearly possible. The anesthesiologist can facilitate intraoperative electrophysiologic monitoring by using those drugs that least alter EEG and evoked potentials, by giving careful attention to technical details, and by keeping the pharmacologic and physiologic state of the patient relatively constant during critical monitoring periods.

References

1. Clark, D. L., and Rosner, B. S. Neurophysiologic effects of general anesthetics: I. The electroencephalogram and sensory evoked responses in man. *Anesthesiology* 38:564, 1973.
2. Cooper, R., Osselton, J. W., and Shaw, J. C. *EEG Technology* (3rd ed.). London: Butterworths, 1980.
3. Dawson, G. D. Cerebral responses to electrical stimulation of peripheral nerve in man. *J. Neurol. Neurosurg. Psychiatry* 10:137, 1947.
4. Dolce, G., and Kunkel, H. (Eds.). *CEAN: Computerized EEG Analysis.* Stuttgart: Gustaf Fischer Verlag, 1975.
5. Drummond, J. C., Tung, H. C., and Bickford, R. G. The effects of sedative agents on magnetic motor evoked potentials. *J. Clin. Neurophysiol.* 4:366, 1988.
6. Friedman, W. A., and Grundy, B. L. Are sensory evoked potentials useful in the operating room? *J. Clin. Monit.* 3:38, 1987.
7. Friedman, W. A., Theisen, G. J., and Grundy, B. L. Electrophysiologic Monitoring of the Nervous System. In R. K. Stoelting, P. G. Barash, and T. J. Gallagher (Eds.), *Advances in Anesthesia,* Vol. 6. Chicago: Year Book Medical, 1988. Pp. 231–289.
8. Gibbs, F. A., Gibbs, E. L., and Lennox, W. G. Effect on the electro-encephalogram of certain drugs which influence nervous activity. *Arch. Intern. Med.* 60:154, 1937.
9. Greenberg, R. P., Becker, D. P., Miller, J. D., and Mayer, D. J. Evaluation of brain function in severe human head trauma with multimodality evoked potentials. *J. Neurosurg.* 47:163, 1977.
10. Grundy, B. L. Monitoring of sensory evoked potentials during neurosurgical operations: Methods and applications. *Neurosurgery* 11:556, 1982.
11. Grundy, B. L. Intraoperative monitoring of sensory-evoked potentials. *Anesthesiology* 58:72, 1983.
12. Grundy, B. L., and Friedman, W. Electrophysiological evaluation of the patient with acute spinal cord injury. *Crit. Care Clin.* 3:519, 1987.
13. Grundy, B. L., Heros, R. C., Tung, A. S., and Doyle, E. Intraoperative hypoxia detected by evoked potential monitoring. *Anesth. Analg.* (Cleve.), 60:437, 1981.
14. Grundy, B. L., Jannetta, P. J., Procopio, P. T., et al. Intraoperative monitoring of brain-stem auditory evoked potentials. *J. Neurosurg.* 57:674, 1982.
15. Grundy, B. L., Lina, A., Procopio, P. T., and Jannetta, P. J. Reversible evoked potential changes with retraction of the eighth cranial nerve. *Anesth. Analg.* (Cleve.) 60:835, 1981.
16. Grundy, B. L., Nash, C. L., and Brown, R. H. Arterial pressure manipulation alters spinal cord function during correction of scoliosis. *Anesthesiology* 54:249, 1981.
17. Grundy, B. L., Nash, C. L., and Brown, R. H. Deliberate hypotension for spinal

fusion: Prospective randomized study with evoked potential monitoring. *Can. Anaesth. Soc. J.* 29:452, 1982.

18. Grundy, B. L., Sanderson, A. C., Webster, M. W., et al. Hemiparesis following carotid endarterectomy: Comparison of monitoring methods. *Anesthesiology* 55:462, 1981.

19. Jasper, H. H. The ten twenty electrode system of the International Federation. *Electroencephalogr. Clin. Neurophysiol.* 10:371, 1958.

20. Kaplan, B. J., Friedman, W. A., Alexander, J. A., and Hampson, S. R. Somatosensory evoked potential monitoring of spinal cord ischemia during aortic operations. *Neurosurgery* 19:82, 1986.

21. Levy, W. J., York, D. H., McCaffrey, M., and Tanzer, F. Motor evoked potentials from transcranial stimulation of the motor cortex in humans. *Neurosurgery* 15:287, 1984.

22. Merton, P. A., Hill, D. K., Morton, H. B., and Marsden, C. D. Scope of a technique for electrical stimulation of human brain, spinal cord, and muscle. *Lancet* 2:597, 1982.

23. Nuwer, M. R. (Ed.). *Evoked Potential Monitoring in the Operating Room.* New York: Raven, 1986.

24. Peterson, D. O., Drummond, J. C., and Todd, M. M. Effects of halothane, enflurane, isoflurane, and nitrous oxide on somatosensory evoked potentials in humans. *Anesthesiology* 65:35, 1986.

25. Remond, A. (Ed.). *EEG Informatics. A Didactic Review of Methods and Applications of EEG Data Processing.* Amsterdam, Elsevier, 1977.

26. Richey, E. T., and Namon, R. *EEG Instrumentation and Technology.* Springfield, Ill.: Thomas, 1976.

27. Rosner, B. S., and Clark, D. L. Neurophysiologic effects of general anesthetics: II. Sequential regional actions in the brain. *Anesthesiology* 39:59, 1973.

28. Sloan, T. B., Ronai, A. K., Toleikis, J. R., and Koht, A. Improvement of intraoperative somatosensory evoked potentials by etomidate. *Anesth. Analg.* 67:582, 1988.

29. Stockard, J., and Bickford, R. The Neurophysiology of Anaesthesia. In E. Gordon (Ed.), *A Basis and Practice of Neuroanaesthesia* (2nd ed.). Amsterdam: Excerpta Medica, 1981.

30. Sundt, T. M., Jr., Sharbrough, F. W., Piepgras, D. G., et al. Correlation of cerebral blood flow and electroencephalographic changes during carotid endarterectomy: With results of surgery and hemodynamics of cerebral ischemia. *Mayo Clin. Proc.* 56:533, 1981.

31. Zentner, J., and Ebner, A. Nitrous oxide suppresses the electromyographic response evoked by electrical stimulation of the motor cortex. *Neurosurgery* 24:60, 1989.

4

Cerebral Damage and Pharmacologic Intervention

FREDERICK G. MIHM

JAMES E. COTTRELL

JOHN HARTUNG

IRA KASS

AUDREE A. BENDO

A. ELISABETH ABRAMOWICZ

Barbiturates

Few areas of anesthesia or intensive care are as controversial as barbiturate treatment of severe brain injuries. Differences of opinion exist because of limited useful information and because of different interpretations of the available data. Many clinicians caring for severely brain-damaged patients with poor prognoses are routinely using barbiturates, hoping that benefit will be gained in an otherwise hopeless situation. Meanwhile, researchers in the field, and those not directly involved with the care of severely brain-damaged patients, demand more solid experimental proof before endorsing the clinical use of barbiturates for brain protection. With these problems in mind, we will review the current state of barbiturate treatment for intracranial hypertension and focal and global ischemia, both from the researcher's perspective (potential beneficial and harmful effects, animals studies) and from the position of the clinician (current mortality, morbidity, and barbiturate experience in stroke, postcardiac arrest, head trauma, Reye's syndrome, and near-drowning).

I. **Potential beneficial effects.** Anesthetic barbiturates effect a significant decrease in cerebral metabolic requirement for oxygen ($CRMO_2$) and cerebral blood flow (CBF). Knowledge of these actions led to the barbiturates' use in animal models of cerebral ischemia. Barbiturates without anesthetic properties are unable to protect the brain [192]. The potential beneficial effects of barbiturates that may result from actions that may be unrelated to concomitant changes in $CMRO_2$ and CBF include the following: decreased free radical activity, decreased edema, beneficial anesthesia state, and anticonvulsant activity.

A. **$CMRO_2$.** Pierce and colleagues [160] documented in humans that an anesthetic dose of thiopental will decrease the $CMRO_2$ by 52%. Since the brain has limited oxygen and energy reserves (with complete ischemia, oxygen and adenosine triphosphate [ATP] are exhausted in 10 seconds and 5 minutes, respectively), it is logical that an injured

59

brain might benefit from a drug that reduces oxygen consumption. Michenfelder [128] has shown in dogs that the flat electroencephalogram (EEG) produced by administration of barbiturates provides a physiologic endpoint for maximal $CMRO_2$ depression. This implies that barbiturates affect only the cells' electrical activity and not the more vital cellular processes (e.g., sodium-potassium pump). Since many drugs that depress $CMRO_2$ do not protect the brain [81], additional mechanisms of action have been sought to explain why barbiturates sometimes do protect.

B. Increased cerebrovascular resistance (CVR). Barbiturates are potent cerebral vasoconstrictors. Pierce and colleagues [160] have shown that anesthetic doses of thiopental will increase CVR and thereby decrease CBF by 48%. Barbiturates do not produce ischemia, however, because the decrease in $CMRO_2$ is always more profound than the decrease in blood flow. Cerebral vasoconstriction by barbiturates may produce two effects: a decrease in intracranial pressure (ICP) and a favorable redistribution of blood flow to more ischemic areas ("inverse steal").

1. **Decreased ICP.** The potent vasoconstriction induced by barbiturates will increase CVR, which decreases total cerebral blood volume (CBV) and thereby lowers ICP.

Barbiturates $\rightarrow$ CVR $\uparrow$ $\rightarrow$ CBV $\downarrow$

Barbiturates have been effectively used to lower ICP in neurosurgical patients [173] and in patients who have head trauma [51,121], Reye's syndrome [120], and near-drowning [130]. Many of these patients fail to respond to routine therapy (hyperventilation, osmotic diuretics, and steroids).

   a. When barbiturates are used to treat increased ICP, care must be taken to ensure hemodynamic stability so that cerebral perfusion pressure (CPP) is not unduly compromised. CPP is the difference between mean arterial pressure (MAP) and intracranial pressure: CPP = MAP − ICP. Several studies show that CPP will increase while ICP decreases in most patients who are properly managed [173,174].

   b. The response to thiopental is rapid (1–10 min), but it is only of short duration (30–90 min) if administered by intermittent bolus [51]. The dose of thiopental needed to maintain maximal cerebral vasoconstriction is not known, but suggested infusion rates range from 0.06 to 0.30 mg/kg/min. The exact infusion rate is difficult to determine because of the nonlinear kinetics of this drug (see sec. **II.B.2**).

2. **"Inverse steal" or "Robin Hood phenomenon."** Another important effect of cerebral vasoconstriction is a beneficial redistribution of blood flow from normal (or near normal) areas of the

brain to severely ischemic areas. This inverse steal or Robin Hood phenomenon can be easily understood by examining the effects of high and low arterial carbon dioxide tension ($PaCO_2$) on a brain that has an area of local ischemia (Fig. 4-1).

a. In the area of focal ischemia, the cerebral vessels are in a state of "vasomotor paralysis," where maximal vasodilatation exists secondary to local tissue acidosis. Cerebral vessels in this area cannot respond further to vasodilators (e.g., high $PaCO_2$, isoflurane) and will not respond to vasoconstrictors (e.g., low $PaCO_2$, barbiturates). In a condition of high $PaCO_2$ (Fig. 4-1A), the normal areas of the brain will vasodilate, resulting in shunting of blood away from the ischemic area where the vessels were already maximally vasodilated ("intracerebral steal"). With a low $PaCO_2$ (Fig. 4-1B), which is analogous to barbiturate treatment, normal vessels vasoconstrict, shunting blood toward the ischemic area, which is unresponsive to other interventions (inverse steal).

b. Barbiturates have been shown to cause an inverse steal in areas of focal ischemia and in areas of heterogenous regional blood flow seen after global ischemia [109]. It is unclear what beneficial role cerebral vasoconstriction plays in some ischemic injuries, however, since hyperventilation after stroke in human beings has not been beneficial [47].

C. Decreased free radical activity. Barbiturates can decrease free radical activity associated with ischemic brain injuries.

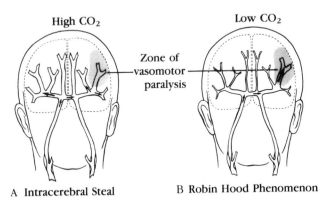

Fig. 4-1. Effect of carbon dioxide (CO_2) on blood flow through ischemic brain. Ischemia causes a zone of vasomotor paralysis in which the vessels are already maximally dilated. *A.* When the CO_2 is high, vessels in this ischemic area cannot dilate further and a condition of intracerebral steal results: Blood is shunted away from the ischemic zone to areas of normal brain where vessels have dilated in response to the elevation in CO_2. *B.* Conversely, when the CO_2 is low, the Robin Hood phenomenon, or inverse steal, causes blood to go from areas of normally perfused brain where the vessels can constrict in response to a decrease in CO_2 to the zone of vasomotor paralysis in which the vessels do not respond to changes in CO_2.

1. **Definition.** Free radicals are chemical forms containing an unpaired electron in their outer orbit. Whether or not they carry a charge, this unpaired electron makes the molecule highly reactive. Free radicals may represent a final common pathway of cell destruction. They are frequently intermediates of stable parent compounds, and they may be produced by a wide variety of agents or conditions [39]. The following are associated with free-radical activation.

   a. Doxorubicin hydrochloride (Adriamycin)
   b. Bleomycin
   c. Daunorubicin
   d. Chloroform
   e. Halothane
   f. Paraquat
   g. Aging
   h. Granulocytes
   i. Hyperoxia
   j. Hypoxia
   k. Radiation

2. **Activators.** Radiation therapy [122] and chemotherapeutic agents (daunorubicin, bleomycin, doxorubicin hydrochloride) [115] are known to damage tissue by forming free radicals. The liver toxicity produced by halogenated anesthetic drugs (chloroform, halothane) may be caused by reactive intermediate compounds (i.e., free radicals) [36]. Granulocytes and macrophages phagocytize, or "kill," and produce inflammation by release of the oxygen free radical, superoxide [14]. The process of aging may actually be linked to a loss of control of free radical activity, which normally occurs in small amounts in aerobic cells [115]. Oxygen toxicity of the lung probably occurs secondary to superoxide formation, which is enhanced by the herbicide paraquat. Even ischemia with resultant hypoxia can produce oxygen-free radicals that may ultimately destroy the cell [71,77].

3. **Role of oxygen.** Oxygen has a key role in initiating free radical activity. Normally in the aerobic cell, most oxygen is consumed by a bivalent pathway in the respiratory chain (Fig. 4-2). This means that two electrons are added simultaneously as water is formed. However, 5% of oxygen consumption is handled by a univalent pathway, where one electron is added at a time, creating the superoxide radical. All aerobic cells have the enzymes superoxide dismutase, catalase, and peroxidase, which convert superoxide first to hydrogen peroxide and then ultimately to water.

   These enzyme systems are helped by various naturally occurring antioxidants, the so-called free radical scavengers: glutathione, alpha-tocopherol, ascorbic acid, and cholesterol. If the enzyme systems are overloaded (secondary to activators), superoxide and hy-

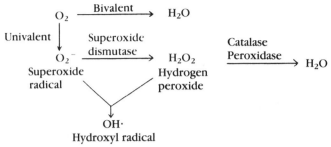

Fig. 4-2. Oxygen-free radicals. Oxygen picks up a bivalent charge and forms water (H_2O). When oxygen acquires a univalent charge, it is transformed into a superoxide radical that can be transformed by superoxide dismutase to hydrogen peroxide (H_2O_2) or can combine directly with H_2O to form the hydroxyl radical (OH·). Hydrogen peroxide is transformed to H_2O by the action of catalase and peroxidase.

drogen peroxide will accumulate and combine to form the reactive hydroxyl radical. These free radicals destroy cells by attacking the lipid moieties within the cell wall. A chain reaction of lipid peroxidation (with production of lipid free radicals) will eventually disrupt the cell [77].

4. **Role of barbiturates.** Thiopental has been shown in vitro to decrease free radical lipid peroxidation induced by ultraviolet irradiation [59]. In a model of middle cerebral artery occlusion in cats, free radical activity was depressed by methohexital [72]. One of the few studies comparing different barbiturates demonstrated that thiopental was a significantly more potent free radical scavenger than phenobarbital and methohexital [186]. The significance of barbiturate suppression of free radicals is unknown, although some authors suggest that this suppression may be the main beneficial effect of these drugs.

D. **Decreased edema formation.** Barbiturates may affect edema formation after ischemic injuries. These brain injuries result in edema of two types: vasogenic edema, produced by infarction, and cytotoxic edema, produced by ischemia without infarction [70,152].

1. **Vasogenic.** The normal anatomy of a cerebral capillary includes tight junctions between the endothelial cells that make up the blood-brain barrier (Fig. 4-3A). If an insult produces infarction, these tight junctions fail and vasogenic edema forms from leakage of protein-rich plasma into the interstitial spaces of the brain (Fig. 4-3B). This type of edema can increase total brain volume and frequently leads to increased ICP and further damage.

2. **Cytotoxic.** Ischemia, on the other hand, may not cause immediate cell death, but it may be so severe that the cellular energy stores (ATP) fall and the ATP–dependent sodium-potassium pump fails. In this situation, sodium (with water), which was maintained outside

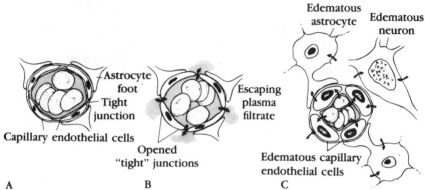

Fig. 4-3. Cerebral capillary endothelial cells. *A.* Endothelial cells of cerebral capillaries are joined by tight junctions. *B.* These tight junctions can open, permitting the escape of plasma filtrate into the surrounding brain parenchyma and causing vasogenic edema. *C.* In cytotoxic edema, the capillary endothelial cells, astrocytes, and neurons themselves become edematous from absorption of interstitial and intravascular fluid. (From R. A. Fishman, *N. Engl. J. Med.* 293:708, 1975. Reprinted by permission.)

the cell, leaks into the cell, causing the cellular swelling typical of cytotoxic edema (Fig. 4-3C). Note that the fluid shift with this kind of edema is primarily extracellular to intracellular, and, therefore, total brain volume may not increase. It is for this reason that vasogenic edema is associated with increased ICP and cytotoxic edema is not [70].

Even though cytotoxic edema may not cause secondary brain damage by increasing ICP, it may be partly responsible for the "no-reflow" phenomenon. The no-reflow phenomenon refers to regional nonperfusion of the brain in the postinsult period after systemic circulation has been reestablished. Other factors that may contribute to this phenomenon include viscosity changes, red cell and platelet aggregation, and potassium flux [98,145,208]. Capillary endothelial swelling from cytotoxic edema may "pinch" the capillary lumen in ischemic regions (Fig. 4-4). The increased resistance to flow caused by these capillary endothelial cells may occur while arterioles to the same region are maximally vasodilated (vasomotor paralysis).

In summary, ischemic injuries may result in two types of edema (Fig. 4-5). If necrosis occurs with the initial insult, vasogenic edema will form with subsequent further injury from increased ICP. In areas in which ischemia is not severe enough to cause infarction, cytotoxic edema and the no-reflow phenomenon may ensue, resulting in further irreversible damage. Cerebral edema after ischemic injury peaks at 48 hours [153]. It appears logical, then, that treatment (e.g., barbiturates) might be most effective if given continuously

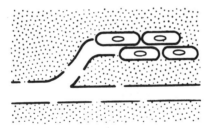

Fig. 4-4. No-reflow capillaries. Swelling of the cerebral capillary endothelial cells occurs after an ischemic insult, which prevents blood flow through that area once reperfusion has been established and exacerbates the initial injury. (From M. S. Christensen, *Acta Anaesthesiol. Scand.* [Suppl. 62]:8, 1976.)

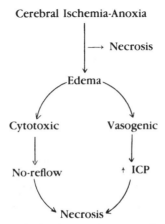

Fig. 4-5. Necrosis after cerebral ischemia or anoxia. The ischemic or anoxic insult causes necrosis both directly and indirectly through cytotoxic and vasogenic edema. Cytotoxic edema leads to necrosis because of the no-reflow phenomenon. Vasogenic edema causes necrosis by an increase in intracranial pressure (ICP).

during the 48 hours after injury and not as a one-time administration.

3. **Barbiturates.** Barbiturates have been shown to decrease edema formation after cryogenic lesions [49,185] and ischemic insults (middle cerebral artery occlusion in monkeys [181] and carotid ligation in gerbils [114]. Barbiturates also decrease potassium efflux from ischemic cells [10], and this decreased efflux may have a beneficial effect on cytotoxic edema. It is unclear whether this effect of barbiturates has a separate mechanism or is simply a combined effect of decreased $CMRO_2$ (and thereby protection of ATP stores for the sodium-potassium pump) and the inverse steal (vasoconstriction of normal areas increases regional perfusion pressure in damaged areas). Barbiturates may also decrease edema through an osmotic effect [3,15].

E. Anesthesia. The anesthetic state induced by high doses of barbiturates may be beneficial in several ways. Amnesia, immobilization, decreased total body oxygen consumption (VO_2), and complete analgesia are part of this state.

1. **Immobilization.** Immobilization by itself (muscle relaxants) has been shown to ameliorate ischemic injuries. The mechanism is not understood [26].

2. **Decreased VO_2.** The reduction of total body oxygen consumption may enhance oxygen delivery to more vital organs (e.g., brain, heart). This may be the reason that immobilization is effective. Muscle relaxants also reduce VO_2 by 30 to 40%.

3. **Analgesia.** High doses of barbiturates produce complete analgesia so that noxious stimuli, which can otherwise result in dangerous increases in ICP and catecholamines, are therefore avoided.

F. Anticonvulsant. Seizures are very expensive metabolic events. If seizures are controlled by a barbiturate, then the oxygen supply to the brain will not be as severely taxed. Not all barbiturates share the same pharmacologic properties. The anticonvulsant activity of phenobarbital is more effective than other commonly used barbiturates.

II. Potential harmful effects. Barbiturates have no known direct tissue toxicity [193]. In spite of this, the use of high doses of barbiturates is not necessarily a benign treatment. Hypotension, loss of the ability to perform neurologic examination, allergic reactions, polyuria, and withdrawal symptoms may occur.

A. Hypotension. By far the most significant complication of the use of barbiturates results from inadequate management of the hemodynamic effects of these drugs. Hypotension may occur in any patient receiving barbiturates, and may be particularly harmful in head-injured patients because CPP may be compromised even though ICP is reduced. Barbiturates act directly on the heart and on the arterial and venous circulation (Fig. 4-6).

1. **Systemic vascular resistance (SVR).** Traditionally, barbiturates were thought to constrict the arterial circulation, causing an increase in SVR [20,66,68,190]. However, in the high doses administered to critically ill patients, barbiturates may produce either no change or a decrease in SVR.

2. **Heart rate.** Chronotropic effects of barbiturates are variable. Heart rate can increase up to 15 to 30% in healthy persons, but may be variable or decrease in critically ill patients.

3. **Venous pooling, inotropic effects.** Regardless of their effect on systemic arterial tone and heart rate, hypotension may result after administration of barbiturates because of decreased inotropic effects and venous pooling of blood. Barbiturates cause dose-

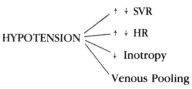

Fig. 4-6. Causes of hypotension after administration of barbiturates. These include an increase or decrease in systemic vascular resistance (SVR), an increase or decrease in heart rate (HR), a decrease in inotropy, and venous pooling.

dependent depression of myocardial contractility as measured by the changes in the first derivative of the left ventricular function curve [64,179,190]. Cardiac index may be decreased up to 15 to 25% by negative inotropic effects, but is equally influenced by venous pooling that can reduce right- and left-ventricular filling pressures.

4. **Assessment, treatment.** Both the venous pooling and negative inotropic effects of barbiturates can be reversed by the appropriate administration of fluids and positive inotropic agents [177,179]. Rational management of hypotension caused by barbiturates depends on the measurement of intravascular filling pressures, cardiac output, and systemic vascular resistance with a thermodilution pulmonary artery catheter.

B. **Loss of neurologic examination.** Another effect of treatment with barbiturates is loss of the ability to perform a neurologic examination because of drug-induced central nervous system (CNS) depression. However, in most clinical circumstances where barbiturates have been used, the patient is already in a coma and the neurologic examination is either insensitive or obviated by other routine therapy (e.g., muscle relaxants). In fact, for comatose patients who have increased ICP, an ICP monitor is a better indicator of the patient's status than are the late neurologic findings associated with herniation of the brain.

1. **"Ultrashort" barbiturates.** The use of ultrashort-acting barbiturates should minimize the duration of drug-induced CNS depression. Unfortunately, the ultrashort barbiturates may be long-acting when given in large doses. For example, thiopental, like some other drugs metabolized by the liver, can be given in quantities sufficient to saturate the hepatic enzyme system. This saturation results in zero-order kinetics, which greatly increases the apparent half-life of the drug [191].

2. **Nonlinear kinetics.** Thiopental in low doses behaves as a drug with first-order kinetics and has a half-life of about six hours. If we plot the log of the drug concentration ($\log C_P$) on the Y axis, we find that drugs exhibiting first-order kinetics produce decreasing concentrations over time that fall along a straight line (Fig. 4-7). The slope of this line defines the rate of elimination (half-life) of the

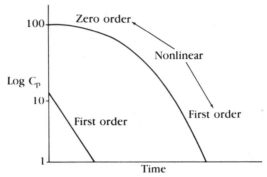

Fig. 4-7. Pharmacokinetics of drug metabolism. Most drugs follow first-order kinetics but the metabolism of large doses of barbiturates follows zero-order kinetics (p = plasma concentration).

drug and is constant at all concentrations of the drug. In high doses, however, the rate of decline of the concentration of thiopental is not linear, but falls very slowly over the range of zero-order kinetics. The apparent half-life of thiopental at these concentrations may be 50 to 60 hours. The rate of elimination progressively increases with time, however, and eventually returns to the first-order half-life of six hours [191].

3. **Implications.** These findings have important implications for barbiturate therapy and the problem of obviating the neurologic examination. It may be possible to minimize the time for recovery from the effects of the drug as the pharmacokinetics of high doses of barbiturates are better understood and as we clarify the amount of drug needed for maximal benefit.

C. **Allergy.** Mild allergic reactions to barbiturates have occurred, but true anaphylaxis is a rare event. A few cases of thiopental anaphylaxis have been reported. It is treated by standard regimens (epinephrine, steroids, antihistamines) [63].

D. **Polyuria.** Purely anecdotal experience has led some investigators to associate polyuria with barbiturate treatment. However, diabetes insipidus is a frequent secondary problem of neurosurgical patients, especially those who have head trauma, and is independent of barbiturate treatment.

E. **Withdrawal syndrome.** Barbiturate withdrawal syndrome may occur if a patient is treated with barbiturates for many days, although withdrawal symptoms associated with this type of barbiturate therapy have not been confirmed. In addition, there is evidence to suggest that neither withdrawal symptoms nor tolerance develops in patients treated for several days to two weeks [40; Mihm, unpublished data]. To avoid the possibility of seizures when discontinuing the barbiturates, another anticonvulsant drug (phenytoin) can be substituted.

III. Animal studies
A. Focal ischemia
1. **"Pro" studies.** Many experiments have demonstrated beneficial effects of barbiturates in focal ischemia. In vitro studies in the hippocampal brain slice [22] have demonstrated that thiopental protects after 10 minutes of anoxia. These studies documented in vitro protection without the effects of blood flow. Barbiturate treatment before, or up to two hours after, middle cerebral artery (MCA) occlusion in monkeys [24,91,126], dogs, cats, and baboons decreases neurologic morbidity as measured by neurologic function or infarction size [89,183]. Other studies of focal ischemia have produced similar results (MCA and internal carotid artery occlusion in dogs [83,184], common carotid artery occlusion in gerbils [123], embolization in monkeys [138]. An additional study suggests that delay of treatment for three or more hours after this type of injury reduces the effectiveness of barbiturates in neurologic injury [55].
2. **"Con" studies.** There are few contradictory studies on focal ischemia, and most have significant methodologic errors. One such study showed increased mortality in treated animals (60 vs. 14%), but this may have been because of inadequately managed hypotension that offset the potential beneficial effect of barbiturates [24].

B. Global ischemia.
Global ischemia is a difficult experimental model to create. The few studies carried out have generated much debate and conflicting opinion.
1. **"Pro" studies.** The first two studies reported impressive results. Wright [215] found that intracarotid injection of pentobarbital or thiopental in cats significantly increased ischemic tolerance. Goldstein [81] compared ischemic tolerance in dogs given local anesthesia ($FIO_2 = 0.21$ and 1.0), local anesthesia with 5% CO_2, morphine, or pentobarbital. Only animals anesthetized with pentobarbital tolerated global ischemia (aortic cross-clamp for 10 minutes) without severe morbidity or death. Thiopental given after global ischemia in monkeys was shown to ameliorate neurologic deficits over a seven-day period [25]. In a study of incomplete global ischemia and hypoxia (trimethaphan, 4% oxygen, flat EEG), methohexital treatment after the insult provided dramatic improvement as compared to control animals [216]. In addition, there have been many global hypoxia (asphyxia) experiments that document the benefit of barbiturate pretreatment [31,84].
2. **"Con" studies.** Goldstein's ischemic model was repeated. Following the same protocol, pentobarbital did not have beneficial effects [194]. The explanation for the different results is not clear; however, it has been suggested that N_2O use may have prevented replication of results [84]. Since depression of $CMRO_2$ by barbiturates parallels

decreased electrical activity [126], it has been postulated that barbiturates would not be beneficial in global injuries once electrical activity had ceased [129,148]. A study of global hypoxia (clamped endotracheal tube) attempted to prove this hypothesis. Unfortunately, this protocol included inadequate management of the hemodynamic effects of barbiturates, however, which affected the results [188]. There is evidence that, in spite of a flat EEG, barbiturates did appear to help [216], perhaps by another mechanism.

The study by Bleyaert [25] has been criticized for the ischemic model used and for the variable results reported. In this model, changing supportive care in the control group (immobilization and controlled ventilation) significantly decreased the group's neurologic deficit [26]. A repeat of this study [82] could not substantiate Bleyaert's original results, but N_2O was used. An animal model of cardiac arrest in cats showed no neurologic improvement after postarrest treatment with thiopental [44], although the treated group did survive longer, perhaps because of controlled seizures [200]. In a recent hypoxic mouse survival model [132], survival time was not extended after intraperitoneal barbiturates when ambient temperature was maintained at 36°C [85].

C. **Problems in clinical application.** Animal studies of focal and global ischemia answer some questions, but leave more unanswered. The clinical relevance of these studies deserves some discussion.

1. **General problems.** What animal models parallel a given clinical state? Some feel that data from focal ischemia models (e.g., MCA occlusions) can only be applied to humans who have clinical stroke, while global ischemia models relate only to humans who have cardiac or respiratory arrest or near-drowning. However, it must be realized that MCA occlusion in a small animal produces a massive hemispheric infarction with increased ICP, so the injury cannot be equated to the injury of a patient who suffers a small ischemic injury in the internal capsule. It must also be remembered that human survivors of global insults, such as cardiac arrest, commonly suffer focal neurologic deficits (hemiparesis, cortical blindness, aphasia) while many other areas of the brain function normally [41,149].

2. **Specific problems.** Additional problems in interpreting animal studies include the following.

   a. **Species.** Small animals have significant physiologic differences from large animals and human beings (P_{50} of hemoglobin, adaptation to hypoxia, etc.). They are also prone to unique diseases that may alter outcome (e.g., rodent respiratory disease) [57]. In large animals, there are major anatomic differences in the blood supply to the brain that may influence results in nonprimate models [126].

b. Anesthesia. Interactions of anesthetic drugs with drugs used as treatment must be evaluated and avoided when possible.

(1) A correlation of the effects of N_2O on barbiturate-induced "protection" studies has been done. In eight studies where substantial N_2O was used, six showed no protection. In 4 studies where curtailed N_2O was used, equivocal results were reported, and in 21 studies where N_2O was not used, 18 showed protection [84] (Table 4-1).

c. Neurologic examination. Performing an adequate neurologic examination is difficult in animals. In rodents, even a hemiparesis is difficult to identify. In large animals including primates, higher cognitive function cannot be tested. In addition, the normal course of functional deficits may vary significantly from human injuries [209].

d. Models. Models of global cerebral ischemia vary (choke collar, ventricular fibrillation, aortic and vena caval occlusion), but all have problems with immediate survival. Many ischemia models require major surgical procedures that can add to morbidity and mortality. Less invasive models of ischemia need to be studied [97].

e. Intensive care. Inappropriate postinsult life support is a fault of many studies. Intensive care of a large animal is very demanding and requires significant expertise and manpower, particularly if the study period lasts for three to seven days to allow appraisal of long-term neurologic outcome.

IV. Human studies. Although many questions remain, barbiturates are being used to treat human brain injuries. The clinical experience with barbiturates includes stroke, cardiac arrest, head trauma, Reye's syndrome, near-drowning, and various anesthetic situations including open ventricle procedures during cardiopulmonary bypass.

A. Stroke

1. General information. Over 200,000 people suffer strokes every year in the United States. Stroke is the general term for neurologic deficits in four major categories: thrombosis, embolism, intracerebral hemorrhage, and ruptured aneurysm. Over 80% of strokes are ischemic (thromboembolic) [167].

2. Current mortality and morbidity. Treatment for a completed ischemic stroke is supportive, but short-term mortality is more than 40% [172]. Significant permanent neurologic deficits will occur in about 60% of the long-term survivors [172]. Barbiturate therapy has not been shown to improve mortality or morbidity in patients who have completed strokes [17,37,205] (Table 4-2).

3. Barbiturate experience. The use of barbiturates in stroke is limited. Since most stroke patients are conscious, barbiturate treatment

Table 4-1. Use of nitrous oxide associates negatively with barbiturate protection ($n = 33$, $X^2 = 10$, $P < 0.01$)

	Barbiturate protection			
	Evident		Not evident	
Use of N_2O	Investigator(s)	Year	Investigator(s)	Year
None	Arnfred and Secher	1962	Snyder et al.	1979
	Wright and Ames	1964	Abramson et al.[f]	1983
	Wilhjelm and Arnfred	1965	Brain	1986
	Wilhjelm	1965		
	Goldstein et al.	1966		
	Secher and Wilhjelm	1968		
	Cockburn et al.	1969		
	Yatsu et al.	1972		
	Hoff et al.	1973		
	Smith et al.	1974		
	Hoff et al.	1975		
	Moseley et al.	1975		
	Michenfelder et al.	1976		
	Steen and Michenfelder	1978		
	Tamura et al	1979		
	Chang et al.	1985		
	Todd et al.	1985		

Curtailed	Nussmeier et al.	1986	Ward et al.[g]	1985
	Wells et al.[a]	1963		
	Corkill et al.[b]	1976		
	Bleyaert et al.[c]	1978		
Substantial	Michenfelder and Theye[d]	1973	Michenfelder and Theye[d]	1973
	Corkill et al.[e]	1978	Steen et al.	1979
			Todd et al.	1982
			Gisvold et al.	1984
			Aldrete and Cubillos	1984
			Gisvold et al.[h]	1984

[a] N_2O used only after insult.
[b] N_2O used during surgical preparation only.
[c] N_2O discontinued before insult.
[d] This paper reports two separate experiments and is therefore listed twice.
[e] One could interpret the results of this paper as not showing protection, but the authors claim otherwise.
[f] Dr. Jastremski informed us (personal communication) that analysis of finished findings revealed that statistical significance in favor of protection was "almost reached" in the most severely arrested group. Perhaps this paper should be classified as showing protection.
[g] Used N_2O in operating room but not in ICU.
[h] This study used hemodilution, hypertension, hypothermia, and dexamethasone in addition to pentobarbital and N_2O. Treated animals woke up sooner, but there was no statistically significant difference between groups on neural deficit score — especially if the treatment group animal that was excluded from the analysis of postinsult deterioration is included.

(From J. Hartung, and J. E. Cottrell, Nitrous oxide reduces thiopental-induced prolongation of survival in hypoxic and anoxic mice. *Anesth. Analg.* 66:47–52, 1987.)

Table 4-2. Outcome of stroke, cardiac arrest, head trauma, Reye's syndrome, near-drowning, and immersion accidents in 100 typical patients

Outcome	Thrombo-embolic stroke	Cardiac arrest (survivors in coma)[a]	Head trauma (Glasgow coma scale ≤ 8)	Reye's syndrome (stages IV and V)	Near-drowning (coma)	Immersion accidents (survivors of near-drowning)[b]
Normal	24	8	25		45	80
Permanent neurologic deficit	36	37	25		20	10
Death	40	55	50	60–100	35	10

[a] When 32 survivors in coma were treated with thiopental (30–50 mg/kg), the outcome was as follows: 15 (48%) normal; 1 (3%) permanent neurologic damage; 15 (48%) death.
[b] Out of 200 immersion accidents, 100 result in drowning, 100 in near-drowning.

not only results in loss of the ability to perform a neurologic examination, but also may require intubation and mechanical ventilation. Many institutions use barbiturates for focal ischemia associated with neurosurgical procedures, particularly if there is an opportunity to treat patients before the insult. Three centers have published their limited experience with various stroke injuries.

   a. A randomized controlled study of 35 patients with thromboembolic stroke reported a 40% decrease in mortality in patients treated with thiopental, 10 gm (2 gm q8h for 5 doses). However, there were significant design problems with this study (control patients were treated with glycerol and dextran), and the control group had an unacceptably high mortality (80%) [57].
   b. Seven patients undergoing cerebral aneurysm surgery requiring temporary or permanent occlusion of a major artery were treated with pentobarbital (15–20 mg/kg initially, then 15 mg/kg/day for two days). Although two patients died, four of the five survivors had no neurologic deficits, suggesting to the authors that these patients had benefited from barbiturate treatment [90].
   c. Four patients undergoing treatment of surgically inaccessible cerebral aneurysms were treated with pentobarbital after iatrogenic thrombosis occurred (sterotaxic injection of a methyl methacrylate–iron mixture). All patients died with fatal ICP elevations after five days of barbiturate treatment [164].

B. Cardiac arrest
   1. General information. With the expanded use of cardiopulmonary resuscitation (CPR) and advanced cardiac life support (ACLS), it is now possible to save approximately 20% of the 350,000 people who will have a cardiac arrest each year [141]. Communities with large numbers of lay persons trained in basic life support and a rapid response system report that more than 40% of patients with documented ventricular fibrillation out of hospital can be successfully resuscitated [4a]. However, many "survivors" of cardiac arrest go on to die a cerebral death in the hospital or survive with a significant neurologic deficit [50].
   2. Current mortality/morbidity. Approximately 30% of the survivors of cardiac arrests will die a cerebral death (i.e., they will never recover consciousness) [21,187]. The subgroup of patients who do not recover consciousness shortly after successful CPR have a particularly poor prognosis (Table 4-1). Patients in a coma one hour after CPR have a high mortality (55%) and a very small chance (8%) of leaving the hospital with normal brain function [16,187,213]. At the present time, postcardiac arrest care is strictly supportive, maintaining cardiac and pulmonary function with a "watch-and-wait" attitude as far as the brain is concerned.

3. Barbiturate experience. Some authorities have expressed great enthusiasm for the treatment of survivors of cardiac arrest who remain in a coma after resuscitation. The results of animal studies suggest that this kind of brain insult should be treated within 1 to 2 hours to achieve maximal benefit [25,55].

   a. Other than several case reports and one controlled study, only one prospective study has been reported using thiopental-bolus treatment. This study followed the optimistic results observed in an uncontrolled study of 32 patients who remained in a coma after successful CPR and were treated with thiopental (30–50 mg/kg) as a single-dose treatment [33]. The good outcome of this study (48% normal, 3% permanent neurologic damage, 48% dead) led to the large prospective randomized and controlled study including 262 patients in a coma after successful CPR [30]. There was no statistically improved outcome in thiopental-treated patients versus control patients (20 vs. 15% good recovery, 2 vs. 5% severe neurologic damage, 77 vs. 80% dead). While this study perhaps has answered the question of bolus-barbiturate treatment after cardiac arrest, it may have only documented the inadequacy of the duration of treatment, not that barbiturates should not be used for this problem.

   b. A feasibility trial was performed at Stanford in patients who had ischemic or traumatic brain injuries to evaluate an aggressive treatment regimen using thiopental as a 15 mg/kg loading dose followed by a continuous infusion for 2 to 3 days. The continuous infusion of thiopental was administered to keep the cortical EEG isoelectric (to achieve maximal $CMRO_2$ depression) since this represents the only known physiologic endpoint other than control of ICP. Fourteen patients who had various brain injuries have been treated with total doses of thiopental ranging from 0.2 to 0.6 gm/kg. Four of these patients were postcardiac arrest; two survived with complete neurologic recovery and two died [165]. Hemodynamic stability was maintained during the infusions by close monitoring and rational supportive care. There was no cardiac arrest or death during the drug infusion nor did the infusion have to be stopped because of intractable hypotension. This trial established the feasibility of continuous treatment of patients with large doses of barbiturates during the entire "postresuscitative disease" period [143].

C. Open ventricle procedures during cardiopulmonary bypass grafts (CPBG). Open-ventricle procedures are associated with embolic phenomenon that cause post–cardiopulmonary bypass deficits. A recent study [151] infused an average of 39.5 mg/kg of thiopental to maintain electroencephalographic silence during normothermic cardiopulmonary bypass for correction of cardiac valvular abnormalities.

By the tenth postoperative day, all neuropsychiatric abnormalities had resolved in the thiopental-treated group (89 patients) but persisted in 7.5% of those treated with fentanyl only (7 of 93 control patients). Those receiving large doses of barbiturate, however, required vaso-pressors and experienced greater difficulty in coming off bypass.

D. Head trauma

1. General information

a. Incidence. An estimated 30,000 people die each year in the United States from head injuries [136]. This number can be expected to increase with the growing popularity of motorcycles, mopeds, and bicycles.

b. ICP. Increased ICP, a frequent secondary event in the head-injured patient, may cause additional brain damage either by herniation with trauma to various parts of the brain (cingulate gyrus, temporal lobe, or cerebellar tonsils) or by decreasing CBF below the critical range necessary for neuronal viability. A progressive cycle of increasing cerebral compression may develop because of edema with resultant ischemia and necrosis. This secondary complication frequently leads to demise or severe disability. Although not always an accompaniment of severe head trauma (25% incidence of normal ICP) [38], significant intracranial hypertension (>30 mmHg) will almost double mortality [111]. Increased ICP does not always correlate with detectable neurologic deterioration, however, most patients will suffer more brain damage when there is a significant rise in ICP [51]. Therefore, controlling ICP has become the main goal in treating head-injured patients. Although the reason for using barbiturates is to decrease ICP, their other effects may also be important.

c. Glasgow coma scale (GCS). This scoring system [100] has clarified the definition of severe head trauma as a score ≤8 (Table 4-3), allowing reasonable comparisons among different series of patients when patient populations are demographically comparable. The GCS is an attempt to standardize classification of outcome in a manner that will help clarify prognosis and many of the unresolved issues in the management of head-injured patients [110].

2. Current mortality and morbidity.

The current mortality from severe craniocerebral trauma has been surprisingly constant at 50% [54,101]. Approximately 25% of severely brain-injured patients will fully recover to normal brain function (see Table 4-2).

a. A recent study reported a mortality of 32% [19]. However, this study included a younger patient population and excluded patients with a coma score of 3. The morbidity in this study was also improved, suggesting that aggressive management favorably affected the outcome.

Table 4-3. Glasgow coma scale

Eye opening	
Spontaneous	4
To speech	3
To pain	2
None	1
Verbal response	
Oriented	5
Confused conversation	4
Incomprehensible words	3
Incomprehensible sounds	2
Nil	1
Best motor response	
Obeys	6
Localizes	5
Withdraws	4
Abnormal flexion	3
Extensor response	2
Nil	1

b. Aggressive management is facilitated by monitoring ICP to direct therapeutic interventions. Treatment regimens for intracranial hypertension vary significantly among institutions, but all include some combination of the following modalities:

(1) Controlled ventilation ($PO_2 > 80$ mmHg)

(2) Blood pressure control

(3) Hyperventilation ($PCO_2 = 25 - 30$ mmHg)

(4) Immobilization

(5) Fluid restriction

(6) Surgery (clot evacuation)

(7) Osmotherapy

(8) Diuretics

(9) Normothermia/hypothermia

(10) Cerebrospinal fluid (CSF) drainage

3. **Barbiturate experience.** Barbiturates received wide attention after they were shown to decrease ICP effectively in neurosurgical patients [173]. The following studies have been published using barbiturates in head trauma (Table 4-4).

a. Overgaard and colleagues [155] reported a series of 201 patients treated nonaggressively by today's standards (no steroids, intubation, osmotherapy, or ICP monitoring). All patients were treated with phenobarbital (150–400 mg/day). Since 62 patients were awake or able to obey commands (GCS > 8), only the results for the remaining 139 severely injured patients are listed in Table 4-4. It is interesting that the mortality and morbidity in this group

Table 4-4. Outcome of six studies using barbiturates in head trauma

Study	n	Mortality (%)	Significant morbidity (%)	Good recovery (%)
Overgaard and colleagues [155]	139	40	30	30
Rockoff and colleagues [164]	45	36	20	44
Bruce and colleagues [38]	85	9	4	88
Rea and Ruckswold [162]	27	52	15	33
Schwartz and colleagues [170]	28	57	21	21
Ward [210]	27	52	37	11

n = number.

of patients treated with barbiturates and without conventional therapy were as good or better than most conventional protocols.

b. Rockoff and colleagues [164] reported on the use of pentobarbital in 45 of 172 patients who had ICP elevations of greater than 40 mmHg for 15 minutes. Aggressive conventional therapy (controlled hyperventilation, steroids, osmotherapy, paralysis) was also used. Pentobarbital was given over 3 to 10 days (3–5 mg/kg initially, then 100–200 mg qlh) and the resulting mortality (36%) in this group was excellent (Table 4-4). This group of patients had fewer mass lesions than those in the nonbarbiturate series, which might favor a better outcome; however, this does not entirely explain the favorable results [121,164].

c. The most impressive results in head trauma were reported by Bruce and colleagues [38] in 85 patients (aged 4 months to 18 years) who had severe brain injuries. Their complicated protocol included conventional therapy (ICP monitoring, hyperventilation, paralysis) for all patients and additional therapy (steroids, mannitol, furosemide, hypothermia, pentobarbital, and thiopental) according to specific guidelines. The low mortality (9%) and morbidity (4%) were gratifying but may have been due in part to the young population and the low incidence of mass lesions in this group (Table 4-4) [110].

d. Rea [162] evaluated the use of high-dose barbiturate therapy in patients with severe head trauma and uncontrolled intracranial hypertension. The study suggested a decreased mortality rate with the use of barbiturates to control ICP.

e. In two prospective randomized studies [170,210], barbiturate therapy in head-injured patients was not shown to decrease morbidity and mortality. Schwartz and colleagues [170] also reported that pentobarbital was less effective than mannitol in controlling ICP.

E. Reye's syndrome

1. General information. Although Brian and colleagues [34] described a syndrome of encephalopathy and fatty liver in 1929, Reye and Johnson are credited with the description of this distinct clinical syndrome in 1963 [102,163].

More than 1000 cases from all over the world had been reported by 1976, but the true incidence is probably much higher than this number indicates. A seasonal variation of peaks in January and June has been noted along with an association with certain viral infections [168]. A significant outbreak of the disease occurred at the time of the influenza-B epidemic of 1973–1975 (1 case of Reye's syndrome per 1700 cases of influenza B) [27,87]. Although the illness generally involves children aged 4 to 15 years, three adults have been reported to have the disease [13]. In recent years there has been an unexplained decrease in the incidence of Reye's syndrome [86]. In the United States there has been a steady decline from 550 cases reported in 1980 to less than 100 cases per year since 1985. While some have attributed this to the cessation of salicylate use, other countries (e.g., Australia) that have not used salicylates for 25 years have experienced a similar decline [154].

a. Clinical course. The clinical course begins with a mild antecedent illness (upper respiratory infection, gastroenteritis, varicella) followed within a week by persistent vomiting and a progressive encephalopathy. Over a period of hours to days, the encephalopathy can progress from combative behavior and hallucinations to decreased responsiveness, coma with abnormal posturing, and, finally, loss of brainstem function and death [142].

b. Diagnosis. The diagnosis is made on the basis of a compatible clinical history and the following: hepatic injury evidenced by elevations of SGOT/SGPT to twice normal, negative toxicology screen, and normal CSF examination. Although they are not necessary for the diagnosis, prolonged prothrombin time, elevated blood ammonia, and hypoglycemia are also consistent with the diagnosis [45]. Reye's syndrome must be distinguished from several inborn errors of metabolism (errors of ureagenesis, defects of fatty acid metabolism, and organic acidemias) that have recently been identified [123]. There should be a high degree of suspicion for a metabolic defect in any child with a recurrent "syndrome."

c. Clinical staging. Two staging systems have been devised for Reye's syndrome [96,118]. The more elaborate classification of Lovejoy has been widely accepted and includes five stages with associated EEG findings (Table 4-5). Morbidity appears increased

Table 4-5. Reye's syndrome staging

Stage	Symptoms
I	Lethargy, vomiting
II	Disorientation, combativeness, hyperventilation, hyperreflexia
III	Coma, decorticate rigidity, hyperventilation
IV	Coma, decerebrate rigidity, fixed pupils, brainstem signs
V	Coma, apnea, seizures, flaccidity

Table 4-6. Aggressive therapy for Reye's syndrome

Hepatic coma	Cerebral edema
Citrulline	Intubation/hyperventilation
Arginine	Fluid restriction
L-Dopa	Osmotherapy
Exchange transfusion	Paralysis
Dialysis	CSF drainage
Total body washout	Hypothermia

CSF = cerebrospinal fluid.

in patients who pass rapidly through stages I to II and who have high ammonia levels > 200 μg/ml and/or a metabolic acidosis.

2. Current morbidity and mortality

  a. Reye's syndrome frequently has an unpredictable course, making evaluation of various treatments tenuous. In the first few years after its recognition, supportive therapy included administration of glucose, neomycin, and dexamethasone, resulting in an overall mortality of 60 to 100% [27,29,130,169].

  b. Aggressive therapy developed along two lines: management of hepatic coma and treatment of cerebral edema. Soon a large list of specific treatments existed (Table 4-6). When the etiology of the encephalopathy was determined to be a direct insult to the brain and not an hepatic encephalopathy, treatment became focused on preventing an increase in ICP from cerebral edema. None of the treatments has undergone controlled trials in Reye's syndrome. However, since the direct insult to the brain appears to be reversible, the effectiveness of aggressive therapy in reducing cerebral edema and ICP is currently believed responsible for the improved mortality and morbidity. Even with aggressive therapy, mortality for all patients varies from 0 to 82%, with a 3 to 15% incidence of neurologic morbidity [6,27,28,62,96,108,113,118, 142,169,176,204]. In the subgroup of patients in stages IV and V coma, mortality is still high (see Table 4-2) [62,113,204].

3. Barbiturate experience

a. The limited role of barbiturates in the treatment of Reye's syndrome dramatically changed when Marshall [120] reported seven patients with stages IV and V coma who were treated with pentobarbital after standard measures (hyperventilation, steroids, mannitol) had failed to control ICP. All seven patients had ICP ≥30 mmHg for at least 30 minutes before administration of barbiturates. Pentobarbital was given in a dose of 3 to 5 mg/kg initially, followed by 2.0 to 3.5 mg/kg every hour as long as the MAP was greater than 60 mmHg and the pentobarbital blood level was <25 μg/ml. Patients were treated for 5 to 13 days, and all made a complete recovery except one who had a neurologic deficit.

b. Currently, barbiturates have been given last place in the order of treatments for raised ICP in Reye's syndrome [202].

F. Near-drowning

1. General information

a. Approximately 7000 to 9000 drowning-related deaths occur each year in the United States. Drowning is the second leading cause of death in young children. About 50% are under 16 years of age [52]. By definition, near-drowning indicates at least temporary survival (24 hours) after asphyxia secondary to submersion in a fluid medium [158].

b. Hypoxia occurs because of asphyxia, aspiration, and ischemia after cardiac arrest. Most persons aspirate, but the volume of water aspirated is generally small (20 ml/kg). Although there are differences between salt-water and fresh-water aspiration, the resultant hypoxemia and respiratory failure are clinically indistinguishable [79]. An important distinction can be made between warm- and cold-water drowning, however, since hypothermia associated with the latter offers some protection to the brain and may account for survival after prolonged submersion [178].

2. Current morbidity and mortality

a. Serious immersion accidents (loss of consciousness in water) result in a mortality of 20 to 80% [157]. Mortality rates are highest in the adult population and in fresh-water immersions. About half of all immersion accidents are drownings (death within 24 hours). The other half are near-drownings in which the victims survive past the first day (see Table 4-2). The subgroup of patients who are comatose on arrival at the hospital has a poorer prognosis. Patients in deep coma who are areflexic and flaccid have a 70% mortality [53].

b. Current therapy for near-drowning victims reflects advances in cardiopulmonary resuscitation and brain-oriented intensive care. There is not much controversy about initial resuscitative efforts, subsequent controlled ventilation with positive end-expiratory pressure, and other general supportive measures. Patients who have significant brain dysfunction may be treated with steroids (not of value for the pulmonary lesion) and hyperventilation. ICP monitoring has been recommended for severely affected patients in combination with the use of osmotic agents, CSF drainage, and hypothermia to help prevent and control intracranial hypertension [52,88,130].

3. Barbiturate experience

 a. Before the acceptance of the effectiveness of barbiturates for lowering ICP, their role in near-drowning was limited to treating seizures when they occurred [79].

 b. Conn [53] recently reported a series of 96 children whose aggressive treatment after near-drowning was based on their neurologic function at the time of arrival at the hospital. Patients were categorized awake ("A"), blunted consciousness ("B"), and coma ("C"). The treatment regimen for "C" patients included administration of barbiturates (phenobarbital) for four days, regardless of the ICP. The morbidity and mortality for this group were not better than for a smaller group reported by Modell [88], in which no barbiturates were used. The groups in coma were not necessarily comparable, however, and only half of Conn's patients received barbiturates. Conn's study was prospective but not randomized or controlled.

 c. The role of barbiturates in near-drowning is unclear, but many institutions use barbiturates in this clinical situation just as they do for head trauma and Reye's syndrome patients.

G. Anesthesia. Anesthesiologists may be involved in the care of patients who have a variety of brain injuries. They should be familiar with the special considerations for anesthetizing patients who have increased ICP and those who require cerebral protection.

 1. ICP. Anesthesia for patients who have intracranial hypertension may involve the use of barbiturates. Because of its rapid action (within 60 seconds), thiopental is most commonly used [173]. The dose for maximal cerebral vasoconstriction is not known, but measurement of ICP provides a valuable guide to therapeutic efficacy. Repeated doses may be necessary if increases in ICP persist or recur. There may be an advantage to continuous infusion of barbiturates to prevent elevations in ICP instead of treating increases after they occur, but this is not currently popular because of concern about hemodynamic instability and prolonged recovery from anesthesia.

2. Cerebral protection

 a. Patients frequently require anesthesia for a surgical procedure that may compromise oxygenation of the brain. Barbiturates are a reasonable choice of anesthetic, especially since this situation represents an opportunity to protect the brain before injury. Barring contraindications to its use, barbiturate anesthesia may be indicated in patients undergoing cerebral aneurysm clip-ligation, carotid endarterectomy, aortic arch repair, cardiopul-monary bypass (in patients who have cerebrovascular disease), and mitral or aortic valve replacement (when there is increased risk for air embolism). Although the need to have an awake patient at the end of the operation will limit the amount of drug that can be given, this goal can be achieved in experienced hands [95].

b. In general, the anesthesiologist and the surgeon should agree beforehand that the potential benefits of barbiturate anesthesia will offset the anticipated need for invasive monitoring and post-operative ventilatory and circulatory support. The type of barbitu-rate, amount of drug, method of administration (single dose vs. continuous infusion), and duration of treatment (24–72 hours) are controversial. Many people use small single doses (e.g., thio-pental 3–5 mg/kg) since this dose causes flattening of the EEG. No further reduction in $CMRO_2$ is achieved and the possible avoidance of hypotension is gained, although this hemodynamic stability is not assured. Other clinicians recommend larger single doses (thiopental 30 mg/kg), which may enhance free radical scavenging, but a bolus dose ignores the fact that the period of postinsult injury may last from 24 to 72 hours. A more rational approach would be to adjust the dose to a physiologic endpoint (e.g., flat EEG) and to use a continuous infusion for 24 to 48 hours.

V. Treatment guidelines
A. Which barbiturate?

1. **Currently used barbiturates.** Several drugs (thiopental, pento-barbital, phenobarbital, methohexital, thiamylal) have been used experimentally and clinically, but there are few comparative studies available. Therefore, the choice of drug must be based on the physical and pharmacologic properties of the individual drugs and the circumstances in which they are to be used.

2. **Physical criteria and pharmacologic properties.** The passage of drugs across the blood-brain barrier requires low protein drug binding, low degree of ionization, and high lipid solubility. There are important differences among the pharmacologic properties of the three most commonly used barbiturates (phenobarbital, pento-barbital, thiopental) [171,175] (Table 4-7).

   a. Phenobarbital. Even though it has a low degree of protein binding, phenobarbital is highly ionized and has a comparatively low lipid solubility. Although it may not cross the blood-brain

Table 4-7. Pharmacologic properties
of the three most commonly used barbiturates

Barbiturate	Plasma protein binding (%)	pKa	% Nonionized (pH 7.4)	Partition coefficient (lipid/H$_2$O)
Phenobarbital	20	7.3	44	3
Pentobarbital	35	8.1	83	39
Thiopental	65	7.6	61	580

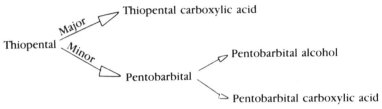

Fig. 4-8. Metabolism of thiopental along the major pathway to thiopental
carboxylic acid and along the minor pathway to pentobarbital, which is then further
metabolized to pentobarbital alcohol and pentobarbital carboxylic acid.

barrier as readily as pentobarbital and thiopental, phenobarbital
has unique anticonvulsant properties, and this may be an important benefit to some patients.

   b. **Pentobarbital and thiopental.** Both pentobarbital and thiopental are significantly less ionized and more lipid soluble than
phenobarbital. Thiopental has a more rapid onset of action than
pentobarbital and although thiopental may not share the unique
anticonvulsant actions of phenobarbital, its effectiveness in status
epilepticus is well-known [35].

   Thiopental is biotransformed to a pharmacologically active
compound, pentobarbital (Fig. 4-8) [119]. While thiopental's major metabolic pathway produces thiopental carboxylic acid, an
inactive metabolite, significant (i.e., pharmacologic) amounts of
pentobarbital are produced when high doses of thiopental are
used. Pentobarbital is metabolized exclusively to inactive compounds.

   At the present time, thiopental appears to be the drug of choice
because of its pharmacologic and physical properties. Direct
administration of pentobarbital is a reasonable alternative. Until
we understand more about the mechanisms of their beneficial
actions in specific brain injuries, the selection of a barbiturate
will remain empiric.

B. Monitoring

   1. **Blood levels.** Blood levels of barbiturate should be measured
every 6 to 8 hours during treatment. This is essential because of its

nonlinear kinetics and the possibility of hepatic dysfunction in some persons. It should be clear that even with a constant rate of infusion, a steady-state condition cannot be achieved with a drug like thiopental. Therefore, serial blood levels provide essential feedback for proper adjustment of dose.

2. ICP monitoring. ICP monitoring, a technique that offers a high degree of reliability and a low risk of infection, is essential in patients receiving barbiturates for control of increased ICP for the following three reasons.

a. To detect neurologic deterioration when physical signs are obscured by barbiturates.

b. To guide therapeutic decisions.

c. To provide objective information (e.g., ICP, intracranial compliance) to support decisions about when to withdraw treatment.

3. Hemodynamic considerations

a. Hemodynamic monitoring. Adequate hemodynamic monitoring of patients receiving high doses of barbiturates include electrocardiogram (ECG), urinary catheter, and direct measurement of arterial pressure and central venous pressure (CVP). A thermodilution pulmonary artery catheter is indicated for any patient in whom CVP measurements would be unreliable reflections of left-ventricular filling pressures and in hemodynamically unstable patients. Since barbiturates may directly affect all the major components of the cardiovascular system (heart rate, strength of contraction, preload, afterload), these parameters should be assessed individually to guide specific therapeutic interventions.

b. Management of hypotension. The management of hypotension is greatly facilitated by adequate monitoring [177]. It is not necessary to stop the barbiturate infusion.

(1) The first step is to restore intravascular volume. This is particularly important in the patient who has been fluid restricted.

(2) If hypotension persists despite normovolemia, an inotropic drug, such as dopamine, can be used.

(3) In rare instances, the addition of a pure vasopressor, such as phenylephrine, may be necessary.

(4) As with any critically ill patient, the adequacy of perfusion should be assessed continually by physical examination, physiologic measurements (urine output, cardiac output), and biochemical tests (blood gases, pH, lactate).

C. Drug administration

1. Dose versus efficacy. The dosage of a drug can be determined when the pharmacology of the drug is understood and when there are clear endpoints indicating achievement of the desired therapeutic effect(s). With barbiturates, however, not only are the pharmacokinetics poorly understood, but the important therapeutic effects (except for the changes in $CMRO_2$ and ICP) are unknown or clinically unmeasurable.

   a. ICP is easily measured, and, if reducing ICP is the only desired effect, then the dose can be adjusted according to response.

   b. Since the EEG becomes isoelectric when there is maximal reduction of $CMRO_2$, this monitor can be used to determine the dose needed for maximal metabolic depression.

   c. The dose to effect the potential benefits of barbiturates (free radical scavenging activity, improved perfusion) is unknown but may be equivalent to the large doses required to produce maximal depression of $CMRO_2$.

2. Dose regimens

   a. Intraoperative control of ICP, thiopental, 1 to 3 mg/kg; may repeat every 20 to 30 minutes.

   b. Prolonged control of ICP: pentobarbital.

      (1) Loading dose: 3 to 5 mg/kg.

      (2) Maintenance: 100 to 200 mg every 30 to 60 minutes or 2 mg/kg/hr as continuous infusion.

      (3) Titrate to maximum blood level of 40 μg/ml.

      (4) Stop treatment after 72 hours if ICP < 20 mmHg and compliance is normal.

   c. "Maximal benefit" dose: thiopental.

      (1) Loading dose: 15 mg/kg.

      (2) Maintenance: 0.2 mg/kg/min as continuous infusion.

      (3) Endpoints

         (a) Isoelectric EEG.

         (b) Maximal blood level of 60 to 80 μg/ml.

      (4) Stop treatment after 48 hours.

VI. Other drugs and techniques. The recent efforts to develop clinically useful techniques of cerebral protection (therapy before the ischemic episode) and amelioration (therapy after the episode) are based on experimental and anecdotal evidence that, under proper circumstances, will increase the brain's tolerance to global and focal ischemia. Attempts to define these circumstances have been hampered, however, by the difficulty in applying animal data to the human situation and by the complexity, risk, and expense of certain of the therapeutic modalities. In addition to the barbiturates, a number of other drugs and procedures are currently under investigation.

   A. Hypothermia. Hypothermia lowers the cerebral metabolic oxygen requirement by 7 to 13% for each degree centigrade that the temperature is reduced, thus enhancing the brain's ability to tolerate ischemia. Consequently, the brain can withstand complete ischemia for 4 minutes at 38°C, for 8 minutes at 30°C, for 16 minutes at 22°C, and for more than 30 minutes at 16°C. Few complications are associated with hypothermia of several hours' duration (as long as the temperature remains above 28°C to avoid arrhythmias) since brief periods of hypothermia do not entail significant metabolic alterations in the absence of shivering, poor tissue perfusion, or prolonged circulatory arrest. Liver, kidney, and endocrine function are decreased during hypothermia, but return to normal within 24 hours after rewarming. The action of narcotics and muscle relaxants is prolonged with cooling.

Shivering during cooling and rewarming increases oxygen consumption by 50 to 200% and may be accompanied by anaerobic metabolism, progressive metabolic acidosis, and cardiac depression. Either thorazine (2.5 mg IV) or incremental doses of meperidine (10 mg IV) can be used to treat shivering in the postoperative period.

Rewarming after prolonged hypothermia for 1 to 3 days, however, has been accompanied by systemic acidosis, hemodynamic collapse, and death [196]. Hypothermia to 29°C for this period causes an increase in peripheral vascular resistance, areas of hypoperfusion of the skeletal muscle and cerebral cortex [195], and the accumulation of acid metabolites. The vascular beds that had closed down during hypothermia reopen with rewarming, introducing the previously sequestered acid metabolites to the systemic circulation and causing cardiovascular collapse. These events documented in animal models may represent the "rewarming shock" noted clinically after prolonged hypothermia [69].

Decreasing the body temperature also causes an increase in CO_2 solubility, pH, and CO_2-combining power, as well as a decrease in buffer capacity. The higher pH and lower temperature produce a leftward shift of the oxygen-hemoglobin dissociation curve. This greater affinity of oxygen by hemoglobin is partially counteracted by the increased solubility of oxygen at lower temperatures.

The desired temperature is attained by surface cooling. The thermal blanket control is returned to the warm mode when the esophageal temperature falls to 33°C, because the temperature will drift downward another 2 to 3° to the desired level of 31°C. To achieve profound hypothermia, extracorporeal circulation is required.

The combination of barbiturates with a moderate degree of hypothermia (34–36°C) may be even more effective than either barbiturates or hypothermia alone, since a modest reduction in temperature has been shown in the hypoxic mouse model to retard depletion of ATP and accumulation of lactic acid and to prolong survival time. The effects of barbiturates and hypothermia are additive [8] in view of the fact that barbiturates affect cellular function as reflected by the EEG, while hypothermia preserves cellular integrity (protein synthesis, pump function).

B. Naloxone. Research continues to identify other drugs effective against focal ischemic insults. The neurologic deficit resulting from unilateral occlusion of the right common carotid artery in gerbils has been modified by the intraperitoneal or subcutaneous administration of the narcotic antagonist naloxone [93]. Morphine given after ligation of the common carotid artery in gerbils that had not had a stroke was associated with development of a neurologic deficit that could be reversed by intraperitoneal injection of naloxone.

C. Gamma-hydroxybutyrate, phenytoin. Other drugs may exert a protective effect when given before or after a period of complete global ischemia. Gamma-hydroxybutyrate decreases the cerebral metabolic rate [214] and enhances hypoxic tolerance (in combination with glucagon), but it has been shown in dogs to reduce CBF to a greater extent than metabolic rate [9], limiting the degree of protection. In the hypoxic mouse model, phenytoin conferred protection that was greater than with gamma-hydroxybutyrate but less than with barbiturates. The mechanism of phenytoin's effect may be related to its limitation of potassium release from ischemic neurons due to membrane stabilization [7]. This correlates with the postulated role released potassium plays in the irreversible neuronal damage that occurs during and after ischemia.

D. Other anesthetic and adjuvant drugs

    1. Midazolam. In humans, 0.15 mg/kg of midazolam causes a 30% decrease in CBF [74]. Induction of anesthesia with midazolam is not associated with an increase in ICP [80] in patients with brain tumors.

    Animal studies have demonstrated a 25 to 30% decrease in $CMRO_2$ and CBF [73,92,150] associated with a decrease in frequency and an increase in the amplitude of the EEG. Large doses of midazolam (above 10 mg/kg) in dogs [73] did not further lower the $CMRO_2$ nor was burst suppression of the EEG achieved. This plateau effect is probably due to the saturation of the benzodiazepine receptors [73].

    In animal studies, midazolam has been shown to prolong survival in hypoxic mice [150] and to improve the mortality and neurologic outcome after incomplete global ischemia in rats [18]. In an in vitro study, midazolam (100 μM) prevented the irreversible loss of neuronal transmission and attenuated the fall of ATP caused by anoxia [1].

    2. Isoflurane. Since isoflurane produces an isoelectric EEG and suppresses brain metabolism at a dose (approximately 2.0 MAC) that is tolerated hemodynamically, cerebral protection similar to thiopental was anticipated [147]. In a mouse hypoxemia study, survival time was extended when isoflurane was used in noncardiorespiratory depressant concentrations [146]. Furthermore, during incomplete global ischemia, cerebral energy stores (ATP, PCr, and the calculated energy charge) were maintained at higher levels and lactate levels were lower in the isoflurane exposed animals than in dogs exposed to N_2O [146].

In a focal ischemia primate model produced by middle cerebral artery occlusion (MCAO), Nehls [144] reported that thiopental therapy was associated with better neurologic outcome and significantly less cerebral infarction than comparable doses of isoflurane. The study was repeated by Milde [132] and failed to demonstrate a significant difference in neurologic outcome and infarct size in the thiopental- and isoflurane-treated animals. Both studies required the use of adjuvant drugs to maintain arterial blood pressures. In addition, the trend toward better neuropathology (reported as mean lesion size) was noted in the thiopental treated animals, $5.1 \pm 2.2\%$ versus $8.5 \pm 1.8\%$ (SEM). This calculated difference was not statistically significant. Nehls [144] used vasodilators to treat hypertension in thiopental-treated animals and phenylephrine to raise arterial blood pressure in isoflurane-treated animals. Despite the use of vasodilators, the thiopental group had significantly higher blood pressure throughout the period of ischemia. The use of vasodilators and the higher CPPs in the thiopental treated group may have influenced the outcome. In Milde's study [132] equivalent arterial blood pressures were maintained in both thiopental- and isoflurane-treated animals, but large doses of phenylephrine were required, especially in the isoflurane-treated animals, which may have also influenced the outcome.

The extent to which the use of vasodilators and vasopressors may have influenced outcome in either study is difficult to assess, as the indirect vascular effects of both the adjuvant drugs and experimental drugs cannot be isolated from the direct effects of the experimental drugs on the brain [139]. An in vitro study [22] using the rat hippocampal brain slice preparation demonstrated protection by 1.5% isoflurane after 7 minutes of anoxia, but not after 10 minutes of anoxia. Thiopental demonstrated protection after 10 minutes of anoxia. Therefore, in this model, where vascular effects were eliminated, both agents demonstrated a direct protective effect on neurons. However, thiopental provided greater protection in vitro.

3. **Etomidate.** Etomidate reduces $CMRO_2$ by 50% and should also be helpful for cerebral ischemia. ATP and PCr are better maintained and lactate levels are reduced after focal ischemia in the presence of etomidate [133]. Animal studies have also shown protection with etomidate after focal ischemia [18,206,212]. Etomidate does vasoconstrict cerebral vessels significantly more rapidly than the time it takes to suppress cerebral metabolism [135].

4. **Sodium channel blocker.** Lidocaine, a sodium channel blocker, has been used to protect after focal ischemia. Large doses (160 mg/kg) produced protection, but cardiopulmonary bypass for hemodynamic support was necessary [12]. Smaller doses of lidocaine (25 mg/kg) were of no benefit during ischemia in animals [211].

5. **N-Methyl-d-aspartate (NMDA) inhibitors.** Recent studies have implicated the action of glutamate, an excitatory neurotransmitter, as a possible cause of anoxic and ischemic brain damage [166,182]. Blockers of the N-Methyl-d-aspartate (NMDA)–type glutamate receptor have been shown to reduce damage in vivo and in vitro [48,103,182]. MK801, a potent NMDA blocker that crosses the blood-brain barrier, has been shown to be protective in vitro [103] and in vivo [75,156]. These results must be viewed with caution since recent experiments did not find improved neurologic outcome when MK801 was given after ischemia [112]. NMDA blockers may prove useful in reducing ischemic damage, however, more studies are needed to establish their efficacy. These agents, of which PCP and ketamine are other examples, have profound negative behavioral effects. A new non-NMDA glutamate receptor antagonist, NBQX, has recently shown promise in a laboratory model of global ischemia.

6. **Calcium channel blockers**

   a. **Nimodipine.** Calcium entry has been implicated as an initiator for the cascade of cellular events that leads to permanent neurologic damage [105,180]. High intracellular calcium may cause phospholipase activation and breakdown of membranes, increase free radical formation, stimulate metabolism, and increase thromboxane, which may further decrease oxygen availability by vasoconstriction. In vitro studies in the rat hippocampal brain slice have demonstrated protection after 10 minutes of anoxia with cobalt and O mM Ca-high magnesium solutions both of which reduce calcium entry.

   In focal ischemic animal models, nimodipine has also afforded protection even when given after the anoxic-ischemic event [191a,195a]. Human studies after stroke from cerebral aneurysmal rupture disease and cerebral ischemic disease have demonstrated the positive effects of nimodipine in decreasing neurologic injury even though nimodipine was given after the stroke [2a,78,159]. The protective effect is believed to be secondary to dilation of penetrating arterioles [199]. Angiographic evidence of vasospasm was not lessened when nimodipine was used even though neurologic improvement was noted [159].

   In vitro studies utilizing the hippocampal slice have been unable to demonstrate protection with nimodipine [104]. Since this preparation superfuses the tissue directly, independent of the vasculature, effects of this agent on the vasculature would not be observed. It was concluded from these studies that nimodipine did not have a direct protective effect on neurons and that its clinical efficacy is probably due to its action on the vasculature (Table 4-8).

b. Flunarizine. This calcium entry blocker has been shown to improve ischemic damage in the hippocampus [61] and to improve histologic outcome in a long-term survival model of ischemia in rats [60]. Pilot studies in humans [94] have demonstrated an overall favorable effect on neurologic symptoms following acute stroke. This has led to the initiation of several human studies in Europe that will look for positive effects of flunarizine following stroke and cardiac arrest [99].

c. Magnesium. In vitro studies in the rat hippocampal brain slice have demonstrated protection after 10 minutes of anoxia with high magnesium concentration solutions [104]. Animal studies have demonstrated protection [203], but interference with insulin release will probably prevent its clinical usefulness [210a].

Animal studies have demonstrated protection after magnesium administration during spinal cord ischemia [203]. There are two major problems with the use of magnesium clinically. There is limited permeability of the intact blood-brain barrier to magnesium [189], thereby preventing effective concentrations in the brain. Magnesium also has the potential to cause profound hypotension if blood levels reach sufficient concentrations.

7. Free radical scavenger. Free radicals are produced during ischemia and are damaging to neurons [58]. After disappointing results

Table 4-8. Percentage recovery of evoked population spike

	Mean	Standard error	n
Dentate granule cells			
Untreated	0	0	5
Nimodipine (10^{-7})	11	11	5
Nimodipine (10^{-5})	12	12	5
Magnesium (10 mM)	76[a]	5	5
CA 1 pyramidal cells			
Untreated	4	3	6
Nimodipine (10^{-7})	5	5	5
Magnesium (10 mM)	35[b]	10	8
Cobalt (2 mM)	64[a]	12	5

n = number.
[a] $P < 0.005$, compared with untreated group from the same region.
[b] $P < 0.05$.

with glucocorticoid administration subsequent to cardiac arrest in humans [99a], a large, randomized, controlled trial has shown that methylprednisolone reduced spinal cord deficits if administered within eight hours of injury [28a]. Super oxide dismutase, alpha-tocopherol, and ascorbic acid are some of the agents that have also been shown to scavenge free radicals [42,43,58]. Alpha-tocopherol in vitro [2] and in vivo [198] has been shown to reduce anoxic or ischemic damage. The effects of barbiturates on free radicals have been discussed in detail earlier in the chapter.

Summary

Evidence that cerebral ischemic damage after stroke [197] and cardiac arrest may be potentially reversible has spurred efforts to identify pharmacologic and mechanical means to decrease cerebral infarction. While there has been progress, restraint is indicated in applying unsubstantiated and risk-laden modalities in the name of therapeutics.

References

1. Abramowicz, A. E., Kass, I. S., Cottrell, J. E., and Chambers, G. The effect of midazolam and gabaergic inhibition on anoxic damage in the rat hippocampal slice. *Anesthesiology* 69:A587, 1989.
2. Acosta, D., Kass, I. S., and Cottrell, J. E. Effect of a-tocopherol and free radicals on anoxic damage in the rat hippocampal slice. *Exp. Neurol.* 97:607, 1987.
2a. Allen, G. S., Ahn, H. S., Preziosi, T. J., et al. Cerebral arterial spasm — a controlled trial of nimodipine in patients with subarachnoid hemorrhage. *N. Engl. J. Med.* 308:619, 1983.
3. Allman, F. D., Talamo, J., and Rogers, M. C. Increased serum osmolality following pentobarbital anesthesia — A possible mechanism for lowering ICP. *Crit. Care Med.* 8:227, 1980.
4. Altura, B. T., and Altura, B. M. Barbiturates and aortic and venous smooth muscle function. *Anesthesiology* 43:432, 1975.
4a. American Heart Association. Standards and guidelines for cardiopulmonary resuscitation and emergency cardiac care. *J.A.M.A.* 255(21) 2841–3044, 1986.
5. Ames, A., Wright, R. L., Kowada, M., et al. Cerebral ischemia: II. The no-reflow phenomenon. *Am. J. Pathol.* 52:455, 1968.
6. Aoki, Y., and Lembroso, C. T. Prognostic value of electroencephalography in Reyes syndrome. *Neurology* 23:333, 1973.
7. Artru, A. A., and Michenfelder, J. D. Anoxic cerebral potassium accumulation reduced by phenytoin: Mechanism of cerebral protection? *Anesth. Analg.* 60:41, 1981.
8. Artru, A. A., and Michenfelder, J. D. Influence of hypothermia or hyperthermia alone or in combination with pentobarbital or phenytoin on survival time in hypoxic mice. *Anesth. Analg.* 60:867, 1981.
9. Artru, A. A., Steen, P. A., and Michenfelder, J. D. Gamme-Hydroxybutyrate: Cerebral metabolic, vascular, and protective effects. *J. Neurochem.* 35:1114, 1980.
10. Astrup, J., Nordstorm, C. H., and Rehncrona, S. Rate of Rise in Extracellular Potassium in the Ischemic Rat Brain and the Effect of Preischemic Metabolic Rate. In O. H. Ingvar and N. Lassen (Eds.), *Cerebral Function, Metabolism and Circulation.* Copenhagen: Munksgaard, 1977. Pp. 376–377.

11. Astrup, J., Skovsted, P., Gjerris, F., and Sorensen, H. R. Increase in extracellular potassium in the brain during circulatory arrest. Effects of hypothermia, lidocaine, and thiopental. *Anesthesiology* 55:256, 1981.

12. Astrup, J., Sorrensen, P. M., and Sorensen, H. R. Inhibition of cerebral oxygen and glucose consumption in the dog by hypothermia, pentobarbital and lidocaine. *Anesthesiology* 44:263, 1981.

13. Atkins, J. N., and Haponik, E. F. Reye's syndrome in the adult patient. *Am. J. Med.* 67:672, 1979.

14. Babior, B. M., Kipnes, R., and Cornutte, J. Biologic defense mechanisms: The production by leukocytes of superoxide, a potential bactericidal agent. *J. Clin. Invest.* 52:741, 1973.

15. Bandaranayake, N. M., Nemoto, E. M., and Stezoski, S. W. Rat brain osmolality during barbiturate anesthesia and global brain ischemia. *Stroke* 9:249, 1978.

16. Bates, D., Caronna, J. J., Cartlidge, N. E. F., et al. A prospective study of non-traumatic coma: Methods and results in 310 patients. *Ann. Neurol.* 2:211, 1977.

17. Bauer, R. B., Meyer, J. S., Fields, W. S., et al. Joint study of extracranial arterial occlusion: Progress report of controlled study of long-term survival in patients with and without operation. *J.A.M.A.* 208:509, 1969.

18. Baughman, V. L., Hoffman, W. E., Miletich, D. J., and Albrecht, R. F. Neurologic outcome following regional cerebral ischemia with methohexital, midazolam and etomidate. *Abstr. Anesthesiology* 67:A582, 1987.

19. Becker, D. P., Miller, J., Ward, J. D., et al. The outcome from severe head injury with early diagnosis and intensive management. *J. Neurosurg.* 47:491, 1977.

20. Becker, K. E., and Tonnesen, A. S. Cardiovascular effects of plasma levels of thiopental necessary for anesthesia. *Anesthesiology* 49:197, 1978.

21. Bell, J. A., and Hodgson, J. F. Coma after cardiac arrest. *Brain* 97:361, 1974.

22. Bendo, A. A., Kass, I. S., and Cottrell, J. E. Anesthetic protection against anoxic damage in the rat hippocampal slice. *Brain Res.* 403:136, 1987.

23. Berman, W., Pizzi, F., Schut, L., et al. The effects of exchange transfusion on intracranial pressure in patient with Reyes syndrome. *J. Pediatr.* 87:887, 1975.

24. Black, K. L., Weidler, M. D., Jallad, N. S., et al. Delayed pentobarbital therapy of acute focal ischemia. *Stroke* 9:245, 1978.

25. Bleyaert, A. L., Nemoto, E. M., Safar, P., et al. Thiopental amelioration of brain damage after global ischemia in monkeys. *Anesthesiology* 49:390, 1978.

26. Bleyaert, A. L., Safar, P., Nemoto, E. M., et al. Effect of postcirculatory-arrest life support on neurological recovery in monkeys. *Crit. Care Med.* 8:153, 1980.

27. Bobo, R. C., Schulbert, W. K., and Partin, J. C. Reyes syndrome: Treatment by exchange transfusion with special reference to the 1974 epidemic in Cincinnati, Ohio. *J. Pediatr.* 87:881, 1975.

28. Boutnos, A., Hout, T., Menezes, A., and Bell, W. Management of Reyes syndrome: A rational approach to a complex problem. *Crit. Care Med.* 5:234, 1977.

28a. Bracken, M. B., Shepard, M. J., Collins, W. F., et al. A randomized, controlled trial of methylprednisolone or naloxone in the treatment of acute spinal-cord injury. *N. Engl. J. Med.* 322:20, 1990.

29. Bradford, W. D., and Latham, W. C. Acute encephalopathy and fatty hepatomegaly. *Am. J. Dis. Child.* 114:152, 1967.

30. Brain Resuscitation Clinical Trial I Study Group. Randomized clinical study of thiopental loading in comatose survivors of cardiac arrest. *N. Engl. J. Med.* 314:397, 1986.

31. Brann, A. W., and Montalvo, J. M. Barbiturates and asphyxia. *Pediatr. Clin. North Am.* 17:851, 1970.

32. Branston, N. M., Hope, T., and Symon, L. Barbiturates in focal ischemia of primate cortex: Effects on blood flow distribution, evoked potential and extracellular potassium. *Stroke* 10:647, 1979.

33. Breivik, H., Safar, P., Sands, P., et al. Clinical feasibility trials of barbiturate therapy after cardiac arrest. *Crit. Care Med.* 6:228, 1978.
34. Brian, W. R., Hunter, D., and Turnbull, H. M. Acute meningo-encephalitis of childhood. *Lancet* 1:221, 1929.
35. Brown, A. S., and Horton, J. M. Status epilepticus treated by intravenous infusions of thiopental sodium. *Br. Med. J.* 1:27, 1967.
36. Brown, B. R. Anesthetic Hepatic Toxicity: A Scientific Problem? ASA Refresher Courses number 106B, 1979.
37. Browne, T. R., and Roskanzer, D. C. Treatment of strokes I and II. *N. Engl. J. Med.* 281:594, 650, 1969.
38. Bruce, D. A., Raphaely, R. C., Goldberg, A. I., et al. Pathophysiology, treatment and outcome following severe head injury in children. *Childs Brain* 5:174, 1979.
39. Butterfield, J. D., and McGraw, C. P. Free radical pathology. *Stroke* 9:443, 1978.
40. Carlon, G. C., Kahn, R. C., Goldiner, P. L., et al. Long-term infusion of sodium pentothal: Hemodynamic and respiratory effects. *Crit. Care Med.* 6:311, 1978.
41. Caronna, J. J., and Finkelstein, S. Neurological syndromes after cardiac arrest. *Stroke* 9:517, 1978.
42. Casthely, P. A., Dluzneski, J., Jones, R., et al. Comparison of superoxide dismutase, thiopental and nimodipine for maintenance of somatosensory evoked responses during aortic cross-clamping and declamping in dogs. *J. Cardiothoracic Anesthesia* II:792, 1988.
43. Casthely, P. A., Dluzneski, J., Jones, R., et al. Superoxide dismutase and hemodynamic changes following aortic cross-clamp release. *J. Cardiothoracic Anesthesia* II:450, 1988.
44. Chadwick, J. S., Todd, M. M., Shapiro, H. M., et al. Neurologic outcome following cardiac arrest in thiopental treated cats. *Anesthesiology* 53:156, 1980.
45. Chin, J. Influenza surveillance. Reye's syndrome and viral infections — United States. *Morbid. Mortal.* 23:58, 1974.
46. Christensen, M. S. Prolonged artificial hyperventilation in cerebral apoplexy. *Acta Anaesthesiol. Scand.* 8, 1976.
47. Christensen, M. S., Paulson, O. B., Olesen, J., et al. Cerebral apoplexy (stroke) treated with or without prolonged artificial hyperventilation: Cerebral circulation, clinical course, and cause of death. *Stroke* 4:568, 1973.
48. Clark, G. D., and Rothman, S. M. Blockade of excitatory amino acid receptors protects anoxic hippocampal slices. *Neuroscience* 21:665, 1987.
49. Clasen, R. A., Pandolfii, S., and Casey, D. Furosemide and pentobarbital in cryogenic cerebral injury and edema. *Neurology* 24:642, 1974.
50. Cobb, L. A., Warner, J. A., and Trobaugh, G. B. Sudden cardiac death: Outcome of resuscitation, management, and future directions. *Mod. Concepts Cardiovasc. Dis.* 69:37, 1980.
51. Collice, M., Rossada, M., Bedushi, A., et al. Management of Head Injury by Means of Ventricular Fluid Pressure Monitoring. In J. W. F. Beks, D. A. Bosch, and M. Breck (Eds.), *Intracranial Pressure III.* New York: Springer, 1976. Pp. 101–109.
52. Conn, A. W., Edmonds, J. F., and Barker, G. A. Near-drowning in cold fresh-water: Current treatment regimens. *Can. Anaesth. Soc. J.* 25:259, 1978.
53. Conn, A. W., Montes, J. E., Barker, G. A., and Edmonds, J. F. Cerebral salvage in near-drowning following neurological classification by triage. *Can. Anaesth. Soc. J.* 27:201, 1980.
54. Cooper, P. R., Moody, S., Clark, K., et al. Dexamethasone and severe head injury: A prospective double-blind study. *J. Neurosurg.* 51:307, 1979.
55. Corkill, G., Chikovani, O. K., McLeish, I., et al. Timing of pentobarbital administration for brain protection in experimental stroke. *Surg. Neurol.* 5:147, 1976.
56. Cote, J., Simard, D., and Rouillard, M. Repercussion sur le debit sanguin cerebral d'une perfusion de thiopental. *Can. Anaesth. Soc. J.* 26:269, 1979.

57. Davis, J. N. The use of small animals to study the effects of hypoxia. *Adv. Neurol.* 26:167, 1979.
58. Demopoulos, H. E., Flamm, E. S., Pietronigro, D. D., and Seligman, M. S. Free radical pathology and antioxidants in regional cerebral ischemia and central nervous system trauma. In J. E. Cottrell and H. Turndorf (Eds.), *Anesthesia and Neurosurgery.* St. Louis: Mosby, 1986. Pp. 246–279.
59. Demopoulos, H. B., Flammn, E. S., Seligman, M. L., et al. Antioxidant effects of barbiturates in model membranes undergoing free radical damage. *Acta Neurol. Scand.* 56:7, 1977.
60. Deshpande, J. K., and Wieloch, T. Flunarizine, a calcium entry blocker, ameliorates ischemic brain damage in the rat. *Anesthesiology* 64:215, 1986.
61. Deshpande, J. K., and Wieloch, T. Amelioration of ischemic brain damage following post ischemic treatment with flunarizine. *Neurol. Res.* 7:27, 1985.
62. DeVivo, D. C., Keating, J. P., and Haymond, M. W. Reye's syndrome: Results of intensive supportive care. *J. Pediatr.* 87:875, 1975.
63. Dolovich, J., Evans, S., Rosenbloom, D., et al. Anaphylaxis due to thiopental sodium anaesthesia. *Can. Med. Assoc. J.* 123:292, 1980.
64. Dwyer, E. M., and Wiener, L. Left ventricular function in man following thiopental. *Anesth. Analg.* 48:499, 1969.
65. Eckstein, J. W., Hamilton, W. K., and McCammond, J. M. The effect of thiopental on peripheral venous tone. *Anesthesiology* 22:525, 1961.
66. Elder, J. D., Nagono, S. M., Eastwood, D. W., and Harnagel, D. Circulatory changes associated with thiopental anesthesia in man. *Anesthesiology* 16:394, 1955.
67. Etsten, B., and Li, T. H. Effects of anesthesia upon the heart. *Am. J. Cardiol.* 6:706, 1960.
68. Etsten, B., and Li, T. H. Hemodynamic changes during thiopental anesthesia in humans: Cardiac output, stroke volume, total peripheral resistance, and intrathoracic blood volume. *J. Clin. Invest.* 34:500, 1955.
69. Fay, T. Early experiences with local and generalized refrigeration of the human brain. *J. Neurosurg.* 16:239, 1959.
70. Fishman, R. A. Brain edema. *N. Engl. J. Med.* 293:706, 1975.
71. Flamm, E. S., Demopoulos, H. B., Seligman, M. L., et al. Free radicals in cerebral ischemia. *Stroke* 9:445, 1978.
72. Flamm, E. S., Seligman, M. L., and Demopoulos, H. B. Barbiturate Protection of the Ischemic Brain. In J. E. Cottrell and H. Turndorf (Eds.), *Anesthesia and Neurosurgery.* St. Louis: Mosby, 1980. Pp. 248–266.
73. Fleischer, J. E., Milde, H. M., Moyer, T. P., and Michenfelder, J. D. Cerebral effects of high-dose midazolam and subsequent reversal with Ro. 15-1788 in dogs. *Anesthesiology* 68:234, 1988.
74. Foster, A., Juge, O., and Morel, D. Effects of midazolam on cerebral blood flow in human volunteers. *Anesthesiology* 56:453, 1982.
75. Foster, A. C., Gill, R., and Kemp, J. A. Protector of N-methyl-D-aspartate induced neuronal degeneration by systemic administration of MK-801. *Br. J. Pharmacol.* 89:870, 1986.
76. Frank, L., and Massaro, D. The lung and oxygen toxicity. *Arch. Intern. Med.* 139:347, 1979.
77. Fridovich, I. Hypoxia and Oxygen Toxicity. In S. Fahn (Ed.), *Advances in Neurology.* New York: Raven, 26:255, 1979.
78. Gelmers, H. J., Gorter, K., DeWeerdt, C. J., and Wiezer, J. A. A controlled trial of nimodipine in acute ischemic stroke. *N. Engl. J. Med.* 318:203, 1988.
79. Giammona, S. T. Drowning pathophysiology and management. *Curr. Probl. Pediatr.* 1:1, 1971.
80. Giffin, J. P., Cottrell, J. E., Shwiry, B., et al. Intracranial pressure, mean arterial pressure, and heart rate following midazolam or thiopental in humans with brain tumors. *Anesthesiology* 60:491, 1984.

81. Goldstein, A., Wells, B. A., and Keats, A. S. Increased tolerance to cerebral anoxia by pentobarbital. *Arch. Int. Pharmacodyn. Ther.* 161:138, 1966.
82. Grisvold, S. E., Safar, P., Hendricks, H. J. L., et al. Thiopental treatment after global brain ischemia in pigtailed monkeys. *Anesthesiology* 60:88, 1984.
83. Hankinson, H., Smith, A. L., Nielsen, S. L., et al. Effect of thiopental on focal ischemia in dogs. *Surg. Forum* 25:445, 1974.
84. Hartung, J., and Cottrell, J. E. Nitrous oxide reduces thiopental-induced prolongation of survival in hypoxic and anoxic mice. *Anesth. Analg.* 66:47, 1987.
85. Hartung, J., and Cottrell, J. E. On hot mice, cold facts and would-be replication. *Anesth. Analg.* 69(3):408–410, 1989.
86. Heubi, J. E., Partin, J. C., Partin, J. S., and Shubert, W. K. Reye's syndrome: Current concepts. *Hepatology* 7:155, 1987.
87. Hochberg, F. H., Nelson, K., and Janzen, W. Influenza type B related encephalopathy: The outbreak of Reyes syndrome in Chicago. *J.A.M.A.* 231:817, 1975.
88. Hoff, B. H. Multisystem failure: A review with special reference to drowning. *Crit. Care Med.* 7:310, 1979.
89. Hoff, J. T. Resuscitation in focal brain ischemia. *Crit. Care Med.* 6:245, 1978.
90. Hoff, J. T., Pitts, L. H., Spetzler, R., et al. Barbiturates for Protection from Cerebral Ischemia in Aneurysm Surgery. In D. H. Ingvar and N. Lassen (Eds.), Cerebral Function, Metabolism and Circulation. *Acta Neurol. Scand.* 56:158, 1977.
91. Hoff, J. T., Smith, A. L., and Hankinson, H. L. Barbiturate protection from cerebral infarction in primates. *Stroke* 6:28, 1975.
92. Hoffman, W. E., Miletich, D. J., and Albrecht, R. F. The effect of midazolam on cerebral blood flow and oxygen consumption and its interaction with nitrous oxide. *Anesth. Analg.* 65:729, 1986.
93. Hosobuchi, Y., Baskin, D. S., and Woo, S. K. Reversal of induced ischemic neurologic deficit in gerbils by the opiate antagonist naloxone. *Science* 215:69, 1982.
94. Hulser, P. J., Bernhart, H., Marbach, C., and Kornhuber, H. H. Treatment with an i.v. calcium overload blocker (Flunarizine) in acute stroke: A pilot study. *Eur. Arch. Psychiatr. Neurol. Sci.* 237:253, 1988.
95. Hunter, A. R. Thiopental supplemented anaesthesia for neurosurgery. *Br. J. Anaesth.* 44:506, 1972.
96. Huttenlocher, P. R. Reyes syndrome: Relation of outcome to therapy. *J. Pediatr.* 80:845, 1972.
97. Jackson, D. L., and Dole, W. P. Total cerebral ischemia: A new model system for the study of post cardiac arrest brain damage. *Stroke* 10:38, 1979.
98. Jamison, R. L. The role of cellular swelling in the pathogenesis of organ ischemia. *West. J. Med.* 120:205, 1974.
99. Janssen, P. Personal communication, 1988.
99a. Jastremski, M., Sutton-Tyrell, K., Vaagenes, P., et al. Glucocorticoid treatment does not improve neurological recovery following cardiac arrest. *J.A.M.A.* 262:3427, 1989.
100. Jennett, B., and Bond, M. Assessment of outcome after severe brain damage. A practical scale. *Lancet* 1:480, 1975.
101. Jennett, G., Teasdale, S., Galbraith, J., et al. Severe head injuries in three countries. *J. Neurol. Neurosurg. Psychiatry* 40:291, 1977.
102. Johnson, G. M., Scurletis, T. D., and Carroll, N. B. A study of sixteen fatal cases of encephalitis-like disease in North Carolina children. *N.C. Med. J.* 24:464, 1963.
103. Kass, I. S., Chambers, G., and Cottrell, J. E. The N-Methyl-D-aspartate antagonists aminophosphonovaleric acid and MK-801 reduce anoxic damage to dentate granule and CA1 pyramidal cells in the rat hippocampal slice. *Exp. Neurol.* 103:116, 1989.
104. Kass, I. S., Cottrell, J. E., and Chambers, G. Magnesium and cobalt, not nimodipine, protect neurons against anoxic damage in the rat hippocampal slice. *Anesthesiology* 69:710, 1988.

105. Kass, I. S., and Lipton, P. Calcium and long term transmission damage following anoxia in dentate gyrus and CA I regions of the hippocampal slice. *J. Physiol. (London)* 378:313, 1986.
106. Keenan. Personal communication.
107. Kennealy, J. A., McLennan, J. E., Loudon, R. G., and McLaurin, R. L. Hyperventilation-induced cerebral hypoxia. *Am. Rev. Respir. Dis.* 122:407, 1980.
108. Kindt, G. W., Waldman, J., Kohl, S., et al. Intracranial pressure in Reye's syndrome: Monitoring and control. *J.A.M.A.* 231:822, 1975.
109. Kofke, W. A., Nemoto, E. M., Hossman, K. A., et al. Brain blood flow and metabolism after global ischemia and post-insult thiopental therapy in monkeys. *Stroke* 10:554, 1979.
110. Langfitt, T. W. Measuring the outcome from head injuries. *J. Neurosurg.* 48:673, 1978.
111. Langfitt, T. W. The Incidence and Importance of Intracranial Hypertension in Head-Injured Patients. In J. W. F. Beks, D. A. Bosch, and M. Breck (Eds.), *Intracranial Pressure III*. New York: Springer, 1976. Pp. 67–72.
112. Lanier, W. L., Perkins, W. J., Rudd, B., et al. Effect of the excitatory amino acid antagonist MK-801 on neurological function following complete cerebral ischemia in primates. *Anesthesiology* 69:A846, 1988.
113. Lansky, L. L., Kalavasky, S. M., Brackett, C. E., et al. Hypothermic total body washout and intracranial pressure monitoring in stage IV Reye's syndrome. *J. Pediatr.* 90:634, 1977.
114. Lawner, P., Lourent, J., Simeone, F., et al. Attenuation of ischemic brain edema by pentobarbital after carotid ligation in the gerbil. *Stroke* 10:644, 1979.
115. Leibovitz, B. E., and Siegel, B. V. Aspects of free radical reactions in biological systems: Aging. *J. Gerontol.* 34:45, 1980.
116. Linko, E., Koskinen, P. J., Sitonen, L., and Ruosteenoja, R. Resuscitation in cardiac arrest: An analysis of 100 consecutive medical cases. *Acta Med. Scand.* 182:611, 1967.
117. Lovejoy, F. H., Bresnan, M. J., Lombroso, C. T., and Smith, A. L. Anticerebral edema therapy in Reye's syndrome. *Arch. Dis. Child.* 50:933, 1975.
118. Lovejoy, F. H., Smith, A. L., Bresnan, M. J., et al. Clinical staging in Reye's syndrome. *Am. J. Dis. Child.* 128:36, 1974.
119. Mark, L. C. Metabolism of barbiturates in man. *Clin. Pharmacol. Ther.* 4:504, 1963.
120. Marshall, L. F., Shapiro, H. M., Ranscher, A., and Kaufman, N. M. Pentobarbital therapy for intracranial hypertension in metabolic coma: Reye's syndrome. *Crit. Care Med.* 6:1, 1978.
121. Marshall, L. F., Smith, R. W., and Shapiro, H. M. The outcome with aggressive treatment in severe head injuries: Part II. Acute and chronic barbiturate administration in the management of head injury. *J. Neurosurg.* 50:26, 1979.
122. McCord, J. M., and Fridovich, I. The biology and pathology of oxygen radicals. *Ann. Intern. Med.* 89:122, 1978.
123. McGraw, C. P. Experimental cerebral infarction effects of pentobarbital in Mongolian gerbils. *Arch. Neurol.* 34:334, 1977.
124. Meldrum, B. S. Metabolic effects of prolonged epileptic seizures and the causation of epileptic brain damage. In F. C. Rose (Ed.), *Metabolic Disorders of the Nervous System*. London: Pitman, 1981. Pp. 175–187.
125. Michenfelder, J. D. Cerebral protection with barbiturates: Relation to anesthetic effect. *Stroke* 9:140, 1978.
126. Michenfelder, J. D. The interdependency of cerebral functional and metabolic effects following massive doses of thiopental in the dog. *Anesthesiology* 41:231, 1974.
127. Michenfelder, J. D., and Milde, J. H. Influence of anesthetics on metabolic functional and pathological response to regional cerebral ischemia. *Stroke* 6:405, 1975.

128. Michenfelder, J. D., Milde, J. H., and Sundt, T. M. Cerebral protection by barbiturate anesthesia. *Arch. Neurol.* 33:345, 1976.
129. Michenfelder, J. D., and Theye, R. A. Cerebral protection by thiopental during hypoxia. *Anesthesiology* 39:510, 1973.
130. Mickell, J. J., Reigel, D. H., Cook, D. R., et al. Intracranial pressure: Monitoring and normalization therapy in children. *Pediatrics* 59:606, 1977.
131. Mihm, F. Unpublished data.
132. Milde, L. N. The hypoxic mouse model for screening cerebral protective agents: A re-examination. *Anesth. Analg.* 67:917, 1988.
133. Milde, L. N., and Milde, J. H. Preservation of cerebral metabolites by etomidate during incomplete cerebral ischemia in dogs. *Anesthesiology* 65:272, 1986.
134. Milde, L. N., Milde, J. H., Lanier, W. L., et al. Comparison of the effects of isoflurane and thiopental on neurologic outcome and neuropathology after temporary focal cerebral ischemia in primates. *Anesthesiology* 69:905, 1988.
135. Milde, L. N., Milde, J. H., and Michenfelder, J. D. Cerebral functional, metabolic, and hemodynamic effects of etomidate in dogs. *Anesthesiology* 63:371, 1985.
136. Miller, J. D., Sweet, R. C., Narayan, R., and Becker, D. P. Early insults to the injured brain. *J.A.M.A.* 240:439, 1978.
137. Modell, J. H., Graves, S. A., and Kuck, E. J. Near-drowning correlation of level of consciousness and survival. *Can. Anaesth. Soc. J.* 27:211, 1980.
138. Moseley, J. L., Laurent, J. P., and Molinari, G. F. Barbiturate attenuation of the clinical course and pathologic lesions in a primate stroke model. *Neurology* 25:870, 1975.
139. Mutch, W. A. C., Malo, L. A., and Ringaert, K. R. A. Phenylephrine increases regional cerebral blood flow following hemorrhage during isoflurane-oxygen anesthesia. *Anesthesiology* 70:276, 1989.
140. Myerburg, R. J. Standards and guidelines for cardiopulmonary resuscitation (CPR) and emergency cardiac care (ECC). *J.A.M.A.* 255:2905, 1986.
141. Myerburg, R. J., Conde, C. A., Sung, R. J., et al. Clinical, electrophysiologic, and hemodynamic profile of patients resuscitated from prehospital cardiac arrest. *Am. J. Med.* 68:568, 1980.
142. Nadler, H. Therapeutic delirium in Reye's syndrome. *Pediatrics* 54:265, 1974.
143. Negovskii, V. A. Introduction: Reanimatology — The Science of Resuscitation. In H. E. Stephenso (Ed.), *Cardiac Arrest and Resuscitation.* St. Louis: Mosby, 1974. Chap. 1.
144. Nehls, D. G., Todd, M. M., Spetzler, R. F., et al. A comparison of the cerebral protective effects of isoflurane and barbiturates during temporary focal ischemia in primates. *Anesthesiology* 66:453, 1987.
145. Nemoto, E. M., Erdman, W., Strong, E., et al. Regional brain PO_2 after global ischemia in monkeys: Evidence for regional differences in critical perfusion pressures. *Stroke* 10:44, 1979.
146. Newberg, L. A., and Michenfelder, J. D. Cerebral protection by isoflurane during hypoxemia or ischemia. *Anesthesiology* 59:29, 1983.
147. Newberg, L. A., Milde, J. H., and Michenfelder, J. D. The cerebral metabolic effects of isoflurane at and above concentrations that suppress cortical electrical activity. *Anesthesiology* 59:23, 1983.
148. Nilsson, L. The influence of barbiturate anesthesia upon the energy state and upon acid-base parameters of the brain in arterial hypotension and in asphyxia. *Acta Neurol. Scand.* 47:233, 1971.
149. Norris, J. R., and Chandrasekar, S. Anoxic brain damage after cardiac resuscitation. *J. Chronic. Dis.* 24:585, 1971.
150. Nugent, M., Antru, A. A., and Michenfelder, J. D. Cerebral metabolic, vascular and protective effects of midazolam maleate. *Anesthesiology* 56:172, 1982.
151. Nussmeier, N. A., Arlund, C., and Slogoff, S. Neuropsychiatric complications after

cardiopulmonary bypass: Cerebral protection by a barbiturate. *Anesthesiology* 64:165, 1986.

152. O'Brien, M. D. Ischemia cerebral edema — A review. *Stroke* 10:623, 1979.

153. O'Brien, M. D., Waltz, A. G., and Jordan, M. M. Ischemia cerebral edema: Distribution of water in brains of cats after occlusion of the middle cerebral artery. *Arch. Neurol.* 30:456, 1974.

154. Orlowski, J. P., Gillis, J., and Kilham, H. A. A catch in the Reye. *Pediatrics* 80:638, 1987.

155. Overgaard, J., Hvid-Hansen, O., Land, A. M., et al. Prognosis after head injury based on early clinical exam. *Lancet* 2:631, 1973.

156. Ozyurt, E., Graham, D. I., Woodruff, G. N., and McCulloch, J. Protective effects of the glutamate antagonist MK-801 in focal cerebral ischemia in the cat. *J. Cereb. Blood Flow Metab.* 8:138, 1988.

157. Pearn, J. Survival rates after serious immersion accidents in childhood. *Resuscitation* 6:271, 1979.

158. Peterson, B. Moribidity of childhood near-drowning. *Pediatrics* 59:364, 1977.

159. Petruk, K. C., West, M., Mohr, G., et al. Nimodipine treatment in poor-grade aneurysm patients: Results of a multicenter double-blind placebo-controlled trial. *J. Neurosurg.* 68:505, 1988.

160. Pierce, E. C., Lambertsen, C. J., Deutsch, S., et al. Cerebral circulation and metabolism during thiopental anesthesia and hypoventilation in man. *J. Clin. Invest.* 41:1664, 1962.

161. Raughman, V. L., Hoffman, W. E., Miletich, D. J., and Albrecht, R. F. Neurologic outcome following regional cerebral ischemia with methoxital, midazolam, and etimonate. *Anesthesiology* 67(3A), Abstr., 1987.

162. Rea, G. L., and Rockswold, G. L. Barbiturate therapy in uncontrolled intracranial hypertension. *Neurosurgery* 12:401, 1983.

163. Reye, R. D. K., Morgan, G., and Baral, J. Encephalopathy and fatty degeneration of the viscera: A disease entity in childhood. *Lancet* 2:749, 1963.

164. Rockoff, M. A., Marshall, L. F., and Shapiro, H. M. High-dose barbiturate therapy in humans: A clinical review of 60 patients. *Ann. Neurol.* 6:194, 1979.

165. Rosenthal, M. H., and Larson, C. P. Protection of the brain from progressive ischemia. *West. J. Med.* 128:145, 1978.

166. Rothman, S. Synaptic release of excitatory amino acid neurotransmitters mediates anoxic neuronal death. *J. Neurosci.* 4:1884, 1984.

167. Sahs, A. L. (Ed.). Stroke Unit: Patient Evaluation, Treatment, and Followup. In *Fundamentals of Stroke Care.* U.S. Government Printing Office, 1976. Pp. 330–339.

168. Safar, P. Brain resuscitation in metabolic-toxic infectious encephalopathy. *Crit. Care Med.* 6:68, 1978.

169. Samaha, F. J., Balu, E., and Berardinelli, J. L. Reye's syndrome: Clinical diagnosis and treatment with peritoneal dialysis. *Pediatrics* 53:336, 1974.

170. Schwartz, M. L., Tator, C. H., Rowed, D. W., et al. The University of Toronto head injury treatment study: A prospective randomized comparison of pentobarbital and mannitol. *Can. J. Neurol. Sci.* 11:434, 1984.

171. Scurr, C., and Feldman, S. (Eds.). *Scientific Foundations of Anesthesia.* Chicago: Year Book, 1974. P. 410.

172. Shafer, S. Q., Bruun, B., and Richter, R. W. The outcome of stroke at hospital discharge in New York City blacks. *Stroke* 4:782, 1973.

173. Shapiro, H. M., Galindo, A., Wyte, S. R., and Harris, A. B. Rapid intraoperative reduction of intracranial pressure with thiopentone. *Br. J. Anaesth.* 45:1057, 1973.

174. Shapiro, H. M., Wyte, S. R., and Loeser, J. Barbiturate augmented hypothermia for reduction of persistent intracranial hypertension. *J. Neurosurg.* 40:90, 1974.

175. Sharpless, S. K. Hypnotics and Sedatives — The Barbiturates. In L. S. Goodman and A. Gilman (Eds.), *The Pharmacological Basis of Therapeutics* (4th ed.). New York: Macmillan, 1970. Pp. 98–120.
176. Shaywitz, B. A., Leventhal, J. M., Kramer, M. S., and Venes, J. L. Prolonged continuous monitoring of intracranial pressure in severe Reye's syndrome. *Pediatrics* 54:595, 1977.
177. Shubin, H., and Weil, M. H. Shock associated with barbiturate intoxication. *Crit. Care Med.* 215:263, 1971.
178. Siebke, H., Rod, T., Breivik, H., and Lind, B. Survival after 40 minutes submersion without cerebral sequelae. *Lancet* 1:1275, 1975.
179. Siegel, J. H., and Sonneblick, E. H. Quantification and prediction of myocardial failure. *Arch. Surg.* 89:1026, 1964.
180. Siesjo, B. K. Cerebral circulation and metabolism. *J. Neurosurg.* 60:883, 1984.
181. Simeone, F. A., Frazer, G., and Lawner, P. Ischemic brain edema: Comparative effects of barbiturates and hypothermia. *Stroke* 10:8, 1979.
182. Simon, R. P., Swan, J. H., Griffiths, T., and Meldrum, B. S. Blockade of N-methyl-D-aspartate receptors may protect against ischemic damage in the brain. *Science* 226:850, 1984.
183. Smith, A. Barbiturate protection in cerebral hypoxia. *Anesthesiology* 47:285, 1977.
184. Smith, A. L., Hoff, J. T., Nielsen, S. L., and Larson, C. P. Barbiturate protection in acute focal cerebral ischemia. *Stroke* 5:1, 1974.
185. Smith, A. L., and Margue, J. J. Anesthetics and cerebral edema. *Anesthesiology* 45:64, 1976.
186. Smith, D. S., Rehncrona, S., and Siesjo, B. K. Inhibitory effects of different barbiturates on lipid preoxidation in brain tissue in vitro: Comparison with the effects of promethazine and chlorpromazine. *Anesthesiology* 53:186, 1980.
187. Snyder, B. D., Ramierez-Lassepas, M., and Lippert, D. M. Neurologic status and prognosis after cardiopulmonary arrest: A retrospective study. *Neurology* 27:807, 1977.
188. Snyder, B. D., Ramirez-Lassepas, M., Sukhaum, P., et al. Failure of thiopental to modify global anoxic injury. *Stroke* 10:135, 1979.
189. Somjen, G., Hilmy, M., and Stephen, C. R. Failure to anesthetize human subjects by intravenous administration of magnesium sulfate. *J. Pharmacol Exp. Ther.* 154:652, 1966.
190. Sonntag, H., Hellerberg, K., Schesk, H. D., et al. Effects of thiopental (trapanal) on coronary blood flow and myocardial metabolism in man. *Acta Anaesthesiol. Scand.* 19:69, 1975.
191. Stanski, D. R., Mihm, F. G., Rosenthal, M. H., and Kalman, S. M. Pharmacokinetics of high dose thiopental used in cerebral resuscitation. *Anesthesiology* 53:169, 1980.
191a. Steen, P. A., Gisvold, S. E., Milde, J. H., et al. Nimodipine improves outcome when given after complete cerebral ischemia in primates. *Anesthesiology* 62:406, 1985.
192. Steen, P. A., and Michenfelder, J. D. Cerebral protection with barbiturates: Relation to anesthetic effect. *Stroke* 9:140, 1978.
193. Steen, P. A., and Michenfelder, J. D. Neurotoxicity of anesthetics. *Anesthesiology* 50:437, 1979.
194. Steen, P. A., Milde, J. H., and Michenfelder, J. D. No barbiturate protection in a dog model of complete cerebral ischemia. *Ann. Neurol.* 5:343, 1979.
195. Steen, P. A., Milde, J. H., and Michenfelder, J. D. The detrimental effects of prolonged hypothermia and rewarming in the dog. *Anesthesiology* 52:224, 1980.
195a. Steen, P. A., Newberg, L. A., Milsw, J. H., and Michenfelder, J. D. Cerebral blood flow and neurologic outcome when nimodipine is given after complete cerebral ischemia in the dog. *J. Cereb. Blood Flow Metab.* 4:82, 1984.

196. Steen, P. A., Soule, E. H., and Michenfelder, J. D. Detrimental effects of prolonged hypothermia in cats and monkeys with and without regional cerebral ischemia. *Stroke* 10:522, 1979.
197. Sundt, T. M., Jr., Grant, W. C., and Garcia, J. H. Restoration of middle cerebral artery flow in experimental infarction. *J. Neurosurg.* 31:311, 1969.
198. Suzuki, J., Fujimoto, S., Mizoi, K., and Oba, M. The protective effect of combined administration of anti-oxidants and perflurochemicals on cerebral ischemia. *Stroke* 15:672, 1984.
199. Takayasu, M., Bassett, J. E., and Darcy, R. G. Effects of calcium antagonists on intracerebral penetrating arterioles in rats. *J. Neurosurg.* 69:104, 1988.
200. Todd, M. M., Chadwick, H. S., Shapiro, H. M., et al. The neurological effect of thiopental therapy following experimental cardiac arrest in cats. *Anesthesiology* 57:76, 1982.
201. Toman, J. E. P. Drugs Effective in Convulsive Disorders. In L. W. Goodman and A. Gilman (Eds.), *The Pharmacologic Basis of Theapeutics* (4th ed.). New York: MacMillan, 1970. P. 209.
202. Trauner, D. A. Treatment of Reye's syndrome. *Ann. Neurol.* 7:2, 1980.
203. Vacanti, F. X., and Ames, A. Mild hypothermia and MG^{++} protect against irreversible damage during CNS ischemia. *Stroke* 15:695, 1984.
204. Van Caille, M., Morin, C. L., and Roy, C. C. Reye's syndrome relapses and neurological sequelae. *Pediatrics* 59:244, 1977.
205. Van Horn, G. Cerebrovascular Disease. In *Disease-A-Month*. Chicago: Year Book, 1973. Pp. 1–35.
206. Van Reempts, J., Borgers, M., Eyndhoven, J. V., and Herman, S. C. Protective effects of etomidate in hypoxic ischemic brain damage in the rat. A morphologic assessment. *Exp. Neurol.* 76:181, 1982.
207. Venes, J. L., Shaywitz, B. A., and Spencer, D. D. Management of severe cerebral edema in the metabolic encephalopathy of Reye-Johnson syndrome. *J. Neurosurg.* 48:903, 1978.
208. Wade, J. G., Amtorp, O., and Sorensen, S. C. No-flow state following cerebral ischemia: Role of increase in potassium concentration in brain interstitial fluid. *Arch. Neurol.* 32:381, 1975.
209. Waltz, A. G. Clinical relevance of models of cerebral ischemia. *Stroke* 10:211, 1979.
210. Ward, J. D., Becker, D. P., et al. Failure of prophylactic barbiturate coma in the treatment of severe head injury. *J. Neurosurg.* 62:383, 1985.
210a. Warner, D. S. Magnesium and the injured brain. *J. Neurosurg. Anesth.* 1:360, 1989.
211. Warner, D. S., Godeisky, J. C., and Smith, M. Failure of preischemic lidocaine administration to ameliorate global ischemic brain damage in the rat. *Anesthesiology* 68:73–78, 1988.
212. Wauquier, A., Ashton, G., Clincke, G., and Niemegeers, C. J. Anti-hypoxic effects of etomidate, thiopental and methohexital. *Arch. Int. Pharmacodyn. Ther.* 249:330, 1981.
213. Willoughby, J. O., and Leach, B. G. Relation of neurological findings after cardiac arrest to outcome. *Br. Med. J.* 3:437, 1974.
214. Wolfson, L. T., Sakurado, O., and Sokoloff, L. Effects of y-butyrolactone on local cerebral glucose utilization in the rat. *J. Neurochem.* 29:777, 1977.
215. Wright, R. L., and Ames, A. Measurement of maximal permissible cerebral ischemia and a study of its pharmacologic prolongation. *J. Neurosurg.* 21:567, 1964.
216. Yatsu, F. M., Diamond, I., Graziano, C., and Lindquist, P. Experimental brain ischemia. Protection from irreversible damage with a rapid-acting barbiturate (methohexital). *Stroke* 43:726, 1972.

II

Intensive Care

5

Respiratory Care of the Neurosurgical Patient

NEAL H. COHEN

The neurosurgical patient presents special problems with respect to respiratory care. In addition to concerns of relevance to all surgical and critically ill patients, the neurosurgical patient has specific needs that must be carefully assessed to ensure adequate oxygen delivery and ventilation without compromising cerebral function. Routine respiratory care must occasionally be modified to fulfill what can be conflicting goals, particularly for the neurosurgical patient who develops a pulmonary complication. When appropriate respiratory care is provided to the neurosurgical patient, morbidity and mortality can be reduced and neurologic outcome improved [60]. An understanding of respiratory physiology is essential to achieve a satisfactory outcome.

I. Respiratory physiology
A. Arterial blood gases.
Arterial blood values provide a direct indication of the adequacy of pulmonary gas exchange both for the spontaneously breathing patient and the neurosurgical patient requiring mechanical ventilatory support. Normal arterial blood gas measured values are

Arterial oxygen tension (PaO_2): 80–100 mmHg
Arterial carbon dioxide tension ($PaCO_2$): 37–43 mmHg
pH: 7.37–7.43

From these measured values, additional data can be calculated to facilitate interpretation of the patient's overall acid-base status, including serum bicarbonate and base excess or deficit. Normal values are

Bicarbonate (HCO_3^-): 23–28 mEq/L
Base excess: ±2 mEq/L

The PaO_2 is a reflection of the adequacy of oxygen delivery (i.e., inspired oxygen concentration) and the ability of the lung to provide for adequate oxygen uptake. It is *not* a reflection of tissue oxygenation. Oxygen delivery is dependent on the amount of oxygen in the blood (bound to hemoglobin and dissolved) and cardiac output.
$PaCO_2$ is a direct reflection of ventilation. If ventilation is "normal," the $PaCO_2$ is in the normal range. Any increase or decrease in the

PaCO$_2$ defines an alteration in ventilation, hypoventilation, or hyperventilation, respectively.

Alterations in arterial blood gas values are defined as follows.

Oxygenation	Hypoxemia	PaO$_2$ < 70 mmHg
Ventilation	Hypoventilation (respiratory acidosis)	PaCO$_2$ > 43 mmHg
	Hyperventilation (respiratory alkalosis)	PaCO$_2$ < 37 mmHg
Acid-base abnormalities	Acidemia	pH < 7.37
	Alkalemia	pH > 7.43
	Metabolic acidosis	HCO$_3^-$ < 23 mEq/L
	Metabolic alkalosis	HCO$_3^-$ > 28 mEq/L

B. Acid-base imbalance. A change in acid-base balance can occur as a result of an alteration in ventilation or due to a metabolic abnormality. The body attempts to compensate for a change in acid-base homeostasis to maintain the pH in the normal range. For example, the neurosurgical patient who hyperventilates as a result of an intracerebral lesion will have a respiratory alkalosis (e.g., PaCO$_2$ < 30 mmHg, pH > 7.47) [24]. In response to this hyperventilation, if sustained, the patient will develop a compensatory metabolic acidosis by excreting bicarbonate (HCO$_3^-$) via the kidney. Similar compensatory mechanisms will occur with other primary acid-base imbalances as listed in Table 5-1.

   1. Respiratory acidosis. A primary respiratory acidosis occurs as a result of hypoventilation with CO$_2$ retention. The increased PaCO$_2$ causes an increase in carbonic acid (H$_2$CO$_3$) and acidemia. Hypoventilation and respiratory acidosis can be caused by the following.

Table 5-1. Compensatory responses to primary acid-base imbalances

Primary acid-base imbalance	Compensatory response
Respiratory acidosis (acute)	HCO$_3^-$ rises 3–4 mEq/L to 32 mEq/L
Respiratory acidosis (chronic)	HCO$_3^-$ rises 0.4 mEq/L for each 1 mmHg increase in PaCO$_2$
Respiratory alkalosis (acute)	HCO$_3^-$ decreases 0.2 mEq/L for each 1 mmHg decrease in PaCO$_2$
Respiratory alkalosis (chronic)	HCO$_3^-$ decreases 0.5 mEq/L for each 1 mmHg decrease in PCO$_2$ to 15 mEq/L
Metabolic acidosis	PCO$_2$ decreases 1.0–1.3 mmHg for each 1 mEq/L decrease in HCO$_3^-$
Metabolic alkalosis	PaCO$_2$ increases 0.5–1.0 mmHg for each 1 mEq/L increase in HCO$_3^-$

HCO$_3^-$ = bicarbonate concentration; PaCO$_2$ = arterial carbon dioxide tension; PCO$_2$ = carbon dioxide tension.

   a. Central nervous system (CNS) depression due to
     (1) Structural lesion
     (2) Pharmacologic depression (e.g., respiratory depressants)
   b. Neuromuscular disorder, (e.g., Guillain-Barré syndrome, myasthenia gravis, diaphragmatic dysfunction)
   c. Chest wall abnormalities
   d. Pleural effusion
   e. Pneumothorax
   f. Airway obstruction
   g. Parenchymal lung disease
   h. Cardiopulmonary arrest
   i. Inappropriate mechanical ventilatory settings or ventilator dysfunction

In response to the respiratory acidosis, HCO_3^- will increase acutely by about 3 to 4 mEq/L. Initially, renal compensation is minimal. However, if the respiratory acidosis is sustained, renal compensation will occur after 6 to 12 hours. The serum HCO_3^- will increase 0.4 mEq/L for each 1 mmHg rise in $PaCO_2$. Associated with the HCO_3^- retention is the development of hypochloremia as chloride is excreted by the renal tubule to preserve electroneutrality.

2. **Respiratory alkalosis.** A primary respiratory alkalosis occurs as a result of hyperventilation and increased CO_2 excretion by the lungs. The causes of hyperventilation include
   a. Hypoxemia
   b. Central nervous system lesion, cerebral edema
   c. Fever
   d. Sepsis
   e. Parenchymal lung disease, particularly during acute phase
   f. Drugs (e.g., salicylates)
   g. Mechanical ventilatory cause (e.g., deliberately increased minute ventilation in a patient with increased intracranial pressure)
   h. Hepatic insufficiency
   i. Hyperthyroidism

In response to the hypocapnia and alkalosis, serum HCO_3^- falls by about 0.2 mEq/L for every 1 mmHg decrease in $PaCO_2$. Renal compensation with acid retention attempts to normalize the pH. Bicarbonate excretion occurs after 7 to 9 days. Chronic respiratory alkalosis is the *only* primary acid-base disturbance for which secondary compensatory mechanisms will return the pH to normal.

3. **Metabolic acidosis.** When a strong acid accumulates in the body or when excessive HCO_3^- is lost, a metabolic acidosis develops. Causes of metabolic acidosis include
   a. Lactic acidosis
   b. Renal failure

   c. Renal tubular acidosis
   d. Ketoacidosis
   e. Toxins (e.g., methanol, ethylene glycol, paraldehyde, salicylates)
   f. Gastrointestinal loss of HCO_3^-
   g. Excessive chloride administration (e.g., hyperalimentation)
      The acidemia is immediately buffered in the body, causing a
   decrease in serum HCO_3^-. Respiratory compensation for the acidosis occurs rapidly; hyperventilation decreases the $PaCO_2$. H_2CO_3
   concentration is reduced and the pH returns *toward* normal, never
   completely returning to 7.40. The respiratory compensation does
   not reach a steady state for 12 to 24 hours.
4. Metabolic alkalosis. A metabolic alkalosis occurs with an increase
   in serum HCO_3^-. The causes of metabolic alkalosis include
   a. Acid loss
   b. Chloride excretion in excess of HCO_3^- loss
   c. Endogenous or exogenously administered alkali (e.g., excessive
      acetate in hyperalimentation fluid)
      In response to the metabolic alkalosis, the patient will hypoven-
   tilate and retain CO_2. The CO_2 retention increases the H_2CO_3,
   shifting the pH toward normal. Compensation is usually incomplete.
   The degree of compensation is dependent on a number of other
   factors. The hypoventilatory response is limited primarily due to the
   potential development of hypoxemia.
5. Mixed acid-base disturbances. Mixed acid-base disturbances
   [37,53] occur when two or more primary disorders exist simultaneously, each eliciting its own compensatory response. Metabolic
   alkalosis and metabolic acidosis may occur together, just as respiratory acidosis may coexist with metabolic acidosis or a respiratory
   alkalosis with a metabolic alkalosis. A *triple* mixed disorder occurs
   when one primary respiratory disorder is superimposed on a coexisting metabolic acidosis and alkalosis (e.g., a patient on continuous gastric suction who has chronic obstructive lung disease and
   develops central hyperventilation and hemorrhagic shock after
   head injury and multiple trauma).
      The complex acid-base disturbances that can occur in the patient
   with multisystem disorders emphasizes the need to carefully analyze arterial blood gas values. The interpretation must take into
   account the overall patient condition and goals of therapy, particularly for the patient with increased intracranial pressure and altered
   intracerebral compliance.
C. Oxygen transport. The goal of respiratory care is to ensure safe and
   adequate gas exchange. Delivery of sufficient oxygen to the tissues is
   not guaranteed by maintaining normal arterial blood gases. Oxygen
   delivery at the cellular level is dependent primarily on oxygen saturation and release from hemoglobin and to a much smaller extent on

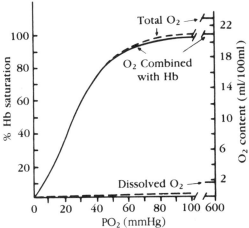

Fig. 5-1. Oxyhemoglobin dissociation curve. The oxyhemoglobin curve describes the affinity of hemoglobin for oxygen. It depicts the percent of hemoglobin that exists as HbO_2 at various levels of O_2 tension. (This standard curve is applicable when pH is 7.4, PCO_2 is 40 mmHG, and temperature is 37°C.) Oxygen content is also shown. This assumes the hemoglobin level is 15 gm/100 ml, and that each gram of hemoglobin when fully saturated combines with 1.34 ml O_2. The dotted line represents O_2 content (HbO_2 plus dissolved O_2.) Note that dissolved O_2 contributes little to O_2 content at ordinary levels of PaO_2. (From H. A. Braun, F. W. Cheney, Jr., and C. P. Loehnen, *Introduction to Respiratory Physiology* (2nd ed.). Boston: Little, Brown, 1980.)

oxygen dissolved in the blood. The relationship between hemoglobin saturation and PaO_2 is described by the oxyhemoglobin dissociation curve (Fig. 5-1) [5,32,64,72]. If a physiologic change occurs, the oxyhemoglobin dissociation curve will shift to the right or left relative to the normal relationship [51]. A rightward shift in the curve decreases the affinity of hemoglobin for oxygen. The P_{50}, which is the PaO_2 at which the hemoglobin is 50% saturated with oxygen, increases from the normal (normal P_{50} is approximately PaO_2 27 mmHg). The rightward shift improves unloading of oxygen at the cellular level. A shift of the oxyhemoglobin dissociation curve to the left has the opposite effect, decreasing peripheral tissue oxygen delivery. The physiologic changes that affect the oxyhemoglobin dissociation relationship are listed in Table 5-2 [42,51,65].

To ensure adequate oxygen content and delivery, optimization of cardiac output, hemoglobin, and oxygen saturation is necessary. A number of compensatory mechanisms exist to ensure homeostasis [33]. For example, in the presence of anemia or hypoxemia, cardiac output will increase to maintain oxygen delivery at a constant level. When this compensatory mechanism is insufficient (e.g., for the patient with myocardial dysfunction), oxygen extraction by the tissues increases, lowering the mixed venous oxygen content and further

Table 5-2. Factors that affect the oxyhemoglobin dissociation curve

Increased oxygen affinity (leftward shift)	Decreased oxygen affinity (rightward shift)
Hypothermia	Hyperthermia
Hypocapnia	Hypercapnia
Alkalemia	Acidemia
Anemia	Increased 2,3-diphosphoglycerate concentration
Reduced 2,3-diphosphoglycerate concentration	
Hypophosphatemia	

stressing a delicately balanced system. Eventually, oxygen extraction is maximized and all compensatory mechanisms fail. Under these circumstances, lactic acidosis will develop as a result of anaerobic metabolism.

II. Respiratory disorders. A number of respiratory abnormalities occur in neurosurgical patients, some as a result of the neurologic abnormality, some due to underlying physiologic abnormalities, and others due to associated injuries.

A. Altered respiratory patterns. Patients with intracranial lesions commonly have altered patterns of respiration [24]. Although Cheyne-Stokes respiration is the most frequently described abnormal breathing pattern, other periodic breathing patterns can occur. If the patient's gas exchange is satisfactory, the altered respiratory pattern does not require specific treatment. If the patient is obtunded and unable to protect the airway, intubation is mandatory.

Central neurogenic hyperventilation occasionally occurs after head trauma or other lesions causing increased intracranial pressure (ICP). The ventilatory pattern is rapid, sustained deep breathing. This breathing pattern often occurs in patients with bilateral CNS lesions, often involving the brainstem [24]. When central neurogenic hyperventilation occurs, the prognosis is poor. The hyperventilation often precipitates other problems, including severe alkalemia, pH often > 7.60. The high pH predisposes the patient to intense cerebral vasospasm and cerebral lactic acidosis. It also can create malignant ventricular arrhythmias due to profound electrolyte shifts. These patients become extremely hypermetabolic with increased oxygen consumption and inability to maintain a positive nitrogen balance despite high caloric intake.

Management of the patient who has central neurogenic hyperventilation includes endotracheal intubation for airway protection and pulmonary hygiene. Careful monitoring of respiratory function for signs of fatigue and hypercapnia is essential. Addition of mechanical dead space is *absolutely* contraindicated because it increases the work of breathing without affecting the acid-base status. If either the metabolic demands become too great or the pH becomes too alkalemic, then paralysis, sedation, and maintenance of $PaCO_2$ between 25 and 30 mmHg using controlled mechanical ventilation are indicated to reduce the metabolic rate and the alkalosis. The use of muscle relaxants, controlled ventilation, and sedation may also help lower ICP.

B. **Neurogenic pulmonary edema.** Acute pulmonary edema can develop in association with anterior hypothalamic compression, intraventricular hemorrhage, rupture of an anterior communicating artery aneurysm, or intracranial lesions remote from the hypothalamus. Intracranial hypertension may or may not be present. Although the exact cause is unknown, a possible mechanism for neurogenic pulmonary edema is catecholamine release caused by cerebral hypoxia, which increases systemic vascular resistance and shifts blood to the relatively low-pressure pulmonary vasculature [8,20,71,73]. This shift causes an acute increase in left atrial and pulmonary venous pressures with disruption of pulmonary capillary endothelial integrity and efflux of protein-rich fluid into the alveoli. Therapy of neurogenic pulmonary edema includes fluid restriction, diuretic administration, and mechanical ventilation (and positive end-expiratory pressure [PEEP]), as well as control of intracranial hypertension [8,20,71,73]. Vasodilators have also been recommended for use when systemic vascular resistance remains elevated [44].

C. **Aspiration pneumonitis.** The neurosurgical patient who is obtunded and unable to protect the airway is at significant risk for aspiration. Aspiration of gastric contents can occur after head injury, during diagnostic evaluations (particularly when transporting the patient with an unprotected airway), and during endotracheal intubation. The greatest risk for the patient is aspiration of gastric contents with pH $<$ 2.5 [1,6,7,35,62], although aspiration pneumonitis can occur after aspiration of other, particularly particulate matter as well [1,6,7].

The clinical signs of aspiration can be minimal. In many patients, however, the clinical presentation includes hypoxemia, tachycardia, and cyanosis with associated expiratory rhonchi and wheezes developing within six hours [1,6,7,48,77]. X-ray findings may also be minimal, although infiltrates or atelectasis may be apparent. Careful monitoring with a pulse oximeter and serial arterial blood gases are essential to determine the physiologic extent and progression of the disease process.

Initial therapy should be supportive. If the patient's airway is not protected, endotracheal intubation should be performed to minimize the risk of further aspiration. Supplemental oxygen and mechanical ventilatory support should be provided as necessary to ensure adequate gas exchange.

Prophylactic antibiotics have not been shown to decrease mortality or prevent secondary infection and may increase the risk of development of a nosocomial pneumonia from resistant organisms [3,43]. Bacterial pneumonia does not usually develop. Serial sputum gram stains should be obtained to look for bacterial superinfections. Steroids do not appear to be useful, unless they happen to have been given prior to aspiration [9,17,21,76]. Pulmonary atelectasis or lobar collapse can develop if the patient aspirates a foreign body, such as a tooth. Bronchoscopy will be required to remove the obstruction.

D. **Respiratory failure after high cervical cord injuries.** Successful resuscitation at the scene of the accident has increased the number of survivors after high cervical cord injuries. Unfortunately, the prognosis for long-term rehabilitation and survival remains poor for patients who have cord injuries at the level of C6 or above [11,68]. Initial aggressive supportive care must be provided, however, since resolution of spinal cord edema and return of ventilatory function may occur in a small percentage of patients.

Initial therapy is directed toward ensuring adequate gas exchange and providing supportive care. Serial quantitative assessment of pulmonary function should be performed to detect return of adequate ventilatory effort. Once respiratory effort returns, weaning can be attempted using intermittent mandatory ventilation [IMV], pressure support ventilation, or intermittent T-piece trials of spontaneous ventilation [47]. For patients without diaphragmatic function, phrenic nerve stimulation has occasionally been successful [27]. For other patients, chronic mechanical ventilatory support will be required, using positive pressure ventilation or devices such as a cuirass or a rocking bed. For long-term airway maintenance for patients requiring positive pressure ventilation, a tracheostomy is essential.

Additional supportive care requirements must also be addressed from the outset. Adequate nutrition must be provided either enterally through a feeding tube or parenterally to maintain positive nitrogen balance. Meticulous attention to infection control policies must be maintained to minimize the risk of infections, particularly for the patients with permanent indwelling urinary catheters.

Autonomic instability, manifest as hypotension, bradycardia, and hypothermia, occurs during the first two weeks after injury [68]. Care must be taken to prevent pulmonary edema when giving intravenous fluids to treat hypotension since fluctuation in sympathetic tone may cause wide variations in vascular resistance and cardiac filling pressures.

E. **Acute respiratory failure.** Respiratory failure after head trauma or a neurosurgical procedure is relatively rare, unless there is associated chest trauma, shock, or aspiration. After trauma or severe hemodynamic instability, however, noncardiogenic pulmonary edema or adult respiratory distress syndrome (ARDS) frequently occurs [15,23,45,55]. In the neurosurgical patient, ARDS may initially be indistinguishable from neurogenic pulmonary edema. ARDS is characterized by increased capillary permeability, pulmonary edema, and a low or normal pulmonary capillary wedge (PCW) pressure. Unlike acute cardiogenic pulmonary edema, the colloid osmotic pressure of the edema fluid is high, often at least 60% of the plasma colloid osmotic pressure [45]. The chest x-ray usually reveals patchy or confluent pulmonary infiltrates throughout the lung fields. Initial arterial blood gases indicate hyperventilation with hypocapnia and significant hypoxemia with an extremely wide alveolar-arterial oxygen gradient. Hypercapnia is seldom present until later in the course of the syndrome as the patient tires. Occasionally, hypercapnia will occur early when ARDS is associated with flail chest, head injury, hemopneumothorax, or high cervical spinal cord injury.

The clinical spectrum of ARDS needs not be present immediately after injury. It usually develops within 12 to 24 hours after the insult. Endotracheal intubation and ventilatory support with continuous positive airway pressure (CPAP) or PEEP, high inspired oxygen concentration (FIO_2), and a large tidal volume are usually essential. Steroids have not been demonstrated to be of benefit [45]. Recently, prostaglandins have been used to treat ARDS with promising preliminary results [67]. Pulmonary artery (PA) catheterization can provide valuable information, particularly as a guide to ventilatory management, appropriate level of PEEP, and fluid requirements. The PCW pressure should be maintained at a low normal level, usually about 5 to 8 mmHg. Vasoactive drugs may be needed to maintain the perfusion pressure. The use of inotropic agents must be carefully monitored, however, since they increase myocardial oxygen demand and may aggravate intrapulmonary shunting.

F. **Chronic obstructive lung disease.** The neurosurgical patient with underlying chronic obstructive lung disease presents significant challenges for intraoperative and postoperative management. Preoperative assessment of pulmonary status is often difficult. The patient's history, if available, may provide the only clues to the nature of the patient's pulmonary dysfunction. A history of chronic, productive cough, shortness of breath, wheezing, or use of bronchodilators will be helpful in planning postoperative care. The physical examination, chest x-ray, arterial blood gas, and electrocardiogram should be obtained and reviewed before proceeding with elective surgery. Serum electrolytes, particularly total CO_2, if elevated, may suggest CO_2 retention due to underlying lung disease. If present, preexisting hypercapnia may necessitate *early* institution of mechanical ventilatory support for the patient with increased ICP since the patient has no ability to increase the work of breathing to spontaneously hyperventilate.

Postoperatively, patients with underlying chronic lung disease require careful manipulation of respiratory parameters. Weaning is often prolonged in the patient with preoperative CO_2 retention. Supplemental oxygen is also often necessary to keep the PaO_2 in a safe range without depressing ventilatory drive due to excessive oxygen concentration. The use of PEEP to treat postoperative hypoxemia is also hazardous in the patient with bullous, emphysematous changes because of the risk for pneumothorax.

G. Pulmonary embolism. The neurosurgical patient is at risk for pulmonary emboli due to immobility, dehydration therapy to reduce ICP, and perhaps an associated hypercoagulable state. Pulmonary emboli usually originate from venous thrombosis in the lower extremities and complicate the course in about 20% of multiple trauma victims [13,74]. Less commonly, emboli arise from the pelvic or prostatic venous plexus or the right ventricle [74]. The pathophysiology of pulmonary embolism includes obstruction of pulmonary blood flow, acute pulmonary hypertension and right ventricular failure, reduction of cardiac output, and hypoxia. Hemorrhagic necrosis and infarction of lung tissue may also occur [16,26,61,74].

Massive pulmonary embolism causes immediate acute respiratory failure, shock, cyanosis, tachycardia, extreme anxiety, and, occasionally, anterior chest pain. Physical findings may include jugular venous distention with hepatojugular reflux, wheezing, a right ventricular S_3 gallop, and an accentuated P_2 sound, although a normal physical examination does not exclude pulmonary emboli. The electrocardiogram is nonspecifically abnormal in 85% of cases and occasionally will show changes of left or right bundle branch block or suggest acute cor pulmonale [74]. Sinus or ventricular rhythm disturbances are common. Positive radioactive isotope ventilation and perfusion lung scans are confirmatory [10]. If the results of the lung scan are equivocal, then the patient should undergo pulmonary angiography [10,34].

The diagnosis of smaller pulmonary emboli is more difficult, but should be suspected in any critically ill patient who has unexplained hypoxemia, tachypnea, chest pain, or new electrocardiographic changes [75]. Arterial blood gas analysis, isotopic lung scans, and pulmonary arteriograms usually confirm the diagnosis [10,34,61].

Treatment of pulmonary emboli in the neurosurgical patient is primarily supportive. Gas exchange should be optimized by providing positive pressure ventilation and appropriate supplemental oxygen [61,74]. Anticoagulation is relatively contraindicated after intracranial or spinal cord operation or injury. A vena caval filter may be required to prevent further emboli in the neurosurgical patient with documented venous thrombosis [29].

H. Fat embolism. Fat embolism syndrome, characterized by hypoxia, respiratory distress, neurologic changes, and coagulation abnormalities, occurs in victims of multiple trauma, particularly of long bones [14,30]. Pathologically, small vessels, particularly in the lungs and the brain, are occluded by lipid particles and fibrin clots. The respiratory abnormality is indistinguishable from ARDS and can occur as late as 48 to 72 hours after the initial trauma.

Neurologic signs include confusion, delirium, frank coma, focal or global deficit, or seizures. Petechiae occur in approximately 90% of cases. Lipid deposits may occasionally be seen in the retinal vessels. Disseminated intravascular coagulation (DIC), manifested by thrombocytopenia and elevated fibrin degradation products, as well as prolongation of prothrombin, partial thromboplastin, and thrombin times is a further complication. Treatment is supportive and depends mainly on correction of hypoxia and establishment of cardiovascular stability. The syndrome usually resolves in 4 to 5 days.

I. Cardiogenic pulmonary edema. Congestive heart failure and cardiogenic pulmonary edema can also occur in patients with CNS lesions. They occur most commonly in patients with reduced myocardial compliance (i.e., particularly elderly patients with coronary artery disease and neonates). They can also occur in patients managed with overzealous fluid resuscitation after major trauma, including high spinal cord injury. Another case of cardiogenic pulmonary edema is rapid administration of hyperosmolar fluids, such as mannitol for treatment of increased ICP.

Management of cardiogenic pulmonary edema includes inotropic support (dopamine, dobutamine, digoxin), diuretics (furosemide), and vasodilators (sodium nitroprusside, nitroglycerin, hydralazine). During treatment, careful attention must be paid to the patient's gas exchange, acid-base balance, and electrolytes, particularly potassium.

J. Pulmonary trauma

  1. Pulmonary contusion. Pulmonary contusion caused by blunt chest trauma is frequently associated with head injuries, especially after automobile accidents. Pulmonary contusion can also result from blast injury or any other nonpenetrating chest trauma. It is associated with rib fractures, pneumothorax, myocardial contusion, and aortic laceration. Pulmonary contusion can also occur alone without obvious external evidence of chest trauma, so careful evaluation of the pulmonary status is essential after any injury. The high mortality (up to 50%) from pulmonary contusion reported previously was due primarily to the unrecognized onset of respiratory failure, usually occurring within six hours after injury and often progressing to ARDS [39]. Early initiation of supportive respiratory care has significantly improved survival.

  Characteristics of pulmonary contusion include alveolar capillary damage with intra-alveolar and interstitial hemorrhage and edema. The initial insult is followed by a parenchymal inflammatory response. The chest x-ray usually demonstrates ill-defined infiltrates in the area of trauma to the chest wall. The patient may complain of chest wall pain and/or dyspnea. Hemoptysis may be present. Arterial blood gases usually indicate hypoxemia and a widened alveolar-arterial oxygen gradient. Hypocapnia usually occurs initially. As the work of breathing increases, the patient may develop hypercapnia.

The therapy for pulmonary contusion is supportive. It includes supplemental oxygen, analgesics, and close monitoring of respiratory function. Early endotracheal intubation and institution of CPAP or positive pressure ventilatory support should be considered if the patient's gas exchange deteriorates. Steroids have not been found to be useful [59]. Isolated pulmonary contusion commonly begins to improve radiographically in 48 to 72 hours, but 2 to 3 weeks may be required for complete resolution.

2. **Rib fractures and flail chest.** Rib fractures, common after blunt chest trauma, often go undiagnosed on chest x-ray films. Meticulous physical examination of the chest wall is required in each patient who has sustained blunt chest trauma. Complications of nondisplaced rib fractures include pneumothorax, laceration of intercostal arteries, and flail chest.

Flail chest of the anterior type occurs when the ribs become separated at their costochondral junction, with or without an associated fracture of the sternum. The characteristic paradoxical chest movement may not be evident initially because of tissue edema or hematoma formation. CPAP or mechanical ventilatory support using intermittent mandatory ventilation or pressure support ventilation and PEEP is necessary for those patients who cannot sustain adequate pulmonary function due to the mechanical problems imposed by the paradoxically moving chest wall [59].

3. **Pneumothorax.** Pneumothorax is most often caused by laceration of the lung by a fractured rib. It can also result from the disruption of alveoli when the limits of intra-alveolar pressure are exceeded during chest wall impact or from rupture of the esophagus or tracheobronchial tree. After simple pneumothorax, the initial air leak will usually seal and be self-limiting. If the defect is large and does not seal spontaneously, tension pneumothorax will develop. Immediate decompression of the tension pneumothorax must be accomplished to minimize the cardiovascular and respiratory effects due to the high intrapleural pressure or a cardiac arrest will occur.

If the pneumothorax is caused by a penetrating chest injury that has caused a large open wound (sucking chest wound), the defect should be covered immediately to seal the air leak. A chest tube is inserted in an area distant from the chest wall defect. After hemodynamic stabilization and adequate oxygenation have been ensured, surgical exploration and revision of the chest wound can be performed.

4. **Hemothorax.** Hemothorax can also occur after any blunt chest trauma. Respiratory embarrassment may result from the accumulation of sufficient blood to impair lung inflation. Immediate placement of a chest tube in a dependent position should provide adequate drainage. If the hemorrhage is persistent after chest tube placement, prompt surgical exploration is required. Coagulation studies should be obtained to rule out a hemostatic defect, particularly DIC. Because of the risk of laceration of intercostal arteries, any involuntary movements, such as seizures, must be prevented in neurosurgical patients who have rib fractures.

5. **Ruptured tracheobronchial tree.** Tears within the tracheobronchial tree cause pneumothorax and are often promptly fatal. Placement of a chest tube with suction will not correct the situation because of the large, continuing air leak. Massive mediastinal and subcutaneous emphysema, dyspnea, cyanosis, and hemoptysis develop.

   With a tracheobronchial tear, auscultation of the anterior chest reveals a mediastinal crunching sound synchronous with the cardiac rhythm (Hamman's sign). In rare instances, there may be no communication with the pleura and no pneumothorax. For the patients for whom the airway is secured and the tear controlled, the lesion usually heals within one to three weeks. Granulation tissue may develop during healing and cause airway obstruction. The granulation tissue may require laser excision.

   When a tracheobronchial rupture is suspected, the assistance of an otolaryngologist or thoracic surgeon should be obtained during the attempt to secure the airway since surgical evaluation and intervention are often necessary. Fiberoptic bronchoscopy is also often necessary as part of the evaluation and to facilitate intubation.

6. **Diaphragmatic rupture.** Automobile accidents are responsible for more than 80% of traumatic diaphragmatic ruptures. The left diaphragm is involved in about 95% of cases. Rupture is secondary to the abrupt elevation of intra-abdominal pressure at the time of impact, which causes herniation of stomach, bowel, spleen, or omentum into the chest. Associated rupture of an intestinal viscus is not uncommon. A clinical picture of respiratory distress and shock develops quickly. If the stomach herniates into the chest, the chest x-ray will reveal the stomach gas bubble above the diaphragm. Strangulation of the herniated abdominal contents may occur, particularly if the rupture is initially not suspected. Management of the airway is critical in these patients, since regurgitation and aspiration from the fluid-filled stomach may occur during induction of anesthesia [1,6,77]. Therefore, for any patient suspected of diaphragmatic rupture, care should be taken to protect the patient from aspiration during intubation, including the possibility of performing an awake intubation.

III. Respiratory care. Respiratory care for the neurosurgical patient must be directed toward ensuring an airway, maintaining a safe level of oxygenation, ensuring adequate ventilation, and minimizing the effects of ventilatory support on cerebral homeostasis.

   A. Oxygen administration. All patients with neurologic dysfunction should receive supplemental oxygen until a safe oxygen saturation or PaO_2 is confirmed. Because of changes in level of consciousness and patterns of ventilation, a marginal level of oxygenation should not be tolerated in the neurosurgical or head trauma patient. A PaO_2 of 60 mmHg, while adequate for an otherwise normal healthy patient, should not be accepted for the brain-injured patient. Higher levels of oxygen are probably required for these patients to maintain adequate cerebral oxygenation [4,66]. Although high inspired oxygen concentrations can damage the pulmonary parenchyma, the risk of hypoxemia outweighs any deleterious effects of oxygen when the patient is unstable.

   A variety of oxygen delivery systems are available to provide supplemental oxygen to the spontaneously breathing patient who is able to protect the airway [49].

   1. Nasal prongs. Nasal prongs can deliver inspired oxygen concentrations of 24 to 44%. They are comfortable, inexpensive, and need not be removed during eating. A low flow of oxygen is ensured if the patient's nares are patent. Accurate concentrations of oxygen cannot be guaranteed, since the FiO_2 changes significantly with fluctuations of the patient's ventilatory pattern. Patients who have rapid inspiratory flow rates receive a lower FiO_2 than patients who have slow inspiratory flow rates. When using nasal prongs, the oxygen flow rate should not exceed 6 L/min. No increase in FiO_2 occurs at higher flows. The higher flows are also poorly tolerated because of irritation to the nares.

   2. Open-mask oxygen. Open-mask oxygen delivery systems can provide relatively high oxygen concentrations (FiO_2 0.50–0.60). Because the system uses wider bore tubing, higher levels of water vapor can be delivered. To be efficient, however, the masks must be tight fitting and use high gas flows that can be uncomfortable for the patient.

   3. Mask with reservoir bag. A tight-fitting mask with a reservoir bag can be used to deliver the highest concentrations of oxygen to the nonintubated patient requiring supplemental oxygen. These masks, when properly applied, can deliver oxygen concentrations as high as about 70%. The mask utilizes one-way values to permit exhalation, maintain FiO_2, and prevent rebreathing. If the values are not appropriately applied, the reservoir bag can become a cause for rebreathing. For the patient with neurologic dysfunction, rebreathing of CO_2 is inappropriate, so care must be taken when using these masks. Because the system utilizes narrow bore tubing, humdification of inspired gas is minimal. If the patient has thick, tenacious secretions, inadequate humidification can interfere with clearance of secretions.

4. **Venturi mask.** The Venturi mask is a high-flow delivery system that ensures an accurate and constant concentration of oxygen. These systems provide oxygen concentrations of 24 to 40%. The delivered oxygen concentration is independent of the patient's minute ventilation or inspiratory flow unless the inspiratory flow exceeds the total flow capability of the device. Because of the high flow provided by the Venturi mask systems, care must be taken to ensure adequate humidification.

5. **Mask CPAP.** CPAP can be administered by mask to the patient requiring supplemental oxygen and positive airway pressure. Although this form of treatment is effective in improving oxygenation and preventing alveolar collapse, its use in neurosurgical patients should be *very* limited. Because the goal of the therapy is to increase mean airway pressure, it may adversely affect intracranial compliance. It is also associated with gastric distention, which increases the risk of regurgitation and aspiration of gastric contents.

6. **Delivery of high oxygen concentrations.** When a high inspired oxygen concentration is required, the safest way to ensure oxygen delivery is to secure the patient's airway with an endotracheal tube.

B. **Airway maintenance.** Any neurosurgical patient who is unable to protect the airway or for whom mechanical ventilatory support is required should have the trachea intubated. The indications for intubation are listed in Table 5-3.

1. **Orotracheal intubation.** Orotracheal intubation is the preferred method for securing the airway in the emergency situation. Intubation can generally be accomplished with minimal trauma. To

Table 5-3. Indications for endotracheal intubation

Airway protection
Bronchopulmonary hygiene
Ensured delivery of high oxygen concentration
Mechanical ventilatory support
  $PaCO_2 > 45$ mmHg
  pH < 7.2
  Respiratory rate > 40 breaths/min
  Tidal volume < 3.5 ml/kg
  Dead space/tidal volume rate $(V_D/V_T) > 0.5$
  Vital capacity < 10 ml/kg
Therapeutic hyperventilation

$PaCO_2$ = arterial carbon dioxide tension.

prevent exacerbation of intracranial hypertension, sedation and muscle relaxation should be administered to facilitate intubation. Although a short-acting depolarizing muscle relaxant (succinylcholine 1.5 mg/kg) is most commonly used after pretreatment with a nondepolarizing relaxant, the depolarizing drug should be avoided for patients with ongoing neurologic dysfunction (e.g., Guillain-Barré syndrome, stroke-in-evolution).

Caution must be used when administering sedatives to patients who are hemodynamically unstable. Since patients with increased ICP are often intravascularly volume depleted (secondary to mannitol and diuretic therapy), hypotension and decreased cerebral perfusion pressure can occur after even small doses of sedatives are administered.

Many neurosurgical patients require emergency intubation for airway protection or to institute mechanical ventilation. These patients should be carefully managed with precautions to minimize the risk of regurgitation and aspiration of gastric contents [69].

2. Nasotracheal intubation. Nasotracheal intubation can often be accomplished blindly without the need to instrument the airway or administer sedatives or muscle relaxants. Local anesthesia with a vasoconstricting agent (cocaine or lidocaine with phenylephrine) applied to the nares, nasopharynx, and oropharynx minimize trauma and facilitate passage of the tube in the spontaneously breathing patient. If the intubation is anticipated to be difficult due to anatomic abnormalities, the fiberoptic bronchoscope can be used to guide the intubation.

Nasotracheal intubation has the advantages of improved tolerance and stabilization of the endotracheal tube. Disadvantages of nasotracheal intubation include (1) pressure necrosis of the external nares, (2) obstruction of sinus drainage [40], (3) otitis, and (4) difficult suctioning due to the curvature and generally smaller diameter of the tube. One *absolute* contraindication to nasotracheal intubation is facial or basilar skull fracture with possible disruption of the cribriform plate [69].

3. Tracheostomy. Tracheostomy is required when endotracheal intubation cannot be accomplished due to facial trauma or anatomic considerations [31]. For long-term airway management, however, endotracheal intubation is usually well tolerated. The indications for tracheostomy include (1) multiple facial fractures, (2) long-term airway management for the patient in persistent vegetative state or after high spinal cord injury, and (3) patient comfort and pulmonary hygiene when prolonged ventilatory support is required. Tracheostomy also reduces dead space and so may facilitate weaning of the patient with minimal pulmonary reserve.

Tracheostomy is associated with significant complications [31], including (1) damage to tracheal mucosa with increased risk of subsequent infection, (2) tracheomalacia, (3) tracheal ulceration or stenosis, (4) granuloma formation [38], (5) hemorrhage, and (6) tracheostomy tube displacement with resultant pneumomediastinum or respiratory arrest.

C. Mechanical ventilatory support. Mechanical ventilation will often be required to ensure and control gas exchange for the neurosurgical patient with depressed ventilatory drive, pulmonary disease associated with or secondary to the neurologic deficit, or altered intracranial compliance. To optimize gas exchange with minimal effect on neurologic function requires careful control of mechanical ventilatory parameters. In general, the ventilatory parameters that must be defined include (1) FIO_2, (2) respiratory rate, (3) tidal volume, (4) mode of ventilation, (5) inspiratory flow and waveform, (6) inspiratory pressure limit, and (7) PEEP or CPAP.

When caring for the neurosurgical patient who is being mechanically ventilated, careful manipulation of the ventilatory parameters is essential to prevent rapid increases in airway pressure that might decrease cerebral perfusion pressure and acute changes in minute ventilation that would affect $PaCO_2$ and pH. Oxygenation must also be assured; FIO_2 changes must be made cautiously. The response to ventilatory changes should be closely monitored. Vital signs, including ICP, should be followed as adjustments are made to ventilation. Pulse oximetry can provide immediate data regarding the effects of suctioning, changes in FIO_2, or weaning on oxygenation [50]. Capnography is a useful guide to adequacy of ventilation during weaning and as a monitor of airway obstruction, bronchospasm, ventilator disconnection, and air emboli [70]. Arterial blood gases should be evaluted within 20 to 30 minutes of a ventilator change, particularly when noninvasive monitors of gas exchange are not available.

1. Modes of ventilation. A variety of modes of ventilation are now available, some of which may be useful for the patient with neurologic dysfunction and some of which are at least relatively contraindicated.

   a. Controlled ventilation. The controlled ventilatory mode provides all ventilation from the ventilator. The machine does not respond to patient needs. This mode of ventilation has few, if any, indications. It is only of use for patients with *no* ventilatory drive, including patients who are brain dead, being supported for organ procurement.

   b. Assist-control ventilation. Assist-control ventilation provides controlled mechanical breaths at a rate and tidal volume set on the ventilator. The ventilator is sensitive to patient-generated breaths, providing the same tidal volume to the patient as the controlled breaths when the patient creates a sufficient negative inspiratory pressure to trigger the ventilator. Inappropriate setting of the trigger sensitivity may predispose to hypo- or hyperventilation. Since patients with neurologic disorders often hyperventilate as a result of brain dysfunction, setting the appropriate trigger-sensitivity can be difficult. Nonetheless, some patients with CNS disorders are most appropriately ventilated with this mode of ventilation.

c. **Intermittent mandatory ventilation.** IMV is appropriate for patients who have some spontaneous ventilatory activity. With IMV, the patient receives a preset number of breaths at a preset tidal volume, but is allowed to breathe spontaneously between mandatory breaths at a rate and tidal volume that are voluntarily generated.

Although IMV was originally introduced as a method of weaning patients from the ventilator, it has become a widely accepted mode of primary ventilatory support and may have advantages over assisted or controlled modes [18]. The advantages of IMV may be (1) fewer hemodynamic complications, (2) maintenance of spontaneous respiratory activity, and (3) better patient acceptance.

d. **Pressure support ventilation.** Pressure support ventilation (PSV) is a relatively new mode of ventilation for which the positive pressure breaths are spontaneously triggered [46]. With initiation of the ventilator breath, inspiration begins and continues until a preset airway pressure is achieved. Inspiration is terminated once that pressure is reached. This form of ventilation requires that the patient have spontaneous ventilatory drive. Tidal volume delivered by the ventilator is variable, depending on patient characteristics. Large tidal volume breaths cannot be assured with PSV. PSV has been demonstrated to improve patient comfort and reduce the work of breathing. Mean airway pressure is slightly higher with PSV than IMV. This increased airway pressure may be a disadvantage for the patient with poor intracranial compliance [46]. Because PSV is an assist mode of ventilation, it is not recommended for patients with altered respiratory drive, impaired lung mechanical function, or poor gas exchange.

e. **Inverse ratio ventilation.** Inverse ratio ventilation (IRV) is a mode of pressure-control ventilation in which the inspiratory to expiratory ratio exceeds 1 : 1. It is designed to improve distribution of ventilation while decreasing peak inspiratory pressure and potentially reducing the hemodynamic consequences of positive pressure ventilation [12,41,58]. Although this mode of ventilation cannot be advocated for use for patients with altered intracranial compliance as yet, further study is warranted to determine if the lower airway pressures give it any advantages over conventional modes of ventilation [41].

  f. High-frequency ventilation. A variety of modes of high-frequency ventilation (HFV) have been utilized to ventilate patients with low tidal volumes at high frequencies (60–3000 cycles/min) [19,57]. The theoretical advantage of these modes of ventilation (high-frequency jet ventilation, high-frequency positive pressure ventilation, and high-frequency oscillation) is that airway pressures are lower, resulting in less compromise of the circulation and a lower risk of barotrauma. Recent studies have documented the lack of deleterious cerebrovascular effects of HFV techniques. For both animals and humans, ICP has been noted to be lower with HFV than conventional positive pressure ventilation [2,54].

2. Positive airway pressure. Use of either PEEP [63] with controlled ventilation or CPAP [28] with spontaneous ventilation increases functional residual capacity, improves the ventilation-perfusion relationship, and may reverse hypoxemia in patients who have abnormal intrapulmonary shunting. Application of PEEP may decrease the need to administer high, potentially toxic concentrations of oxygen.

  The use of increased airway pressure to improve oxygenation can have deleterious effects on ICP. When adding expiratory pressure, increments of no more than 3 to 5 cm H_2O should be used. The hemodynamic response, ICP, and neurologic status must be carefully monitored. The aim is to achieve a PaO_2 of about 100 mmHg without exacerbation of neurologic dysfunction. During application of either PEEP or CPAP, patients should be nursed in a 30-degree head-up position with the head in the neutral position [25]. If ICP increases with PEEP, methods to improve intracranial compliance should be instituted, including cerebrospinal fluid (CSF) drainage through an intraventricular catheter and administration of mannitol, steroids, or barbiturates.

3. Weaning. Weaning from mechanical ventilation can be attempted when the patient is stable and the reason for which the patient required ventilation is resolved. In general, weaning should begin when the patient is (1) hemodynamically stable, (2) free of significant pulmonary disease, (3) has normal acid-base and metabolic balance, and (4) is neurologically stable with well-controlled ICP. The patient should not require $FiO_2 > 0.5$ and should have a vital capacity of 15 ml/kg. Resting minute ventilation should not exceed 10 L/min. Under these circumstances the patient will generally have adequate gas exchange and ventilatory reserve and should have a sufficient ability to cough and handle pulmonary secretions [22,56].

The alert patient should be able, on command, to produce a maximal minute ventilation of at least twice the resting minute ventilation and a maximal inspiratory force of at least -20 to -30 cm H_2O. The average tidal volume should be about 5 ml/kg, and the spontaneous respiratory rate should not be greater than 30 breaths per minute. The alveolar-arterial oxygen tension gradient must be less than 300 to 350 mmHg on 100% oxygen, and the dead space/tidal volume ratio $[V_D/V_T]$ should be less than 0.5.

The patient can be weaned from mechanical ventilation using a variety of techniques. Intermittent T-piece trials, IMV [18], and PSV [46] have all been used successfully. When the patient is breathing spontaneously without ventilatory support, CPAP can be continued, as needed, to ensure adequate oxygenation. The CPAP can then be tapered as tolerated.

Extubation of the patient with neurologic dysfunction should be attempted after the patient has been successfully weaned from mechanical ventilation, has a satisfactory gag and cough, and is able to protect the airway. If the patient is not able to maintain adequate pulmonary hygiene or protect the airway, a tracheostomy will be required for long-term airway management.

4. **Monitoring.** The neurosurgical patient with superimposed respiratory failure requires careful monitoring of neurologic function, cardiac function, and adequacy of ventilation and overall respiratory status. Routine neurologic assessment should be ongoing. The Glasgow coma scale (Table 5-4) should be recorded hourly as a sequen-

Table 5-4. Glasgow coma scale

Best verbal response	
None	1
Incomprehensible sound	2
Inappropriate words	3
Confused	4
Oriented	5
Eyes open	
None	1
To pain	2
To speech	3
Spontaneously	4
Best motor response	
None	1
Abnormal extensor	2
Abnormal flexion	3
Withdraws	4
Localizes	5
Obeys	6

tial indication of neurologic improvement or deterioration. ICP monitoring is often required to ensure appropriate control of cerebral perfusion during manipulations of ventilatory parameters. Although ICP can be monitored using a subdural catheter or bolt, an intraventricular cannula is required if CSF needs to be drained to control ICP in the patient requiring high levels of PEEP to maintain adequate oxygenation.

Additional monitoring of the patient's cardiovascular and respiratory status is also required. Routine monitors include a continuous electrocardiogram, routine vital signs (respiratory rate, heart rate, blood pressure, and temperature), and fluid balance (intake and output). Most patients with respiratory failure requiring mechanical ventilatory support will benefit from placement of an intra-arterial catheter to allow direct monitoring of blood pressure and access for arterial blood gas determinations. In addition, a pulse oximeter should be used to noninvasively monitor oxygen saturation [50]. A capnograph is a useful monitor of ventilation, particularly when hyperventilating the patient to reduce ICP, during surgery to diagnose air embolism, and during weaning [70]. For spontaneously breathing patients with periodic breathing patterns, an apnea monitor is useful.

When the neurosurgical patient becomes hemodynamically unstable or is requiring frequent mannitol or diuretic therapy to control the ICP, central venous pressure monitoring is useful to assess the patient's intravascular volume. If the patient has coexisting cardiac disease or if assessment of myocardial function is required, a pulmonary artery catheter should be placed to monitor cardiac output, pulmonary capillary wedge pressure, arterial-mixed venous oxygen content difference ($avDO_2$), and vascular resistance.

References

1. Arms, R. A., Dines, D. E., and Tinstman, T. C. Aspiration pneumonia. *Chest* 65:136, 1974.
2. Barrington, K. J., Ryan, C. A., Peliowski, A., et al. The effects of negative pressure external high frequency oscillation on cerebral blood flow and cardiac output of the monkey. *Pediatr. Res.* 21:166, 1987.
3. Bartlett, J. G., Gorbach, S. L., and Finegold, S. M. The bacteriology of aspiration pneumonia. *Am. J. Med.* 56:202, 1974.
4. Borstrom, L., Johannsson, H., and Siesjo, B. K. The relationship between arterial PO_2 and cerebral blood flow in hypoxic hypoxia. *Acta Physiol. Scand.* 93:423, 1975.
5. Bryan-Brown, C. W. Oxygen Transport and the Oxyhemoglobin Dissociation Curve. In J. L. Berk and J. E. Sampliner (Eds.), *Handbook of Critical Care* (2nd ed.). Boston: Little, Brown, 1982. Pp. 557–578.
6. Bynum, L. J., and Pierce, A. K. Pulmonary aspiration of gastric contents. *Am. Rev. Respir. Dis.* 114:1129, 1976.
7. Cameron, J. L., Mitchell, W. H., and Zuidema, G. D. Aspiration pneumonia: Clinical outcome following documented aspiration. *Arch. Surg.* 106:49, 1973.

8. Casey, W. F. Neurogenic pulmonary oedema. *Anaesthesia* 38:985, 1983.
9. Chapman, R. L., Jr., Downs, J. B., Modell, J. H., et al. The ineffectiveness of steroid therapy in treating aspiration of hydrochloric acid. *Arch. Surg.* 108:858, 1974.
10. Cheely, R., McCartney, W. H., Perry, J. R., et al. The role of noninvasive tests versus pulmonary angiography in the diagnosis of pulmonary embolism. *Am. J. Med.* 70:17, 1981.
11. Cheshire, D. J. E. Respiratory management in acute traumatic tetraplegia. *Paraplegia* 1:252, 1964.
12. Coles, A. G. H., Weller, W. F., and Sykes, M. K. Inverse ratio ventilation compared with PEEP in adult respiratory failure. *Intensive Care Med.* 10:227, 1984.
13. Coon, W. W. Venous thromboembolism: Prevalence, risk factors, prevention. *Clin. Chest Med.* 5:391, 1984.
14. Curtis, A. McB., Knowles, G. D., Putman, C. E., et al. The three syndromes of fat embolism: Pulmonary manifestations. *Yale J. Biol. Med.* 52:149, 1979.
15. DeOliveira, G. G., and DeOliveira-Antonio, M. P. Role of the central nervous system in the adult respiratory distress syndrome. *Crit. Care Med.* 15:844, 1987.
16. Dismuke, S. E., and Wagner, E. H. Pulmonary embolism as a cause of death. *J.A.M.A.* 255:2039, 1986.
17. Downs, J. B., Chapman, R. L., Jr., Modell, J. H., et al. An evaluation of steroid therapy in aspiration pneumonitis. *Anesthesiology* 40:129, 1974.
18. Downs, J. B., Perkins, H. M., and Modell, J. H. Intermittent mandatory ventilation: An evaluation. *Arch. Surg.* 109:519, 1974.
19. Drazen, J. M., Kamm, R. D., and Slutsky, A. S. High-frequency ventilation. *Physiol. Rev.* 64:505, 1984.
20. Ducker, T. B. Increased intracranial pressure and pulmonary edema. I. Clinical study in eleven patients. *J. Neurosurg.* 28:112, 1968.
21. Dudley, W. R., and Marshall, B. E. Steroid treatment for acid aspiration pneumonitis. *Anesthesiology* 40:136, 1974.
22. Feeley, T. W., and Hedley-Whyte, J. Weaning from conventional ventilation and supplemental oxygen. *N. Engl. J. Med.* 292:903, 1975.
23. Fowler, A. A., Hamman, R. F., Good, J. T., et al. Adult respiratory distress syndrome: Risk with common predisposition. *Ann. Intern. Med.* 98:593, 1983.
24. Frost, E. The physiopathology of respiration in neurosurgical patients. *J. Neurosurg.* 50:699, 1979.
25. Frost, E. A. M. Effects of positive end-expiratory pressure on intracranial pressure and compliance in brain-injured patients. *J. Neurosurg.* 47:195, 1977.
26. Fulkerson, W. J., Coleman, E., Ravin, C. E., and Saltzman, H. A. Diagnosis of pulmonary embolism. *Arch. Intern. Med.* 146:961, 1986.
27. Glenn, W. W. L., Hogan, J. F., Loke, J. S. O., et al. Ventilatory support by pacing of the conditioned diaphragm in quadraplegia. *N. Engl. J. Med.* 310:1150, 1984.
28. Greenbaum, D. M., Millen, J. E., Eross, B., et al. Continuous positive airway pressure without tracheal intubation in spontaneously breathing patients. *Chest* 69:615, 1976.
29. Greenfield, L. J. Use and abuse of intracaval devices. *Surgery* 99:383, 1986.
30. Guenter, C. A., and Braun, T. E. Fat embolism syndrome: Changing prognosis. *Chest* 79:143, 1981.
31. Hardy, K. L. Tracheostomy: Indications, technics, and tubes. *Am. J. Surg.* 126:299, 1973.
32. Harken, A. H. The surgical significance of the oxyhaemoglobin dissociation curve. *Surg. Gynecol. Obstet.* 144:935, 1977.
33. Hechtman, H. B., Grindlinger, G. A., Vegas, A. M., et al. Importance of oxygen transport in clinical medicine. *Crit. Care Med.* 7:419, 1979.
34. Hull, R. D., Hirsh, J., Carter, C. J., et al. Pulmonary angiography, ventilation lung scanning, and venography for clinically suspected pulmonary embolism with abnormal perfusion lung scan. *Ann. Intern. Med.* 98:891, 1983.

35. James, C. F., Modell, J. H., Gibbs, C. P., et al. Pulmonary aspiration: Effects of volume and pH in the rat. *Anesth. Analg.* 63:665, 1984.
36. Kaehny, W. D. Pathogensis and Management of Respiratory and Mixed Acid-Base Disorders. In R. W. Schrier (Ed.), *Renal and Electrolyte Disorders* (2nd ed.). Boston: Little, Brown, 1982. Pp. 159–181.
37. Kaehny, W. D., and Gabow, P. A. Pathogenesis and Management of Metabolic Acidosis and Alkalosis. In R. W. Schrier (Ed.), *Renal and Electrolyte Disorders* (2nd ed.). Boston: Little, Brown, 1982. Pp. 115–157.
38. Kirchner, J. A., and Sasaki, C. T. Fusion of the vocal cords following intubation and tracheostomy. *Trans. Acad. Ophthalmol. Otolaryngol.* 77:88, 1973.
39. Kirsh, M. M., and Sloan, H. *Blunt Chest Trauma.* Boston: Little, Brown, 1977.
40. Kronbert, F. G., and Goodwin, W. J., Jr. Sinusitis in intensive care unit patients. *Laryngoscope* 95:936, 1983.
41. Lachmann, B., Jonson, B., Lindroth, M., and Robertson, B. Modes of artificial ventilation in severe respiratory distress syndrome: Lung function and morphology in rabbits after wash-out of alveolar surfactant. *Crit. Care Med.* 10:724, 1982.
42. Lichtman, M. A., Miller, D. R., Cohen, J., and Waterhouse, C. Reduced red cells glycolysis, 2,3-diphosphoglycerate and adenosine triphosphate concentration and increased haemoglobin-oxygen affinity caused by hypophosphataemia. *Ann. Intern. Med.* 74:562, 1971.
43. Lorber, B., and Swenson, R. M. Bacteriology of aspiration pneumonia. A prospective study of community- and hospital-acquired cases. *Ann. Intern. Med.* 81:329, 1974.
44. Loughnan, P. M., Brown, T. C. K., Edis, B., and Klug, G. L. Neurogenic pulmonary oedema in man: Aetiology and management with vasodilators based upon haemodynamic studies. *Anaesth. Intensive Care* 8:65, 1980.
45. Loyd, J. E., Newman, J. H., and Brigham, K. L. Permeability pulmonary edema: Diagnosis and management. *Arch. Int. Med.* 144:143, 1984.
46. MacIntyre, N. R. Respiratory function during pressure support ventilation. *Chest* 89:677, 1986.
47. McMichan, J. C., Michel, L., and Westbrook, P. R. Pulmonary dysfunction following traumatic quadriplegia. *J.A.M.A.* 243:528, 1980.
48. Mendelson, C. L. The aspiration of stomach contents into the lungs during obstetric anesthesia. *Am. J. Obstet. Gynecol.* 52:191, 1946.
49. Menn, S. J., and Tisi, G. M. Oxygen as a drug: Chemical Properties, Benefits, and Hazards of Administration. In G. G. Burton, G. N. Gee, J. N. Hodgkin (Eds.), *Respiratory Care: A Guide to Clinical Practice.* Philadelphia: Lippincott, 1977. Pp. 386–399.
50. Mihm, F. G., and Halperin, B. D. Noninvasive detection of profound arterial desaturation using a pulse oximetry device. *Anesthesiology* 62:85, 1985.
51. Miller, L. D., Oski, F. A., Diaco, J. F., et al. The affinity of haemoglobin for oxygen: Its control and in vivo significance. *Surgery* 68:187, 1970.
52. Mushin, W. W., Rendell-Baker, L., Thompson, P. W., and Mapleson, W. W. *Automatic Ventilation of the Lungs* (3rd ed.). Oxford: Blackwell Scientific Publications, 1980. Pp. 62–131.
53. Narins, R., and Emmet, M. Simple and mixed acid-base disorders: A practical approach. *Medicine* 59:161, 1980.
54. O'Donnell, J. M., Thompson, D. R., and Layton, T. R. The effect of high-frequency jet ventilation on intracranial pressure in patients with closed head injuries. *J. Trauma* 24:73, 1984.
55. Pepe, P. E., Potkin, R. T., Reus, D. H., et al. Clinical predictors of the adult respiratory distress syndrome. *Am. J. Surg.* 144:124, 1982.
56. Pontoppidan, H., Wilson, R. S., Rie, M. A., and Schneider, R. C. Respiratory intensive care. *Anesthesiology* 47:96, 1977.

57. Raju, T. N. K., Braverman, B., Nadkarny, U., et al. Intracranial pressure and cardiac output remain stable during high frequency oscillation. *Crit. Care Med.* 11:856, 1983.
58. Ravizza, A. G., Carugo, D., Cerchiari, E. L., et al. Inversed ratio and conventional ventilations: Comparisons of the respiratory effects. *Anesthesiology* 59:A523, 1983.
59. Richardson, J. D., Adams, L., and Flint, F. M. Selective management of flail chest and pulmonary contusion. *Ann. Surg.* 196:481, 1982.
60. Rose, J., Valtonen, S., and Jennet, B. Avoidable factors contributing to death after head injury. *Br. Med. J.* 2:615, 1977.
61. Sasahara, A. A., Sharma, V. R. K., Barsamian, E. M., et al. Pulmonary thromboembolism: Diagnosis and treatment. *J.A.M.A.* 249:2945, 1983.
62. Schwartz, D. J., Wynne, J. W., Gibbs, C. P., et al. The pulmonary consequences of aspiration of gastric contents at pH values greater than 2.5. *Am. Rev. Respir. Dis.* 121:119, 1980.
63. Shapiro, B. A., Cane, R. D., and Harrison, R. A. Positive end-expiratory pressure therapy in adults with special reference to acute lung injury: A review of the literature and suggested clinical correlation. *Crit. Care Med.* 12:127, 1984.
64. Shappell, S. D., and Lenfant, C. J. M. Physiological Role of the Oxyhaemoglobin Curve. In D. McN. Surgenor (Ed.), *The Red Blood Cell* (2nd ed.). New York: Academic Press, 1975. Pp. 842–871.
65. Sheldon, G. F. Hyperphosphataemia, hypophosphataemia and the oxygen dissociation curve. *J. Surg. Res.* 14:367, 1972.
66. Shinozuka, T., and Nemoto, E. M. Dynamics of cerebrovascular responses to oxygen. *Anesthesiology* 55:235, 1981.
67. Shoemaker, W. C., and Appel, P. C. Effects of prostaglandin F_1 in adult respiratory distress syndrome. *Surgery* 99:275, 1986.
68. Silver, J. R., and Gibbon, N. O. K. Prognosis in tetraplegia. *Br. Med. J.* 4:79, 1968.
69. Stauffer, J. L., Olson, D. E., and Petty, T. L. Complications and consequences of endotracheal intubation and tracheostomy. *Am. J. Med* 70:65, 1981.
70. Swedlow, D. B. Capnometry and capnography: The anesthesia disaster early warning system. *Semin. Anesthesia* V:194, 1986.
71. Theodore, J., and Robin, E. D. Speculations on neurogenic pulmonary edema. *Am. Rev. Respir. Dis.* 113:405, 1976.
72. Thomas, H. M., Lefrak, S. S., Irwin, R. S., et al. The oxyhaemoglobin dissociation curve in health and disease. *Am. J. Med.* 57:331, 1974.
73. Wauchob, T. D., Brooks, R. J., and Harrison, K. M. Neurogenic pulmonary oedema. *Anaesthesia* 39:529, 1984.
74. West, J. W. Pulmonary embolism. *Med. Clin. North Am.* 70:877, 1986.
75. Williams, J. W., Eikman, E. A., and Greenberg, S. Asymptomatic pulmonary embolism: A common event in high risk patients. *Ann. Surg.* 195:323, 1982.
76. Wolfe, J. E., Bone, R. C., and Ruth, W. E. Effects of corticosteroids in the treatment of patients with gastric aspiration. *Am. J. Med.* 63:719, 1977.
77. Wynne, J. W., and Modell, J. H. Respiratory aspiration of stomach contents. *Ann. Intern. Med.* 87:466, 1977.

6

Cardiovascular Therapy

MARK F. NEWMAN

J. G. REVES

ROBERT D. McKAY

I. **Basic considerations.** Tissues of the central nervous system (CNS), like tissues of other organ systems, depend on an adequate supply of oxygen to meet their metabolic requirements. The cardiovascular system (CVS) supplies the CNS with oxygen and other substrates for metabolism. Preservation of cardiovascular function is essential for normal CNS function. Some fundamental considerations regarding the relationship of the CVS and CNS influence the ability of vasoactive drugs to affect the cerebral circulation.

   A. **Autoregulation.** Normal cerebral blood flow (CBF) in conscious adults is approximately 45 to 50 ml/100 gm brain tissue/min. CBF is maintained at this level over a wide range of mean arterial pressure (MAP) by autoregulation (Fig. 6-1). The cerebral perfusion pressure (CPP), MAP minus intracranial pressure (ICP), may be reduced without decreasing CBF until a perfusion pressure of 50 mmHg is reached. At this point, the cerebral vasculature can no longer compensate by dilatation, and further reductions in MAP lead to decreases in CBF with the potential for ischemia. Increases in MAP beyond the upper limit of 150 mmHg lead to increases in CBF with the possibility of edema formation. The entire autoregulation curve is shifted to the right with chronic hypertension [38]. As a result of this shift, the brain is better protected at high MAP but is made more vulnerable to ischemia at low MAP. Autoregulation may become impaired in a variety of intracranial disorders. In the absence of autoregulation, CBF varies linearly with CPP: the higher the CPP, the higher the CBF. The importance of distinguishing between CPP and MAP will be even more apparent when conditions that increase the ICP are encountered.

   B. **Interrelationships among CNS fluid compartments.** There are three fluid compartments in the CNS: brain tissue water, cerebrospinal fluid (CSF), and cerebral blood volume (CBV). These three compartments are contained within the semiclosed, rigid confines of the skull. The Munro-Kellie doctrine describes the relationship between these three compartments: a volume increase in one of the intracranial fluid compartments must be matched by a volume decrease in one or both of the other compartments or ICP will increase. This doctrine is graphically shown in Figure 6-2. Of the three fluid compartments, CBV is most likely to be altered by vasoactive drugs.

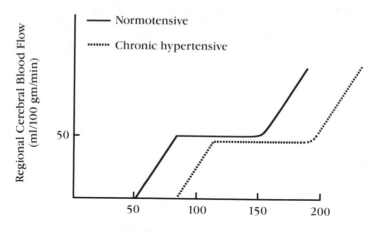

Fig. 6-1. Cerebral autoregulation in both normotensive and chronic hypertensive patients whose actual limits of MAP depend on the degree of hypertension. Autoregulation occurs normally from a MAP of about 50 to 150 mmHg and keeps cerebral blood flow relatively constant at about 50 ml/100 gm/min over this range.

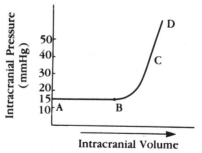

Fig. 6-2. The relationship between changes in intracranial volume and intracranial pressure. The line between A and B on the curve shows that the increase in volume of one of the three intracranial compartments (blood, brain, cerebrospinal fluid) was compensated successfully by a decrease in volume of one or both of the other two compartments. The line between B and C is the knee of the curve, intracranial compliance is decreased. Between C and D, a relatively small increase in intracranial volume leads to a large increase in intracranial pressure. The slope of the curve from B to C is also influenced by the rate at which the intracranial volume is increased.

C. The blood-brain barrier. A barrier exists between the blood and the CNS. The blood-brain barrier is a continuous layer of endothelial cells lining the vascular lumen. These cells are connected by tight junctions, which restrict the intercellular passage of water-soluble drugs, proteins, and ions from blood to brain. The physiochemical properties that govern the ability of a given drug to cross the blood-brain barrier include lipid solubility, ionization, molecular size, and degree of protein binding.

Although alpha-adrenergic, beta-adrenergic, and dopaminergic receptors can be demonstrated in the cerebral circulation, vasoconstricting drugs and inotropic agents seem to have less effect on cerebral vasculature than on other vascular beds [26]. Vasodilators, however, can have a profound effect on the cerebral vasculature. This may be due, in part, to the direct action of many of these agents on vascular smooth muscle without adrenergic receptor mediation.

D. Cardiac output and the CNS

  1. Determinants of cardiac output. Cardiac output is the product of heart rate and stroke volume (CO = HR × SV), but the determinants of cardiac output are a complex interrelation of the positive and negative influences of preload, afterload, heart rate, contractility, and synergy of myocardial contraction (Fig. 6-3). Blood pressure is the product of cardiac output and systemic vascular resistance (BP = CO × SVR).

  2. Cardiac failure

    a. Cardiovascular causes of pump failure are multifold (e.g., hypovolemia, tachyarrhythmia, decreased contractility, increased afterload), but most often a progressive cycle occurs that involves the major determinants of cardiac function and leads to heart failure (e.g., with ischemic heart disease, myocardial ischemia develops → decreased contractility → asynergy of contraction → increased preload → compensatory tachycardia → increased afterload → decreased cardiac output, worsened ischemia, forming a vicious circle).

    Reduced preload (hypovolemia) is a common cause of reduced cardiac output in the neurologic intensive care unit (ICU).

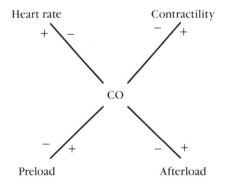

Fig. 6-3. Determinants of myocardial performance affect the cardiac output both positively and negatively. CO = cardiac output.

Hypotension (and presumably decreased cardiac output) in association with head injury almost always results from some other injury, rarely from the head injury per se. Common sites of injury associated with systemic hypotension include intra-abdominal hemorrhage, hemothorax, retroperitoneal hematoma, and hematoma forming from pelvic or femoral fractures. Blood loss from scalp and facial lacerations may be substantial enough to cause hypovolemia and reduced cardiac output. In a child, bleeding into a subgaleal or intracranial hematoma may be of sufficient magnitude to cause low cardiac output on a hypovolemic basis. To assess the patient's intravascular volume, cardiac filling pressure should be measured. With normal heart function, measuring the right atrial pressure is adequate. If there is left ventricular disease and dysfunction, the filling pressure should be assessed with a pulmonary artery catheter to measure the pulmonary artery diastolic or pulmonary artery occlusion pressure.

  b. CNS causes of reduced cardiac output include paralysis of the vasomotor center and subsequent hypotension from cerebral trauma. This hypotension is usually accompanied by bradycardia, agonal gasping respirations, and death. Cardiac dysrhythmias may result from head injury, subarachnoid hemorrhage, or cerebrovascular insufficiency with potential alteration of cardiac output. Spinal cord injury, on the other hand, often causes neurogenic hypotension by sympathetic blockade and predominance of the parasympathetic autonomic system. However, spinal cord injury, like head injury, may be associated with other causes of hypotension (such as hypovolemia) and these causes must be ruled out. (Of assistance in the differential diagnosis is the usual association of neurogenic hypotension with bradycardia, whereas hypovolemic hypotension is usually accompanied by tachycardia.) In cases in which the cardiac output is depressed by both neurogenic and hypovolemic mechanisms, accurate assessment of preload is mandatory.

3. Effect of low cardiac output on the CNS. The effect of reduced cardiac output on the CNS is apparently not pronounced until CPP falls below the autoregulatory threshold value of approximately 50 mmHg. CBF is better preserved during pharmacologically induced hypotension than with decreased cardiac output from hemorrhage [8,15,21,27,28]. Data from anesthetized patients undergoing carotid endarterectomy with continuous electroencephalogram (EEG) monitoring and periodic measurements of CBF show that a regional CBF (rCBF) of less than 18 ml/100 gm/min is almost invariably accompanied by EEG changes of ischemia. The EEG becomes isoelectric at rCBF of 15 ml/100 gm/min, and cell death occurs when rCBF is less than 10 ml/100 gm/min [36]. Data from unanesthetized monkeys suggest that when CBF is less than 12 ml/100 gm/min for two hours or longer, infarction results [29].

II. Pharmacologic intervention for cardiovascular dysfunction. Pharmacologic intervention is necessary to augment cardiovascular function when it is suboptimal in the neurologic ICU patient. Vasoactive drugs may be broadly classified *by use* into four groups: vasoconstrictors, vasodilators, positive inotropic drugs, and negative inotropic and/or chronotropic drugs [31]. Commonly encountered cardiovascular complications requiring therapy with these drugs are presented in section **III.**

A. Vasoconstrictors

    1. Mode of action. Generally speaking, the most commonly used vasoconstrictors are phenylephrine and methoxamine, which cause vasoconstriction by their primary alpha-adrenergic agonist action (Table 6-1). Both are sympathomimetic amines (so named because they mimic the action of norepinephrine and epinephrine) whose spectrum of activity is shown in Figure 6-4 [1]. The other sympathomimetic amines that have significant alpha-adrenergic actions are norepinephrine, metaraminol, ephedrine, mephentermine, and, in higher dosages, epinephrine and dopamine. The relative degree of alpha and beta effects of most sympathomimetic amines depends on

Table 6-1. Some effects of receptor stimulation by catecholamines

Adrenergic receptor	Site	Action
Alpha-1	Postsynaptic receptors that regulate smooth muscle arterioles (systemic and pulmonary circulation)	Vasoconstriction (increased impedance)
	Iris	Dilatation
	Heart	Increased contractility
Alpha-2	Presynaptic receptors that, when stimulated, inhibit the release of norepinephrine of smooth muscle	Vasodilatation
Beta-1	Heart	Increased atrial and ventricular contraction
	Sinoatrial node	Increased heart rate
	Atrioventricular conduction	Increased conduction velocity or rate of conduction
	Kidney	Renin release
Beta-2	Smooth muscle arterioles (systemic and pulmonary)	Vasodilatation (decreased impedance)
	Bronchi	Bronchodilatation
	Heart	Increased rate and contractility

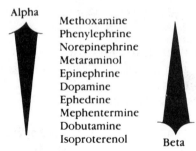

Alpha

Methoxamine
Phenylephrine
Norepinephrine
Metaraminol
Epinephrine
Dopamine
Ephedrine
Mephentermine
Dobutamine
Isoproterenol   Beta

Fig. 6-4. The spectrum of adrenergic activity of sympathomimetic amines. Drugs toward the top of the list possess more alpha-adrenergic agonist properties and those toward the bottom exert beta-adrenergic agonist effects. The proportion of alpha and beta activity changes according to dose: some drugs exhibit more alpha-adrenergic activity than beta-adrenergic activity as dose increases.

the dosage: small doses have less alpha-adrenergic agonism than large dosages [20]. Angiotensin (not readily available in the United States) is a potent nonadrenergic vasoconstrictor. It acts directly on vascular smooth muscle, even in the face of alpha-adrenergic blockade. A comparison of the pharmacologic characteristics of the commonly used vasoconstrictors is shown in Table 6-2.

2. **Hemodynamic effect.** The hemodynamic effects of vasoconstrictors depend on two factors: the specific drug chosen (relative degree of alpha and beta agonism) and the clinical setting (vascular resistance, cardiac function, and integrity of baroreceptor reflexes). All vasoconstrictors increase vascular resistance, which usually results in an increase in systemic and pulmonary artery pressures, particularly when systemic vascular resistance is low. Depending on the original myocardial ventricular function and the amount of beta-1 agonism of the drug, cardiac output may decrease, increase, or remain unchanged. A pure alpha-adrenergic agonist (e.g., phenylephrine) may reduce cardiac output owing to increased resistance, whereas drugs with mixed alpha and beta-1 activity (e.g., ephedrine) increase systemic resistance as well as cardiac output. The response of the heart rate is also variable; it is more likely to decrease if a pure alpha drug is given because of reflex slowing from baroreceptor responses to increased systemic blood pressure, but may increase if the particular drug has significant beta-1 activity.

3. **Cerebral effect.** There is in vitro evidence that cerebral arteries possess alpha-adrenergic receptors [44]. However, clinical doses of alpha-agonist drugs cause little or no cerebrovasoconstriction nor a decrease in CBF. This is confirmed by studies during cardiopulmonary bypass, which show that changes of 25% in MAP with phenylephrine did not increase or decrease CBF as would be expected with intact autoregulation [34]. If autoregulation is lost, or if these

Table 6-2. Comparison of pharmacologic characteristics of commonly used vasoconstrictors

| Generic name | Trade name | Receptor activity | | | | | Onset | Duration | Adult dose (IV) |
| | | Vascular | | Cardiac | | | | |
		Alpha	Beta-2	Beta-1				
Methoxamine	Vasoxyl	++++	0	0			++	+++	0.2–0.5 mg bolus
Phenylephrine	Neo-Synephrine	++++	0	+			++	++	0.1–0.5 μg/kg/min infusion
Norepinephrine	Levophed	++++	0	++			++++	+	0.05–0.15 μg/kg/min infusion
Ephedrine	Ephedrine	+++	+	++			++	++++	2.5–5.0 mg bolus

The number of + denotes increasing activity or time; 0 = no activity.

135

drugs are given in sufficient doses to raise the mean arterial blood pressure beyond the upper limits of autoregulation, CBF may increase significantly. This increase may be associated with a breakdown in the blood-brain barrier, which enhances vasogenic edema formation.

4. Indications

    a. The primary indication for the use of a vasoconstrictor is *decreased* **vascular resistance.** This often an iatrogenic problem caused by the administration of either anesthetics or other drugs with vasodilatory properties.

    b. Alpha drugs are often given to increase blood pressure and therefore correct **low CPP** during and after carotid endarterectomy when BP falls.

    c. Occasionally, vasoconstrictors are essential in the treatment of **hypovolemia** (e.g., uncontrolled hemorrhage) to support blood pressure while volume deficits are being corrected with intravenous fluid therapy.

    d. Rarely, **anaphylactic** and other drug or blood **reactions** necessitate the use of vasoconstrictors to restore systemic resistance and perfusion pressure.

    e. Vasoconstrictors with both alpha and beta-1 agonism are used to **improve cardiac output** and resistance when both are diminished.

    f. Vasoconstrictors are used in conjunction with appropriate cardiac drugs in cardiopulmonary resuscitation to perfuse vital organs (e.g., heart and brain) [5].

5. Contraindications

    a. The primary contraindication to the use of pure alpha-adrenergic drugs is the combination of **elevated vascular resistance** and **myocardial left ventricular failure.** Although the blood pressure may transiently improve in this setting, the increased work of the heart (oxygen consumption) and decreased cardiac output (oxygen supply) will inevitably result in deterioration of cardiac function.

    b. Vasoconstrictors, although effective, are relatively contraindicated in the presence of slight to **moderate hypovolemia** because the degree of actual hypovolemia is masked by the elevated arterial and venous pressure.

    c. With the exception of dopamine, the alpha-adrenergic stimulation by vasoconstrictors causes renal arterial constriction and reduced renal perfusion; therefore, **impaired renal function** is another consideration.

B. Vasodilators

    1. Mode of action. There are three primary modes of action of vasodilators: direct smooth muscle relaxation (e.g., the calcium channel–blocking drugs verapamil and nifedipine), interruption of peripheral alpha-adrenergic stimulation (including gangli-onic blockade, catecholamine depletion, prevention of catechol-amine release, and competitive blockade), and conversion of CNS neurotransmitters (e.g., alpha-methyldopa conversion to alpha-methylnorepinephrine, which causes decreased peripheral nerve firing).

The predominant site of vasodilator action (arterial vs. venous) is of paramount importance. Although this is not completely estab-lished for all drugs in human beings, and overlap exists among the drugs, generally the alpha-adrenergic blocking drugs are mixed arterial and venous dilators, the nitrates are venous dilators, and the other direct-acting drugs are arteriolar dilators. A comparison of the pharmacologic characteristics of commonly used vasodilators is shown in Table 6-3.

2. **Hemodynamic effect.** The hemodynamic effects of vasodilators depend on the site of action of the drug and the status of the circulation. The drugs that cause arteriolar dilatation (e.g., diazoxide and hydralazine) decrease systemic resistance with little change in cardiac preload. Cardiac output will remain unchanged or increase (if a decrease had occurred because of increased systemic resis-tance), and heart rate will remain constant or increase (reflexly if the blood pressure drops significantly and the baroreceptors are func-tional). Drugs that cause venous dilatation (e.g., nitroglycerin) de-crease left ventricular filling pressure, as manifested by reduced pulmonary artery occluded (PAO) pressure. There can be concomi-tant decreases in cardiac output unless optimal filling pressures are maintained. Drugs that have mixed arterial and venous dilatation (e.g., nitroprusside and phentolamine) decrease systemic vascular resistance and blood pressure, and often cause a reflex tachycardia. Cardiac output may or may not decrease depending on whether the filling pressure is maintained. Reflex tachycardia is less of a problem with nitroglycerin (because of venous dilatation), trimethaphan (be-cause of ganglionic blockade), prazosin (because of maintenance of negative feedback presynaptically), and labetalol (because of con-comitant beta blockade) [14].

3. **Cerebral effect.** The direct-acting vasodilators, sodium nitroprus-side, nitroglycerin, diazoxide, aminophylline, hydralazine, and pa-paverine, all produce cerebral vasodilatation. In the absence of hypotension, CBF will increase (Table 6-4). Intracerebral steal may be induced and autoregulation may be impaired with these drugs. Cerebral blood volume may increase and elevate ICP, altering the patient's neurologic status (see Fig. 6-2). However, the increase in ICP observed with sodium nitroprusside, and possibly other cere-bral vasodilators, may be attenuated by a technique of slow ad-ministration under hypocapnic and hyperoxic conditions [22,24]. Trimethaphan and alpha-blocking agents do not demonstrate this

Table 6-3. Comparison of pharmacologic characteristics of commonly used vasodilators

Generic name	Trade name	Mode of action	Prominent vasodilation	CBF	Onset (min)	Duration	Adult dosage (IV)
Sodium nitroprusside	Nipride	Direct	Arteriovenous	↑	0.5	2–4 min	0.2–1.0 μg/kg/min infusion
Nitroglycerin	Nitrostat	Direct	Venous	↑	1–2	10 min	0.4–0.8 mg sublingual or 0.5–5.0 μg/kg/min infusion
Diazoxide	Hyperstat	Direct	Arterial	↑	1–2	4–12 hr	3–5 mg/kg bolus
Nifedipine	Procardia	Calcium channel blocker	Arterial	↑	5–15	2–4 hr	10–20 mg sublingual
Trimethaphan	Arfonad	Ganglionic blockade	Arteriovenous	↑	1–2	4–8 min	10–50 μg/kg/min infusion
Hydralazine	Apresoline	Direct	Arterial	↑	10–20	3–4 hr	5.0–7.5 mg bolus
Phentolamine	Regitine	Alpha-1 and alpha-2 adrenergic blockade	Arteriovenous	?	1–2	20 min	0.5–? μg/kg/min infusion
Labetalol	Trandate	Alpha-1 and beta adrenergic blockade	Arteriovenous	?	2–3	2–4 hr	0.25–1.0 mg/kg bolus
Prazosin	Minipress	Alpha-1 adrenergic blockade	Arteriovenous	?	Not available in a parenteral formulation		
Droperidol	Inapsine	Alpha-adrenergic blockade	Arteriovenous	→	1–2	5–30 min	1.2–2.5 mg bolus
Chlorpromazine	Thorazine	Alpha-adrenergic blockade	Arteriovenous	→	1–2	5–30 min	2.5–5.0 mg bolus

CBF = cerebral blood flow; NC = no change.

Table 6-4. Effects of vasodilators on cerebral blood flow

Increase	Decrease or no change
Sodium nitroprusside	Droperidol
Nitroglycerin	Chlorpromazine
Diazoxide	Labetalol
Hydralazine	Esmolol
Nifedipine	
Trimethaphan	

cerebrovasodilating property to the same extent. Labetalol, the new combination alpha-1 and beta-adrenergic blocking agent, decreases blood pressure with stable CPP, without causing the sedation or loss of effective pupillary exam seen with droperidol, chlorpromazine, or trimethaphan [30].

4. Indications

   a. Treatment of **hypertension** that occurs during or after surgery.

   b. Treatment of **cerebral arterial spasm.**

   c. Reduction of the usual increase in systemic vascular resistance associated with **low cardiac output** and heart failure. Frequently, vasodilators are combined with positively inotropic drugs to treat heart failure, but vasodilators can work alone in some cases.

   d. Vasodilators, specifically nitroglycerin, are indicated for treatment of **myocardial ischemia** associated with an imbalance in oxygen supply and demand, particularly when the filling pressure is elevated. The calcium channel–blocking drugs (verapamil and nifedipine) are effective coronary artery vasodilators useful in preventing coronary artery spasm.

   e. Vasodilators improve forward flow or enhance forward cardiac output in cases of **aortic** and **mitral valvular insufficiency.** In these instances, vasodilator therapy increases cardiac output by lowering the afterload (decreasing impedance) [7]. As with administration of all vasodilators, care must be taken to preserve coronary artery perfusion pressure (diastolic blood pressure) to prevent myocardial ischemia, and to maintain ventricular filling pressure to preserve cardiac output.

5. Contraindications

   a. The greatest contraindication to vasodilators is the presence of **hypovolemia.** Administration to patients who have inadequate blood volume results in decreased cardiac output and hypotension.

   b. Decreased intracranial compliance is a relative contraindication to the use of the direct-acting vasodilators. If possible, they should be used in conjunction with ICP monitoring. The ability of some drugs to reduce MAP and increase ICP can markedly decrease CPP (see Table 6-3).

   c. A relative contraindication to the use of the mixed arterial and venous vasodilators may be the excessive quantity of **infused volume** required to keep the preload at optimal levels. This is a consideration in patients who have renal failure and increased pulmonary or brain water.

   d. Cyanide toxicity is a potential complication of administration of sodium nitroprusside; if it develops the drug must be discontinued [33].

C. Positive inotropic and chronotropic drugs

   1. Mechanism of action. For the most part, drugs that have positive inotropic effects are beta-1 adrenergic agonists. The more beta-1 activity, the more positive the inotropic effect. Drugs that exert their positive inotropic effect by beta-1 stimulation include epinephrine, ephedrine, dopamine, dobutamine, and isoproterenol [37]. Calcium, digitalis glycosides, and amrinone are positive inotropic compounds that work directly on the heart [10]. A comparison of pharmacologic characteristics is listed in Table 6-5.

   2. Hemodynamic effect. As with the other vasoactive drugs, the hemodynamic effects of each positive inotropic drug depend on the particular drug, its dosage, and the clinical setting (cardiovascular status). Sympathomimetic drugs that have nearly pure beta-1 effects (isoproterenol and dobutamine) increase myocardial contractility, heart rate, and cardiac output. Atrioventricular conduction is enhanced, as is automaticity of pacemaker cells (see Table 6-1). They also, through beta-2 effects, cause weak vasodilatation and decrease systemic vascular resistance and blood pressure. The drugs that have mixed alpha and beta activity tend to increase contractility, cardiac output, and systemic resistance. Changes in heart rate are variable, but are usually increased as is blood pressure. The onset and duration of action of all the sympathomimetic amines are rapid and short lived.

   Calcium and digitalis are both nonadrenergically mediated positive inotropic drugs that increase cardiac output and slightly decrease systemic vascular resistance. The positive inotropic effects of calcium occur within 1 minute, whereas it takes 10 to 30 minutes to achieve the inotropic effects of digoxin. Amrinone is a positive inotropic agent with vasodilator properties. Its effect on the heart is not mediated by adrenergic receptors. Although its exact mechanism of action has not been determined, it is a phosphodiesterase inhibitor that increases cardiac cyclic adenosine monophosphate (AMP) and causes enhanced CA^{2+} influx. The hemodynamic effects of amrinone most closely resemble those seen with dobutamine [4]. All inotropic drugs shift the ventricular function curves to the left, as illustrated in Figure 6-5; therefore, cardiac output is augmented at a lower filling pressure, and cardiac work is more efficient.

3. **Cerebral effects.** In addition to alpha receptors, cerebral arteries also possess dopaminergic receptors and beta receptors. Beta receptors react as beta-1 receptors rather than as beta-2 receptors. (Beta-2 receptors are usually found outside the heart.) When used to treat hypotension from low cardiac output, the positive inotropic drugs can restore CPP with an improvement in CBF. Their effects on the cerebral circulation have not been clearly established when administered in the presence of a normal cardiac output. As with the alpha-adrenergic agonists, the positive inotropic agents will increase CBF either if autoregulation is absent or if the upper limits of autoregulation are exceeded.

The effect of dopamine on the cerebral circulation is dose dependent. When low-dose ($< 2\mu g/kg/min$) dopamine was administered intravenously to dogs, CBF was either slightly decreased or unchanged [40]. The administration of moderate doses (2– 6 $\mu g/kg/min$) resulted in an increase in CBF, whereas high-dose (7–20 $\mu g/kg/min$) dopamine caused a decrease in CBF. The latter effect can be blocked by either the alpha antagonist phentolamine or the serotonin receptor antagonist methysergide; the increase in CBF caused by moderate-dose dopamine can be blocked by the dopamine receptor antagonist haloperidol. Epinephrine, which crosses the blood-brain barrier, has been shown to increase CBF, whereas norepinephrine and metaraminol have, in some models, caused a mild reduction in CBF [26].

4. **Indications**

   a. Positive inotropic drugs are used in patients who have **chronically decreased cardiac output** or **failing left ventricular function.** However, positive inotropic drugs are not a substitute for appropriate volume replacement, afterload reduction, or heart rate. The specific drug used depends on the clinical condition. Dopamine or epinephrine is useful when a positive inotropic effect is needed, as in a patient who has low systemic vascular resistance and poor renal perfusion (low urine output). In the presence of increased systemic vascular resistance, normal heart rate, and low cardiac output, dobutamine, amrinone, or isoproterenol is indicated.

   b. Calcium and ephedrine will increase contractility during **brief periods of myocardial dysfunction.** Whenever cardiac output is depressed for prolonged periods, infusions of catecholamines, mechanical assist devices, or both are required to aid the failing heart.

Table 6-5. Comparison of pharmacologic characteristics of positive inotropic drugs

| Generic name | Trade name | Receptor activity | | | Adult dose (IV) | Comments |
| | | Vascular | | Cardiac | | |
		Alpha	Beta-2	Beta-1		
Epinephrine	Adrenalin	++++	+	++	0.05–0.15 μg/kg/min infusion	Relative alpha and beta activity is dose related (beta in low doses and alpha in higher doses)
Dopamine*	Intropin	++	+	++	1–20 μg/kg/min infusion	Relative alpha and beta effects are dose related (like epinephrine), but splanchnic and renal vasoconstriction is spared. Used in patients with compromised renal function
Ephedrine	Ephedrine	+++	0	++	5–10 mg bolus	Beta effects are primarily secondary to release of norepinephrine. Lasts 5–10 min after bolus injection. Tachyphylaxis may occur
Dobutamine	Dobutrex	+	+	+++	1–10 μg/kg/min infusion	Theoretically, primarily beta-1 effects on myocardial contractility and little other beta-1 cardiac effect. Given by infusion

Isoproterenol	Isuprel	0	++++	++++	0.025–0.05 μg/kg/min infusion	Pure beta effects. High doses cause ventricular irritability
Amrinone	Inocor	0	0	0	0.75–1.5 mg/kg bolus followed by 5–20 kg/min infusion	Nonadrenergic intrope. Rapid onset (prolonged elimination) may cause significant decrease in systemic vascular resistance
Calcium	Calcium	0	0	0	1–10 mg/kg/bolus	Rapid-acting positive inotropic drug effects that persist for 5-10 min. Mechanism of action is direct and not beta adrenergic. Useful in patients on propranolol to increase contractility
Digoxin	Lanoxin	0	0	0	0.125–0.25 mg bolus	Had delayed onset on inotropic action and low therapeutic safety ratio that makes acute use inappropriate in most cases. Mechanism of action does not involve beta system

Note: The number of + denotes increasing activity or time; 0 = no activity.
* Dopamine also stimulates dopaminergic receptors, which causes mild renal and splanchnic arterial dilatation.

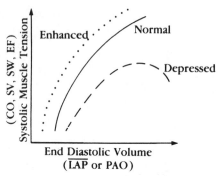

Fig. 6-5. Frank-Starling force-length relationship. Systolic muscle tension is plotted against end diastolic volume. The solid line describes the normal Frank-Starling force-length relationship, the dashed line represents cardiac function with a diseased or depressed ventricle, and the dotted line demonstrates the enhanced force-length relationship of a heart that is stimulated with a positive inotropic drug (e.g., calcium or epinephrine). CO = cardiac output; SV = stroke volume; SW = stroke work; EF = ejection fraction; LAP = mean left atrial pressure; PAO = pulmonary artery occluded pressure.

      c. Positive inotropic agents that have primarily beta or dopaminergic effects (e.g., isoproterenol or dopamine) have been used in the treatment of **cerebral vasospasm.**

   5. Contraindications

      a. Particular drugs should not be used when their primary hemodynamic effects will aggravate the clinical situation. For example, isoproterenol and perhaps dobutamine and dopamine may exacerbate **tachyarrhythmias.** Isoproterenol will increase myocardial oxygen demand and diminish supply; therefore, it is usually contraindicated in patients who have **ischemic heart disease.**

      b. High doses of norepinephrine and epinephrine are likely to decrease nutrient flow to many tissue beds (because of alpha-adrenergic–mediated vasoconstriction) and may contribute to **renal failure** and the state known as "irreversible shock" in patients who have low cardiac output and high systemic vascular resistance.

      c. Digoxin must be used cautiously in previously **digitalized** or **hypokalemic patients** and patients in **renal failure** because of the potential for development of digitalis toxicity and associated arrhythmias.

      d. Although seemingly benign, prolonged or excessive administration of calcium can cause toxicity. If continued inotropic support is warranted, it is prudent to switch to a catecholamine, amrinone, or digoxin rather than to give repeated doses of calcium.

  D. Negative inotropic and chronotropic drugs

   1. Mechanisms of action. Propranolol, metoprolol, and esmolol are negative inotropic and negative chronotropic drugs. All are beta-1 adrenergic blocking drugs of approximately equal potency [12]. Propranolol is also a beta-2 blocker. The major differences include the greater cardioselective (beta-1) effects of metoprolol and esmolol, the greater membrane stabilizing activity of propranolol, and the shorter half-life of esmolol [19]. The clinical significance of these differences is difficult to document, and, indeed, when high dosages of metoprolol and esmolol are used, some beta-2 blockade occurs. A comparison of pharmacologic characteristics of negative inotropic and chronotropic drugs is shown in Table 6-6.

Calcium channel-blocking drugs (verapamil, nifedipine) inhibit calcium conductance of the slow calcium channel of the sarcolemma and affect the electrical and mechanical function of the heart. They exert a negative inotropic effect on the heart by interfering with calcium-mediated excitation contraction. Their primary hemodynamic effect, however, is vasodilatation.

2. **Hemodynamic effect.** Propranolol given intravenously in incremental dosages of 0.25 to 0.5 mg up to 0.1 mg/kg decreases (in a dose-related fashion) heart rate, blood pressure, and cardiac output. With moderate doses, the negative chronotropic effects are more pronounced than the negative inotropic effects. Esmolol produces a dose-related negative chronotropic and inotropic response as a bolus or continuous infusion. It has been used successfully to ameliorate the heart rate and blood pressure changes associated with acute perioperative interventions. The short half-life (nine minutes) of this drug allows for rapid resolution of unwanted side effects [3]. Verapamil causes a dose-related decrease in blood pressure owing to decreased systemic vascular resistance and a variable (usually increased) effect on heart rate and cardiac output. The negative inotropic effect of verapamil (and most calcium channel-blocking drugs) is relatively unimportant clinically and is counteracted by reflex increases in heart rate and, presumably, contractility secondary to its pronounced vasodilatory action.

3. **Cerebral effect.** The negative inotropic drugs apparently do not affect the cerebral circulation significantly. Calcium channel-blocking drugs cause cerebral vasodilatation [13].

4. **Indications**

   a. The primary indication for negative inotropic and chronotropic drugs is to **reduce myocardial oxygen consumption** associated with increases in myocardial contractility and heart rate, particularly in patients who have ischemic heart disease.

   b. Propranolol, esmolol, and verapamil are additionally useful in treating **supraventricular arrhythmias.**

   c. In the neurologic ICU, beta-adrenergic blocking drugs are useful adjuncts to the treatment of **hypertension.**

   d. Calcium channel-blocking drugs (e.g., nimodipine) are effective in treating **cerebral vasospasm.**

Table 6-6. Comparison of pharmacologic characteristics of negative inotropic and chronotropic drugs

Generic name	Trade name	Negative inotropic effect	Negative chronotropic effect	Mechanism of action	Adult dose	Comments
Halothane	Fluothane	++	0	Direct	0.5–1.0 vol% (inhalation)	
Enflurane	Ethrane	+++	0	Direct	1.0–1.5 vol% (inhalation)	
Propranolol	Inderal	++	++++	Beta-1 adrenergic blockade	0.25–0.5 mg (IV)	Used primarily to decrease heart rate and treat arrhythmias
Metoprolol	Lopressor	++	++++	Beta-1 adrenergic blockade	50–100 mg (PO)	Used primarily for medical therapy of hypertension.
Esmolol	Brevibloc	++	++++	Beta-1 adrenergic blockade	500 μg/kg/min × 1 min, then 50–300 μg/kg/min	To decrease heart rate, treat SVT or hypertension
Labetalol	Trandate	+	++	Beta- and alpha-1 adrenergic blockade	0.25–1.0 mg/kg	Primarily for treatment of hypertension
Verapamil	Isoptin	+	0	Ca^{2+} antagonism	0.1 mg/kg (IV)	Used primarily for supraventricular arrhythmias

The number of + denotes increasing activity.
0 = no activity; IV = intravenous administration; PO = oral administration.

5. Contraindications

  a. Low cardiac output is a relative contraindication to the use of negative inotropic and chronotropic drugs. An obvious exception is the patient whose low cardiac output is secondary to an arrhythmia that can be treated with propranolol or verapamil.

  b. Since there is a significant beta-2 blockade effect of propranolol, it should be given cautiously in patients who have **bronchospastic pulmonary disease.**

III. Management of cardiovascular complications of neurologic disorders

  A. Cerebral arterial spasm. The management of patients who have subarachnoid hemorrhage (SAH) from ruptured intracranial aneurysms may be complicated by cerebral arterial spasm and infarction. The incidence of radiographic vasospasm after aneurysmal rupture ranges from 30 to 50%, while 40 to 65% of patients undergoing cerebral aneurysm surgery will demonstrate vasospasm postoperatively [2,39,43]. Vasospasm may also complicate craniocerebral trauma, particularly when SAH is present.

  1. Pathophysiology. Vasospasm has two phases. The early phase is probably due to the hemorrhage itself that either mechanically causes vasoconstriction or precipitates release of catecholamines from sympathetic nerve endings. This early phase is a transient phenomenon. The second or delayed phase of vasospasm occurs on or about day three and is maximum at one week. The delayed phase probably results from the breakdown of the subarachnoid blood and/or the gradual release of serotonin and vasoactive amines from platelets and other blood elements [41]. Prostaglandins may also play a role. Vasospasm decreases CBF to the affected vessels. If CBF is reduced below critical levels, ischemic damage may occur.

  2. Prevention. Aneurysm surgery is frequently delayed for 10 to 14 days after SAH to allow time for resolution of vasospasm. However, delay increases the risk of rebleeding from the aneurysm, maximal at 7 to 14 days. Reserpine and kanamycin have been used to deplete the platelets of serotonin and reduce serotonin blood levels [45]. These drugs, as well as nifedipine and other calcium-channel blockers, have been shown to be effective in the prevention and treatment of experimental vasospasm [43].

  3. Treatment

  a. The circulating blood volume should be increased with balanced salt solutions, blood transfusions, and albumin.

  b. The pharmacologic therapy of vasospasm is based in part on the assumption that autoregulation in the involved vessels is probably not intact [11]. Therefore, CBF will vary directly with the CPP. Drugs that raise the blood pressure, cardiac output, or both have been used alone or in combination with drugs that promote *cerebrovasodilatation,* either by direct action, inhibition of phosphodiesterase, or increase in cyclic AMP (cAMP). Combination therapies include isoproterenol (125 μg/hr) and aminophylline (125 mg/hr). However, these drugs increase myocardial oxygen consumption through increased heart rate and contractility. Myocardial ischemia, irritability, or both may be produced, which has prompted the addition of lidocaine (1–4 mg/min) to these regimens to prevent serious ventricular arrhythmias.

Other drugs being investigated in the treatment of this disorder include the calcium antagonists verapamil and nifedipine, which have been shown to relax isolated constricted cerebral arteries [17]. The new body of information with nimodipine indicates that it improves neurologic outcome in cerebral vasospasm associated with SAH, even though the degree of spasm was not changed [42]. At present, there are no good comparison studies of different treatment modalities in cerebral vasospasm.

B. Hypotension after head injury

1. Pathophysiology. Hypotension after head injury results from either the cerebral injury or hypovolemia secondary to systemic trauma. When head injury is complicated by shock, the mortality is significantly higher. Hypotension in the presence of increased ICP markedly reduces CPP and increases the likelihood of irreversible damage.

2. Treatment

a. The intravascular volume should be expanded rapidly with balanced salt solutions, blood, and albumin. The use of albumin is controversial; it may leak into cerebral tissue if the blood-brain barrier is disrupted. Avoiding volume overload is essential. Measurement of cardiac filling pressures with a right atrial or pulmonary artery catheter is helpful. The goal, however, is not to achieve a specific filling pressure but rather to maintain organ perfusion as monitored by physical examination and measurement of blood pressure, pulse, and urine output and specific gravity (which may be misleading when osmotic or loop diuretics are used). Direct measurement of cardiac output and calculation of systemic vascular resistance may be necessary if left ventricular dysfunction is suspected. Overzealous fluid administration may promote cerebral edema as well.

b. Positive inotropic agents or vasoconstrictors are indicated, depending on the systemic vascular resistance (see Tables 6-2 and 6-5 for drugs and dosages), if cardiac output remains low despite adequate cardiac filling pressures.

c. In a patient who is brain-dead, hypotension warrants treatment if organs are to be donated. Therapy includes vigorous fluid administration and infusion of dopamine. Dopamine increases renal perfusion at doses below 8 μg/kg/min.

C. Autonomic hypotension

1. Pathophysiology. Hypotension may either accompany spinal cord injury or be a preterminal event in the head-injured patient. Hypotension results from loss of sympathetic influence on the heart and systemic circulation, which causes a decrease in cardiac output and systemic vascular resistance.

2. Treatment

a. Raising the legs will augment preload, increase venous return, and enhance cardiac output.

b. Judicious management of fluids is necessary to avoid over-transfusion and congestive heart failure. These patients may be unable to increase heart rate in response to either hypovolemia or hypervolemia.

c. Vasopressors or positive inotropic drugs are required if hemodynamic performance is not improved by replacement of intravascular volume (see Tables 6-2 and 6-5 for drugs and dosages).

d. If the decreased sympathetic nervous system activity causes bradycardia, *atropine* (0.6–0.8 mg IV) is indicated.

D. Hypotension after carotid endarterectomy

1. Pathophysiology. Patients who have carotid artery disease are usually elderly and may have marked cardiovascular dysfunction and reduced carotid sinus baroreceptor function. These factors predispose them to hypotension as well as hypertension in the perioperative period. Hypotension can decrease perfusion of both brain and heart and also cause thrombosis of the operated vessel. The blood pressure should be maintained within the preoperative range.

2. Treatment

a. Intravascular volume is augmented by administering fluids, recognizing that these patients may have left ventricular dysfunction.

b. If hypotension is accompanied by bradycardia, atropine (0.6–0.8 mg IV) should be administered.

c. Vasoconstrictors (see Table 6-2), such as phenylephrine, given by continuous infusion are indicated if perfusion pressure is not restored by increasing heart rate and intravascular volume. Monitoring for myocardial ischemia and renal hypoperfusion is imperative.

d. If phenylephrine is not tolerated or is ineffective, then a mixed alpha- and beta-adrenergic drug such as dopamine is an alternate choice (see Table 6-5 for drugs and dosages).

E. Hypertension

1. Pathophysiology. There are many causes of hypertension. Present in approximately 25% of the adult population in the United States, hypertension is an incremental risk factor in the development of cerebrovascular accidents as well as cardiac disease [16,18]. Patients admitted to the neurologic ICU frequently have hypertension because of their pre-existing disease, head injury, or surgical procedure (especially exploration of the posterior fossa) [9,23,35,40].

2. **Treatment.** Treatment of hypertension in the patient who has intracranial pathology risks intolerable reductions in CPP. The chronically hypertensive patient requires a higher than normal blood pressure for preservation of autoregulation [38]. Left untreated, hypertension may increase CBF, CBV, and ICP; induce hemorrhage into the brain; and promote formation of cerebral edema. There is recent evidence that cerebral ischemia is better tolerated in the treated hypertensive patient than in the untreated patient [16]. Vasodilators (see Table 6-3) and other antihypertensive drugs, such as alpha methyldopa, are useful in controlling chronic hypertension. The goal of treatment in the neurologic ICU is to reestablish blood pressure control with the drugs that the patient took before the acute episode but without significant increases in ICP.

F. **Hypertension after head injury**

1. **Pathophysiology.** CPP is dependent on the difference between MAP and ICP. Therefore, reduction of MAP without a concomitant reduction in ICP may compromise cerebral perfusion. Hypertension often occurs when ICP is elevated (Cushing reflex). Therefore, there may be reluctance to treat hypertension in the head-injured patient for fear of compromising cerebral perfusion. However, ICP monitoring has demonstrated that the systemic arterial pressure is not a reliable indicator of ICP since the Cushing reflex does not occur universally in the presence of intracranial hypertension. Other patients may have hypertension despite normal ICP.

2. **Treatment**

   a. Careful assessment of the hypertensive head-injured patient is necessary. Hypercapnia, distended bladder, pain, anxiety, and other causes should be treated before vasodilator therapy is initiated.

   b. ICP monitoring and direct arterial blood pressure measurement have greatly facilitated the treatment of hypertension coexistent with intracranial pathology by enabling calculation of the CPP at all times.

      (1) The best antihypertensive drugs for these patients are vasodilators that do not dilate cerebral vessels (see Table 6-4). The initial choice in the past was chlorpromazine in interval dosing. The new combination alpha-1 and beta-adrenergic blocking agent, labetalol, is an effective antihypertensive in neurosurgical patients with minimal changes in CPP and decreases in ICP [30]. Trimethaphan, another suitable drug, lowers blood pressure without increasing ICP. Drawbacks to

its use are tachyphylaxis, tachycardia, and cycloplegia. Direct cerebral toxicity of this drug has been reported, but only when MAP is less than 50 mmHg. Propranolol and esmolol may be used as well.

(2) Hydralazine, diazoxide, nitroglycerin, and sodium nitroprusside are cerebrovasodilators and thus may increase ICP when intracranial compliance is decreased. The effect of sodium nitroprusside on ICP may be attenuated by hypocapnic and hyperoxic conditions as well as by administering the drug slowly [22]. Since sodium nitroprusside and trimethaphan must be mixed in 5% dextrose in water, it may be advantageous to make a more concentrated solution to decrease the amount of hypotonic solution administered (Table 6-7). These drugs should only be administered through a calibrated infusion pump.

Table 6-7. Concentrations of vasoactive drugs used at Duke University

Drug	For bolus IV	For infusion IV (infants and children)	Adults
Calcium	1 gm/10 ml (100 mg/ml)	—	—
Dobutamine	—	250 mg/250 ml (1 mg/ml)	500 mg/250 ml (2 mg/ml)
Dopamine	—	200 mg/250 ml (0.8 mg/ml)	400 mg/250 ml (1.6 mg/ml)
Ephedrine	50 mg/10 ml (5 mg/ml)	—	—
Epinephrine	0.1 mg/10 ml (10 μg/ml)	2 mg/250 ml (8 μg/ml)	4 mg/250 ml (16 μg/ml)
Isoproterenol	—	0.5 mg/250 ml (2 μg/ml)	1.0 mg/250 ml (4 μg/ml)
Methoxamine	20 mg/10 ml (2 mg/ml)	—	—
Nitroprusside	—	50 mg/500 ml (100 μg/ml)	50 mg/250 ml (200 μg/ml)
Norepinephrine	—	2 mg/250 ml (8 μg/ml)	4 mg/250 ml (16 μg/ml)
Phenylephrine	1 mg/10 ml (100 μg/ml)	—	10 mg/250 ml (40 μg/ml)
Trimethaphan	—	—	500 mg/250 ml (2 mg/ml)

The carrier fluid is D5W; when large volumes of D5W are contraindicated, the concentrations are increased.

G. Postoperative hypertension

1. Pathophysiology. Postoperative hypertension is common in the neurosurgical patient. Multiple causes include increased ICP (Cushing response), hypothermia, emergence excitement with sympathetic discharge, hypercapnia, and distended bladder. Postoperative hypertension is usually accompanied by increased systemic vascular resistance and cardiac output.

a. After craniotomy. Patients who have undergone debulking of large tumors usually show improvement in intracranial compliance; however, patients who have had a craniotomy for epidural or subdural hematoma may have severe underlying cerebral contusion and edema and therefore still have poor intracranial compliance.

b. After carotid endarterectomy. The combination of a labile cardiovascular system, preexisting hypertension, and altered baroreceptor function is responsible for the high incidence of postoperative hypertension. Impaired baroreceptor function is more likely to contribute to postendarterectomy hypertension if both carotid arteries have been operated. As with hypertension after head injury, controversy exists as to whether the elevated blood pressure should be treated. The argument against therapy is the potential risk of hypotension and cerebral hypoperfusion, particularly with the more potent antihypertensive agents. Patients who have carotid artery disease, however, commonly have ischemic heart disease as well. While hypertension increases the rate-pressure product, pharmacologic treatment to decrease the systolic blood pressure to acceptable levels may produce undesirable diastolic hypotension and jeopardize adequate coronary blood flow.

There is substantial evidence, however, that postendarterectomy hypertension should be treated. Uncontrolled hypertension may lead to cerebral edema (particularly if autoregulation is impaired), myocardial ischemia, or infarction. Hemorrhage from the arteriotomy site may cause a hematoma in the neck, which can impede carotid blood flow and compromise the airway by compressing and displacing the trachea and larynx. Fatal intracerebral hemorrhage within 24 hours after carotid endarterectomy is a complication of hypertension [6].

2. Treatment

a. Hypertension after craniotomy. Therapy and considerations are the same as for hypertension after head injury (see sec. **III.F.2**).

b. Hypertension after extracranial surgery

(1) Vasodilators (see Table 6-3) are used to treat arterial hypertension. Hydralazine, 5.0 to 7.5 mg IV initially supplemented by doses of 4 mg as needed, labetalol in 5- to 10-mg doses, or sodium nitroprusside, 0.2 μg/kg/min up to 10 μg/kg/min, are all effective. Hypotension can be prevented by (a) using a calibrated infusion pump to deliver drugs that are given as a continuous infusion, (b) placing the infusion pump line as close as possible to the IV site to avoid the dead space in long tubing (a pediatric T connector may be useful here), (c) allowing sufficient time for evaluation of drug effect before increasing the dose, (d) basing the end point of therapy on diastolic or mean arterial pressure rather than on systolic pressure, and (e) ensuring adequate intravascular volume.

(2) Tachycardia either before or after therapy with vasodilators should be treated with esmolol 0.5 to 1.0 mg/kg as a bolus, followed by an infusion at 50–300 mg/kg/min [32].

IV. Drug interactions. Patients who have CNS disease usually come to the neurologic ICU with a history of having taken many drugs, some of which involve the cardiovascular system. The purpose of this section is to outline potential interactions between chronic medications and vasoactive drugs administered in the perioperative period (Table 6-8).

A. Digitalis. Digitalis and the synthetic cardiac glycosides are used in the medical treatment of patients who have heart failure and atrial fibrillation. Frequently, they are given in combination with potassium-wasting diuretics that may cause digitalis toxicity manifested as one or a combination of three dysrhythmias: (1) premature ventricular contractions, (2) paroxysmal atrial tachycardia with block, and (3) Wenckebach (Mobitz type I) atrioventricular block. Therefore, close monitoring of potassium in patients receiving digitalis is necessary, particularly if loop or osmotic diuretics are used.

B. Antihypertensive medications. Antihypertensive medications such as alpha methyldopa, hydralazine, prazosin, and clonidine should be continued up to the day of surgery. Pharmacologically controlled hypertensive patients appear to tolerate anesthesia better than partially controlled or uncontrolled patients. There actually may be some danger of rebound hypertension in patients who discontinue antihypertensive therapy (e.g., clonidine withdrawal) [25]. The one group of antihypertensive drugs that should be discontinued two weeks before surgery and replaced with others at that time are the monamine oxidase (MAO) inhibitors. (These drugs also are used as antidepressants and a partial list of them appears in Table 6-8.) MAO inhibitors alter both the function of the normal adrenergic nerve terminal and the synthesis of catecholamines and their metabolites, which may lead to unusual interactions between drugs such as catecholamines and meperidine. Severe hypertension and unpredictable adrenergic drug effects have all been encountered during the perioperative period in patients taking MAO inhibitors.

Table 6-8. Interactions of vasoactive drugs used in the perioperative period with patient medications

Drug group	Representative drugs	Interactive drugs	Complications	Recommendations
Beta-adrenergic blockers	Propranolol, metoprolol	Halogenated anesthetics (methoxyflurane, halothane)	Possible potentiation of myocardial depression	Taper propranolol to 80–160 mg/day as tolerated. Do not discontinue
		Beta-agonist drugs	Resistance (larger doses required for beta effects)	Use calcium or other nonbeta agonist for + inotropic effects. Use atropine for + chronotropic effect
Digitalis	Digoxin (Lanoxin) (many others)	Pre-op diuretics and diuresis during operation	Digitalis toxicity manifest by arrhythmias	Discontinue on day of surgery, monitor serum K^+
Anti-hypertensive medications	Methyldopa, hydralazine, prazosin, clonidine (others)	Anesthetics or drugs that produce vasodilatation	Hypotension	Continue drug, monitor volume status, give volume or alpha-adrenergic agonist if hypotension occurs

Monamine oxidase inhibitors (pargyline and others)	Sympathomimetic amines	Hypertension, unpredictable hemodynamic responses to vasoactive drugs	Discontinue drug 2 weeks before anesthesia
Diuretics	Chlorthiazide, hydrochlorothiazide, furosemide	Anesthetics or drugs that produce vasodilatation — Hypotension	Continue drug, monitor volume status and serum K^+
		Digitalis — Arrhythmias with hypokalemia	Monitor serum K^+
Tricyclic anti-depressants	Amitriptyline, imipramine, nortriptyline, protriptyline (others)	Sympathomimetic amines — Tachycardia, hypertension	Taper if possible, administer adrenergic drugs cautiously

C. Diuretics. Diuretics treat hypertension by counteracting the compensatory sodium retention that accompanies antihypertensive therapy. They also improve congestive heart failure by reducing the blood volume. In high doses, these drugs may cause depletion of extracellular fluid volume, which, combined with vasodilator therapy, can result in postoperative hypotension. Postoperative hypotension is also a problem in patients whose intracranial hypertension is treated with fluid restriction or patients who have hypertension and coronary artery disease and a reduction in plasma volume.

D. Tricyclic antidepressants. Patients are often treated with tricyclic antidepressants because of depression associated with neurologic and major cardiac disease. These drugs have three principal actions: sedation, peripheral and central anticholinergic effects, and inhibition of the amine pump responsible for norepinephrine reuptake at the adrenergic nerve terminal. It is the last action that probably accounts for the antidepressant activity of these drugs. The anticholinergic and adrenergic effects are also responsible for the undesirable cardiovascular sequelae and perioperative drug interaction problems. The anticholinergic effects of tricyclic therapy cause a sustained increase in heart rate and a transient decrease in atrioventricular conduction. Myocardial depression is also a transient feature after initiation of tricyclic antidepressant therapy.

Potential problems from drug interactions include the tachycardia that occurs after the administration of sympathomimetic amines such as epinephrine, norepinephrine, and ephedrine. Patients who require tricyclic antidepressants for the treatment of psychiatric depression should continue taking them, but ideally the drugs should be tapered or discontinued before surgery in all other patients. The use of the combination of halothane and pancuronium is avoided during anesthesia for patients taking tricyclic antidepressants. Tricyclic antidepressants may be reinstituted during the postoperative hospital course for appropriate psychiatric indications.

V. Decision-making. The decision to intervene or, perhaps more importantly, not to intervene in the treatment of cardiovascular lability is crucial to appropriate management. Administration of all drugs entails risks and requires thorough consideration of the indications and contraindications.

To make correct decisions all the time is difficult under ideal conditions and impossible in less than optimal circumstances. The most favorable conditions exist when the physician, through appropriate monitoring, knows the pertinent physiologic data and the probability of success using a particular intervention in a given circumstance. Calm, efficient management of threatened circulatory failure is best achieved by combining thorough understanding of the clinical pathophysiology with knowledge of the pharmacodynamics of vasoactive drugs. Decision schemes or "protocols" are extremely valuable in organizing therapeutic approaches. The

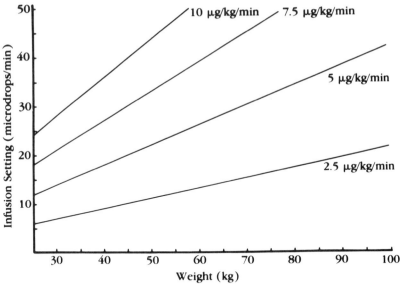

Fig. 6-6. Nomogram for the administration of dopamine (160 mg/250 ml) in patients ranging in weight from 25 to 100 kg. The drug infusion in microdrops/min is shown on the vertical axis and the dose from 2.5 to 10.0 μg/kg/min is plotted as isobars above the weight of the patient. To calculate the correct infusion setting for a patient in whom the desired dosage is 5 μg/kg/min, a vertical line is drawn from the patient's weight to intersect the 5 μg/kg/min line and then drawn horizontally to intersect the infusion setting line. Nomograms for commonly used drugs given by infusion should be constructed to facilitate the accurate administration of vasoactive drugs.

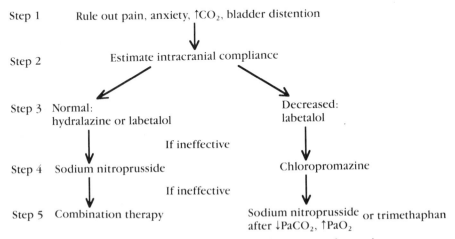

Fig. 6-7 A stepwise protocol for the evaluation and treatment of arterial hypertension in the neurosurgical intensive care patient. If tachycardia is either present initially or develops with therapy, esmolol or propranolol is the treatment of choice.

protocols are based on well-defined physiologic and pharmacologic principles, which aid in the selection of appropriate therapy. It is also helpful to have nomograms for infusion of vasoactive drugs to facilitate rapid and accurate selection of infusion rate (Fig. 6-6) and standardized, institution-wide drug concentrations (see Table 6-7).

An example of a logical progression in decision-making is presented in the steps for treating high blood pressure (Fig. 6-7). Generally, the interventions with the least risk and/or highest probability of success are made first, and interventions with greater risk and lesser probability of success are made later.

References

1. Ahlquist, R. P. Adrenergic receptors and others. *Anesth. Analg.* (Cleve.) 58:510, 1979.
2. Allen, G. S. Cerebral arterial spasm. Part 8: The treatment of delayed cerebral arterial spasm in human beings. *Surg. Neurol.* 6:71, 1976.
3. Askenazi, J., MacCosbe, P. E., Hoff, J., et al. Hemodynamic effects of esmolol, an ultrashort-acting beta blocker. *J. Clin. Pharmacol.* 8:561, 1987.
4. Bottorff, M. B., Rutledge, D. R., and Pieper, J. A. Evaluation of intravenous amrinone: The first of a new class of positive inotropic agents with vasodilator properties. *Pharmacology* 5:227, 1985.
5. Brown, C. G., Birinyi, F., Werman, H. A., et al. The comparative effects of epinephrine versus phenylephrine on regional cerebral blood flow during cardiopulmonary resuscitation. *Resuscitation* 3:171, 1986.
6. Caplan, L. R., Skillman, J., Ojemann, R., et al. Intracerebral hemorrhage following carotid endarterectomy: A hypertensive complication? *Stroke* 9:457, 1978.
7. Cohn, J. N., and Franciosa, J. A. Vasodilator therapy of cardiac failure. *N. Engl. J. Med.* 297:27, 1977.
8. Cottrell, J. E., Gupta, B., and Turndorf, H. Induced Hypotension. In J. E. Cottrell and H. Turndorf (Eds.), *Anesthesia and Neurosurgery.* St. Louis: Mosby, 1980.
9. Davies, M. J., and Cronin, K. D. Post carotid endarterectomy hypertension. *Anaesth. Intensive Care* 8:190, 1980.
10. Doherty, J. E., and Kane, J. J. Digitalis glycosides: Recent advances in clinical pharmacology and treatment. *South. Med. J.* 70:470, 1977.
11. Fleischer, A. S., and Tindall, G. T. Cerebral vasospasm following aneurysm rupture: A protocol for therapy and prophylaxis. *J. Neurosurg.* 52:149, 1980.
12. Frishman, W. Clinical pharmacology of the new beta-adrenergic blocking drugs. Part I. Pharmacodynamic and pharmacokinetic properties. *Am. Heart J.* 97:663, 1979.
13. Giffin, J. P., Cottrell, J. E., Hartung, J., and Skwiry, B. Intracranial pressure during nifedipine-induced hypotension. *Anesth. Analg.* 62:1078, 1983.
14. Graham, R. M., and Pettinger, W. A. Drug therapy. Prazosin. *N. Engl. J. Med.* 300:232, 1979.
15. Gregory, P. C., McGeorge, A. P., Fitch, W., et al. Effects of hemorrhagic hypotension on the cerebral circulation. II. Electrocortical function. *Stroke* 10:719, 1979.
16. Halsey, J. H., Jr., O'Brien, M., and Strong, E. R. Amelioration of cerebral ischemia by prior treatment of hypertension. *Stroke* 11:235, 1980.
17. Hayashi, S., and Toda, N. Inhibition by Ca^{2+}, verapamil and papaverine of Ca^{2+} induced contractions in isolated cerebral and peripheral arteries of the dog. *Br. J. Pharmacol.* 60:35, 1977.

18. Hypertension prevalence and status of awareness, treatment and control in the United States. *Hypertension* 7:457, 1985.
19. Koch-Weser, J. Drug therapy. Metoprolol. *N. Engl. J. Med.* 301:698, 1979.
20. Kones, R. J. The catecholamines: Reappraisal of their use for acute myocardial infarction and the low cardiac output syndromes. *Crit. Care Med.* 1:203, 1973.
21. Mackenzie, E. T., Farrar, J. K., Fitch, W., et al. Effects of hemorrhagic hypotension on the cerebral circulation. I. Cerebral blood flow and pial arteriolar caliber. *Stroke* 10:711, 1979.
22. Marsh, M. L., Aidinis, S. J., Naughton, K. V. H., et al. The technique of nitroprusside administration modifies the intracranial pressure response. *Anesthesiology* 51:538, 1979.
23. Marsh, M. L., Marshall, L. F., and Shapiro, H. M. Neurosurgical intensive care. *Anesthesiology* 47:149, 1977.
24. Marsh, M. L., Shapiro, H. M., Smith, R. W., et al. Changes in neurologic status and intracranial pressure associated with sodium nitroprusside administration. *Anesthesiology* 51:336, 1979.
25. Metz, S., Klein, C., and Morton, N. Rebound hypertension after discontinuation of transdermal clonidine therapy. *Am. J. Med.* 82:17, 1987.
26. Michenfelder, J. D. The Cerebral Circulation. In C. Prys-Roberts (Ed.), *The Circulation in Anaesthesia.* Oxford: Blackwell, 1980.
27. Michenfelder, J. D., and Theye, R. A. Canine systemic and cerebral effects of hypotension induced by hemorrhage, trimethaphan, halothane, or nitroprusside. *Anesthesiology* 46:188, 1977.
28. Miletich, D. J., Gil, K. S. L., Albrecht, R. F., et al. Intracerebral blood flow distribution during hypotensive anesthesia in the goat. *Anesthesiology* 53:210, 1980.
29. Morawetz, R. B., De Girolami, V., Ojemann, R. G., et al. Cerebral blood flow determined by hydrogen clearance during middle cerebral artery occlusion in unanesthetized monkeys. *Stroke* 9:143, 1978.
30. Orlowski, J. P., Shiesley, D., Vidt, D. G., et al. Labetalol to control blood pressure after cerebrovascular surgery. *Crit. Care Med.* 16:765, 1988.
31. Reves, J. G. Vasoactive Drugs and When to Use Them. In S. Thomas (Ed.), *Handbook of Cardiac Anesthesia.* (in press).
32. Reves, J. G., Croughwell, N., Hawkins, E., and Jacobs, J. R. Esmolol for treatment of intraoperative tachycardia and/or hypertension–bolus loading technique. *Anesthesiology* 67:A33, 1987.
33. Reves, J. G., Sheppard, L. C., Wallach, R., and Lell, W. A. Therapeutic uses of sodium nitroprusside and an automated method of administration. *Int. Anesthesiol. Clin.* 16:51, 1978.
34. Rogers, A. T., Stump, D. A., Gravlee, G. P., et al. Response of cerebral blood flow to phenylephrine infusion during hypothermic cardiopulmonary bypass. *Anesthesiology* 69:547, 1988.
35. Satiani, B., Vasko, J. S., and Evans, W. E. Hypertension following carotid endarterectomy. *Surg. Neurol.* 11:357, 1979.
36. Drummond J. C., Shapiro, H. M. Cerebral Physiology. In R. D. Miller (Ed.), *Anesthesia.* New York: Livingstone, 1990. P. 621.
37. Sonnenblick, E. H., Frishman, W. H., and LeJemtel, T. H. Drug therapy. Dobutamine: A new synthetic cardioactive sympathetic amine. *N. Engl. J. Med.* 300:17, 1979.
38. Strardagaard, S., Olesen, J., Skinhoj, E., and Lassen, N. A. Autoregulation of brain circulation in severe arterial hypertension. *Br. Med. J.* 1:507, 1973.
39. Sundt, T. M., Szurszewski, J., and Sharbrough, F. W. Physiological considerations important for the management of vasospasm. *Surg. Neurol.* 7:259, 1977.
40. Von Essen, C., Zervas, N. T., Brown, D. R., et al. Local cerebral blood flow in the dog during intravenous infusion of dopamine. *Surg. Neurol.* 13:181, 1980.

41. Weir, B., Grace, M., Hansen, J., and Rothberg, C. Time course of vasospasm in man. *J. Neurosurg.* 48:173, 1978.
42. Welty, T. E. Use of nimodipine for prevention and treatment of cerebral arterial spasm in patients with subarachnoid hemorrhage. *Clinical Pharmacy* 6:940, 1987.
43. Wilkins, R. H. Attempted prevention and treatment of intracranial arterial spasm: A survey. *Neurosurgery* 6:198, 1980.
44. Wroblewska, B., Spatz, M., Merkel, N., and Bembry, J. Cerebrovascular smooth muscle culture characterization of adrenergic receptors linked to adenylate cyclase. *Life Sciences* 34:783, 1984.
45. Zervas, N. T., Candia, M., Candia, G., et al. Reduced incidence of cerebral ischemia following rupture of intracranial aneurysms. *Surg. Neurol.* 11:339, 1979.

7

Fluid Management

DONALD S. PROUGH

NEAL H. COHEN

Neurosurgical patients present a complex fluid management problem. They require, as do all other surgical patients, sufficient fluid of appropriate electrolyte composition to maintain circulatory and metabolic homeostasis. However, excessive or inappropriate fluid administration may increase intracranial pressure (ICP) sufficiently to reduce cerebral perfusion pressure (CPP), as is evident from the equation:

(CPP = mean arterial pressure − ICP)

This chapter will review the physiologic background for fluid and electrolyte management of neurosurgical patients and will emphasize special fluid and electrolyte problems that arise in these patients.

I. Basic principles of fluid management
A. Provision of maintenance fluids plus abnormal losses
1. **Water and electrolyte requirements.** Neurologic and neurosurgical patients must receive adequate fluids and electrolytes to provide a sufficient proportion of normal maintenance requirements and to replace *abnormal* losses such as those produced by gastric suction or profuse diarrhea. Water administration in patients with neurologic disease is often restricted to a fraction of the normal daily maintenance requirement of approximately 1500 ml/m^2/day. Two convenient formulas for calculating daily and hourly fluid requirements in patients *without* neurologic disease are shown below:

	ml/kg/day	ml/kg/hr
1st–10th kg	100	4
11th–20th kg	50	2
21st–nth kg	20	1

By these formulas, before adjusting for fluid restriction, a 70-kg individual would receive 2500 ml/day or 110 ml/hr.

Usual external losses of water and electrolytes include gastrointestinal (primarily fecal losses of 100–200 ml/day) and insensible losses averaging 500 to 1000 ml/day. Urinary output, normally 1000 to 1500 ml/day, is not counted as a loss when fluid requirements are calculated because of the regulatory capacity of the neuroendocrine system and kidneys. If those systems are functioning normally, an increase in urinary output implies volume expansion rather than increased fluid needs. Insensible losses from cutaneous evaporation and respiratory gas humidification, normally about 800 ml/day, increase as minute ventilation increases in patients who are spontaneously breathing through a natural airway. In contrast, respiratory losses are minimal in patients who are breathing humidified gases through a ventilator circuit. Insensible losses increase by about 10% for every 1°C increase in body temperature above 37°C.

The daily renal excretion of sodium, the principal cation responsible for maintaining the normal osmolality of the extracellular fluid compartment, is 70 to 75 mEq. Replacement with 75 mEq sodium/day (2.5 L of a solution containing 30 mEq/L) prevents a negative sodium balance, although the kidneys are capable of greater sodium conservation if 4 to 7 days are permitted for adaptation. Because the normal kidneys and endocrine system easily accommodate for variations in sodium administration, adult patients commonly receive 0.45% saline, containing 77 mEq sodium (Na^+) per liter. Most of the 3200 mEq of potassium contained in the average 70-kg adult is intracellular; only about 2% is extracellular. Obligatory daily potassium loss in a patient who has normal renal function includes urinary excretion of 25 to 30 mEq and stool losses of 12 mEq, well below the normal daily oral intake of 40 to 120 mEq/day. Parenteral replacement of potassium should be at least 40 to 50 mEq/day (approximately 2.5 L of a solution containing 20 mEq/L) in the patient who has no oral intake.

2. **Sources of water and electrolytes.** Intravenous fluid administration supplements water and electrolytes available from the diet and endogenous metabolism. Although the normal diet provides about 1800 to 2000 ml of water each day, neurologically impaired patients will frequently ingest less because of obtundation, anorexia, inability to swallow, abnormal thirst mechanisms, nausea, and vomiting. In catabolic states, endogenous water production, normally minimal, may increase to as much as 500 to 1500 ml/day, including 150 ml/kg from oxidation of protein and 1080 ml/kg from oxidation of fat.

In neurosurgical patients, water intake is customarily restricted to one-half to two-thirds of normal maintenance amounts to limit the accumulation of cerebral edema. Because of the special hazards of intracranial hypertension and reduced CPP, plans for maintenance and replacement fluid administration should include careful consideration of the distribution volumes of various fluid choices (see sec. **I.B**). Replacement of abnormal water and electrolyte losses should include an estimate or analysis of the electrolyte composition of the lost fluid. Insensible losses, nearly sodium free, can be replaced with free water. Gastrointestinal losses, which generally contain substantial concentrations of sodium and potassium, can be replaced with

0.9% saline, containing potassium 20 mEq/L, if the kidneys and cardiovascular system are functioning well. If losses secondary to pharmacologic diuresis require replacement, 0.45% saline containing
potassium 20 mEq/L is appropriate.

Short-term parenteral fluid therapy usually requires no supplementation of electrolytes other than sodium and potassium. Calcium is readily mobilized from bone in adults. Children, however,
require calcium replacement (calcium gluconate 200 to 300 mEq/kg/
day in divided doses) if they are not receiving adequate oral calcium
intake. Magnesium deficiency, a common occurrence in critically ill
individuals, is unlikely to occur in previously healthy patients during
short-term hospitalization. Phosphate deficiency, which may produce
sufficient weakness to impede weaning from mechanical ventilation,
also becomes a concern in patients who require long-term parenteral
fluid therapy. Calcium, magnesium [6,27], phosphate, zinc, and trace
minerals should be provided for the patient who receives parenteral
fluids without enteral intake for more than 5 to 7 days.

3. **Caloric requirements.** Glucose is commonly included in maintenance fluid therapy, although in amounts that at most will partially
reduce protein catabolism in nonseptic, fasting patients. A fasting
70-kg adult catabolizes 80 gm of protein each day. Administration of
100 gm of glucose (2 L of 5% dextrose solution daily) reduces this
loss by about one-half. Glucose also reduces depletion of liver glycogen, limits mobilization of fatty acids, and minimizes starvation ketosis. In patients who require intensive parenteral nutritional support,
glucose is a primary source of maintenance caloric needs, with fat
generally providing 25 to 33% of necessary calories.

However, glucose administration in patients with potential neurologic ischemia must be carefully controlled to limit hyperglycemia.
Animal and clinical studies clearly demonstrate that hyperglycemia
aggravates ischemic neurologic injury [14,23]. Therefore, it seems
prudent to eliminate glucose from fluids given rapidly for volume
expansion (e.g., for patients with head injury associated with hemorrhage from systemic injuries). In patients at risk for ongoing neurologic injury, such as those receiving intensive monitoring and care
following closed head injury, nutritional support should be rigor-
ously monitored to recognize and correct hyperglycemia.

B. **Distribution volumes of fluid and electrolytes.** Exogenously administered fluid and electrolytes are distributed within total body water,
which in turn consists of three distinct compartments: the plasma volume, the interstitial volume, and the intracellular volume.

The normal distribution of body water for a 70-kg male is summarized
in Figure 7-1. In the average young, lean individual, total body water is
approximately 60% of total body weight (42 L in a 70-kg person). Of that
volume, the intracellular two-thirds (approximately 28 L) contains a low

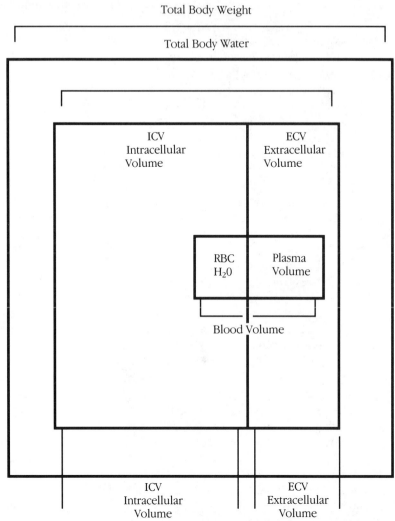

Fig. 7-1. Graphic representation of body compartments. Total body water constitutes 60% of total body weight (42 L in a 70-kg individual); extracellular volume (ECV) equals 20% and intracellular volume (ICV) equals 40% (14 and 28 L respectively); plasma volume is 4% of body weight; plasma volume (part of extracellular volume) and red cell volume (part of intracellular volume) constitute the blood volume. RBC = red blood cells.

concentration of sodium and a high concentration of potassium. The extracellular one-third of total body water consists of the interstitial volume, approximately 11 L, and the plasma volume (PV), about 3 L. Extracellular volume contains higher concentrations of sodium, normally about 140 mEq/L. Although the electrolyte composition of PV and interstitial volume are similar, plasma contains a fourfold greater concentration of albumin, which exerts oncotic pressure that tends to oppose filtration of plasma from the capillary bed.

The distribution of any exogenous fluid can be inferred from the above concepts, according to the following formula:

$$\frac{PV\ increment}{Volume\ infused} = \frac{PV}{Distribution\ volume}$$

Intravenous fluids that contain sodium in concentrations approximately that of serum (i.e., 0.9% saline or lactated Ringer's solution) are primarily distributed within the extracellular volume. Sodium-free water (i.e., 5% dextrose in water) is uniformly distributed across total body water. Saline (0.45%) is distributed proportionately between the extracellular and intracellular spaces; slightly more than one-half (equivalent to 550 ml of 0.9% saline) remains within the extracellular volume while the other half (equivalent to 450 ml of free water) distributes across total body water. Hyperoncotic fluids, such as 25% albumin or 6% hydroxyethylstarch, draw fluid from the interstitium into the PV, with the amount of transcapillary fluid movement dependent on the difference between plasma and interstitial oncotic pressure and the integrity of the capillary membranes. Hypertonic fluids that are distributed primarily extracellularly, such as 20% mannitol or 3% saline, osmotically draw fluid from the intracellular to the extracellular space.

Central nervous system tissue contains, as do other metabolically active tissues, a higher concentration of water than do tissues such as bone and fat. The distribution of water among PV, interstitial fluid (ISF), and intracellular fluid (ICF) in the brain is governed by one important physiologic factor in addition to those operating in nonnervous tissue. The blood-brain barrier, the cerebral capillary membrane, is poorly permeable to sodium and nearly impermeable to protein. In contrast, sodium and protein move freely from capillaries to the interstitial space in peripheral tissues. Therefore, sudden increases in serum sodium concentration will osmotically attract water into the intracranial capillaries both from the brain intracellular and interstitial spaces.

Blood volume, which includes both the PV and the volume of the red cells, normally varies as a function of gender, age, and body fat. Though rarely measured for clinical purposes, blood volume must be estimated when planning blood and fluid replacement and when resuscitating patients in shock. The estimates in Figure 7-2 apply to individuals of varying body habitus.

The average adult five L of blood volume includes two L of red blood cells and three L of plasma. Within the vasculature, the majority of blood volume is in the capacitance (venous) circulation. If the capacitance bed dilates secondary to the administration of anesthetic drugs or to a change from the supine to the sitting or upright position, cardiac filling

	Fat	Thin	Normal	Muscular
Male	6.0	6.5	7.0	7.5
Female	5.5	6.0	6.5	7.0

Fig. 7-2. Blood volume expressed as a percentage of total body weight for individuals of varying body habitus.

pressure will decline and cardiac output may fall. In contrast, the supine or head-down position can redistribute intravascular volume to the central circulation. The resulting increase in jugular venous pressure can increase ICP and reduce CPP in the neurosurgical patient who has reduced intracranial compliance.

C. **Regulation of intravascular volume.** The kidneys, through processes mediated in part by the neuroendocrine system, regulate both the volume and the total solute concentration (osmolality) of the fluid compartments within a narrow range, despite wide variations in water and electrolyte intake. The kidneys can modify volume and solute concentration by three mechanisms: filtration, reabsorption, and secretion. Glomerular filtration changes in response to alterations in blood pressure, atrial pressure, and sympathetic tone. In the distal renal tubule, sodium reabsorption is controlled by aldosterone. In the collecting ducts, water reabsorption is controlled by antidiuretic hormone. Because of the extraordinary flexibility of these control mechanisms, a normal adult can excrete an average daily obligatory solute load in a daily urinary volume varying from 0.5 to 17.0 L. Urinary sodium concentration can be reduced to as little as 2.0 mEq/L in response to sodium depletion, or it can substantially exceed the serum concentration in hypernatremic, hypervolemic patients. Urinary osmolality can vary from 50 mOsm/L in hyponatremic, volume-expanded patients to 1400 mOsm/L if the secretion of antidiuretic hormone is maximal.

II. Surgical considerations
A. Preoperative assessment
1. **Assessment of intravascular volume.** Neurosurgical patients who have evidence of altered intracranial compliance pose a challenge both in assessing the adequacy of intravascular volume and managing perioperative fluids. Insufficient fluid therapy can reduce intravascular volume, cardiac output, and organ perfusion. The opposite extreme, excessive fluid administration, may cause or exacerbate brain swelling, increase ICP, and decrease CPP.

The clinical assessment of intravascular volume status is imperfect. Normal skin turgor, moist mucous membranes, and urinary output of at least 0.5 to 1.0 ml/kg/hr suggest adequate volume expansion. However, substantial intravascular depletion may be present despite apparently normal findings. The "tilt test," often used to assess fluid deficits in adults, refers to an increase of 20 beats per minute in the heart rate and a decline of 20 mmHg in the systolic blood pressure on assuming the upright position. Because compensatory mechanisms can maintain blood pressure in the supine position despite a 30% deficit of intravascular volume, orthostatic stress will often demonstrate otherwise inapparent hypovolemia. In young, previously healthy adults, a positive tilt test implies an intravascular deficit of 20% of total blood volume (approximately 1000 ml). However, elderly patients, chronically bedridden patients, and patients on chronic antihypertensive medications may "tilt" despite a normal or slightly reduced blood volume.

Neurosurgical patients often are mildly hypovolemic. Virtually all elective neurosurgical patients have undergone eight or more hours of preoperative fluid restriction. This deficit amounts to about 800 to 1000 ml of water and 30 mEq of sodium in a 70-kg adult. In patients with reduced intracranial compliance, the sodium deficit can be replaced with only 200 to 300 ml of lactated Ringer's solution or with 0.9% saline; replacement of the water deficit with sodium-free water will tend to exacerbate intracranial hypertension and will contribute little to intraoperative hemodynamic stability.

Many neurosurgical patients have been subjected to fluid restriction in an attempt to limit brain edema, and some patients have received osmotic and loop diuretics to reduce ICP. Osmotherapy, by increasing urinary output, will limit the utility of that monitor of the adequacy of intravascular volume. Patients with acute closed head injury represent a particularly difficult problem because of associated visceral and peripheral injuries. Closed wounds can mask significant blood loss; femoral fractures or retroperitoneal bleeding may sequester 500 to 1500 ml of blood. Blood and fluid losses from open wounds, though visually obvious, are difficult to quantify. The hand and fist rule, a useful guide to quantitating traumatic hemorrhage, states that each hand required to cover a wound or each fist required to fill a wound represents about a 10% blood volume deficit.

2. **Electrolyte imbalance.** Hyponatremia frequently complicates neurologic disease. Hyponatremia always represents a relative excess of total body water in relationship to sodium. Most hyponatremic patients have excess free water accounting for the low serum sodium concentration, despite normal total body sodium stores (Fig. 7-3). Severe or precipitous reductions in serum sodium can increase ICP and precipitate seizures. Exogenous water overload must be differentiated from the syndrome of inappropriate antidiuretic hormone secretion (SIADH) (see sec. **III.C**) and from the "salt-wasting syndrome" that occasionally accompanies acute brain disease [2,9]. Hyponatremia may also occur because of hypovolemia [7]; in effect, a

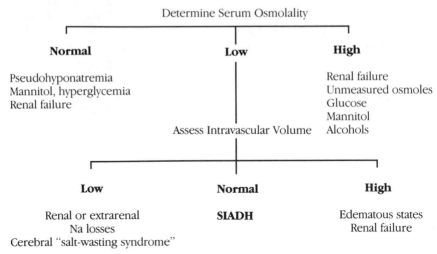

Fig. 7-3. Abbreviated diagnostic approach to hyponatremia. Na = sodium; SIADH = syndrome of inappropriate diuretic hormone.

sufficiently severe sodium deficit will initiate physiologic control mechanisms, including antidiuretic hormone (ADH) release, that sacrifice tonicity to preserve intravascular volume. This situation may occur in patients who have undergone prolonged diuresis without adequate sodium replacement.

Hypernatremia usually reflects a deficit of total body water and normal or less severely reduced total body sodium. Because water constitutes such a large proportion of total body mass, relatively small increases in serum sodium reflect large water deficits. The water deficit (WD) can be estimated from the following equation:

$$WD = \frac{[\text{Measured serum Na}^+ - 140]}{140} \times 0.60 \times \text{weight (kg)}$$

where 140 is the normal serum Na and 0.60 is the average fraction of body weight that represents total body water.

Diabetes insipidus, an occasional complication of closed head trauma and a more common occurrence following pituitary surgery, may result in very rapid water loss and severe hypernatremia. Isolated water deficits must be differentiated from sodium excess, as occasionally occurs with rapid administration of solutions containing concentrated sodium salts (e.g., sodium bicarbonate). Urine and serum electrolytes and osmolalities are useful in differentiating the etiology of hypernatremia.

3. **Effect of underlying diseases.** Nonneurologic disease often influences perioperative fluid and electrolyte management. For exam-

ple, hypertensive patients may be intravascularly volume depleted despite abnormally high systemic blood pressure. Chronic hypertension also alters autoregulation of cerebral blood flow (CBF), increasing both the upper and lower limits (i.e., the autoregulatory curve is displaced to the right, see Fig. 7-4). Such patients may not tolerate low CPP secondary to the often exaggerated hypotension that follows anesthetic induction in patients who have unrecognized hypovolemia.

Impaired myocardial function reduces physiologic tolerance both for excess and for inadequate fluid administration. In particularly fragile patients, a pulmonary artery catheter will allow measurement of intracardiac filling pressures and cardiac output and calculation of peripheral vascular resistance. These data supplement other clinical estimates of fluid requirements. Although the pulmonary capillary wedge pressure (PCWP) is normally 6 to 12 mmHg, systemic hypoperfusion may warrant an increase to 15 to 18 mmHg. Further increases are unlikely to produce further increments in cardiac output and may precipitate pulmonary edema. If a central venous pressure (CVP) catheter is used, the normal range of 4 to 8 mmHg provides a guide to fluid requirements. Quantitation of cardiovascular function in patients who have both limited cardiac reserve and impaired

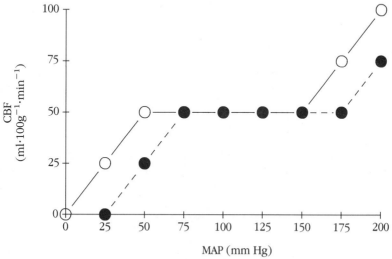

Fig. 7-4. The normal cerebral autoregulatory curve (open circles connected by solid lines) is associated with unchanged cerebral blood flow between a mean arterial pressure (MAP) (or cerebral perfusion pressure) ranging from 50 to 150 mm Hg. In chronically hypertensive individuals, however, the autoregulatory curve is shifted rightward (closed circles, dotted lines). Therefore, CBF begins to decline at a higher level of mean arterial pressure, but also remains constant until mean arterial pressure is increased to a greater level than in normal patients.

intracranial compliance facilitates precise management of CPP through the use of a rational combination of fluids, osmotic diuretics, vasodilators, and vasopressors.

B. Intraoperative management

1. Fluid management. Preoperative fluid deficits and intraoperative blood and fluid losses must be adequately replaced during neurosurgical procedures while avoiding the complications of injudicious fluid administration, such as increased cerebral edema and ICP, reduced CPP, or worsened cerebral ischemia. In most neurosurgical patients, fluids, such as lactated Ringer's solution or 0.9% saline, that contain sodium in a concentration similar to that of serum are administered in a volume sufficient to maintain peripheral perfusion while avoiding hypervolemia. Usually, less fluid is given than would be administered for nonneurologic surgery. For the patient who has underlying cardiovascular or renal disease, invasive hemodynamic monitoring may facilitate management.

Unless hypoglycemia is likely, dextrose-containing solutions are best avoided during neurosurgical procedures because of the risk of exacerbating ischemic damage. Dextrose in combination with free water (D5.45% saline or D5W) is contraindicated because the free water will rapidly equilibrate throughout all intracranial fluid compartments. The resulting brain edema may interfere with surgical exposure or, if the skull is closed, compromise cerebral perfusion.

Fluid therapy is most challenging during prolonged surgical procedures or surgical management of multiple trauma. If tissue trauma is severe or if hemorrhage has been prolonged, patients develop a marked reduction in functional extracellular volume as a result of internal redistribution of fluids ("third space" losses; Fig. 7-5). Although the extent of tissue manipulation in most routine neurosurgical procedures is small, third-space fluid losses during prolonged surgery and in patients with severe associated systemic trauma can be sufficient to decrease intravascular volume, reduce peripheral perfusion, and impair renal function. The sequestered extracellular fluid can be cautiously replaced with lactated Ringer's solution or with 0.9% saline [20]. In the absence of diuretic therapy, a urinary output of 0.5 to 1.0 ml/kg/hr suggests adequate replacement, as do hemodynamic stability and cardiac filling pressures within the normal range. Although some clinicians prefer colloid-containing solutions in neurosurgical patients, such solutions appear to exert negligible effects on brain water and ICP [1].

Recent experimental evidence and a limited amount of clinical data suggest that hypertonic, hypernatremic fluids might be valuable for acute fluid resuscitation of patients who have both limited intracranial compliance and hypovolemia. [19,26]. Small volumes of hypertonic, hypernatremic solutions (most recent data describe the use

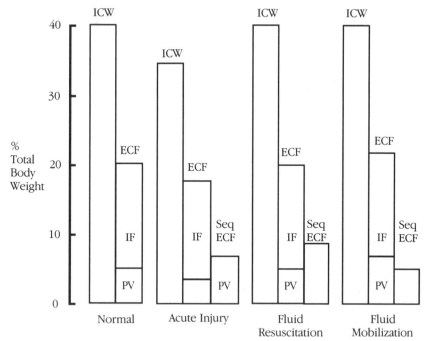

Fig. 7-5. Fluid sequestration during injury, resuscitation, and fluid mobilization. ICW = intracellular water; ECF = extracellular fluid; IF = interstitial fluid; PV = plasma volume.

of approximately 7.5% saline) effectively restore cardiac output following the loss of substantially larger volumes of blood or other fluids [19]. Because the hemodynamic improvement is no more prolonged than that following conventional isotonic fluid resuscitation, the primary utility of hypertonic fluids will likely be for acute hemodynamic stabilization.

2. **Hyperosmotic diuretic agents.** The intraoperative management of patients often includes intravenous administration of hyperosmotic diuretics. If the blood-brain barrier is intact, mannitol, urea, and glycerol decrease ICP by increasing plasma osmotic pressure, thereby reducing brain interstitial and intracellular volume [17]. Osmotic diuretics may also lower cerebrospinal fluid (CSF) pressure by reducing the rate of CSF production. Because in some patients these drugs initially increase cerebral blood volume and ICP, they are usually given in conjunction with other maneuvers to decrease intracranial volume (such as steroids, hyperventilation, or CSF drainage). Hyperosmotic drugs have been associated with "rebound" increases in ICP in patients with disruption of the blood-brain barrier.

Mannitol, the most commonly used osmotic agent, produces few acute complications. Mannitol is given as a rapid intravenous infusion in a dose of 0.25 to 1.50 gm/kg. Although larger doses may provide a longer duration of action, they do not reduce ICP more effectively. Large doses, because they markedly increase intravascular volume, risk pulmonary edema in patients who have impaired myocardial function. Protracted osmotic diuresis may produce dehydration, electrolyte disturbances, and impaired renal function. Prolonged use mandates careful monitoring of serum electrolytes and osmolality.

3. **Other diuretics.** The loop diuretics furosemide and ethacrynic acid reduce ICP, both by inducing diuresis and by directly diminishing CSF formation. [8,21]. Although commonly used intraoperatively, loop diuretics are less frequently used in the management of chronically increased ICP. Because the loop diuretics do not increase intravascular volume, they represent an appropriate alternative to osmotic diuretics when ICP must be reduced in patients with left ventricular dysfunction who may not tolerate the transient increase in intravascular volume associated with mannitol. In such patients, diuresis may also indirectly lower ICP by improving oxygenation and carbon dioxide elimination.

C. Postoperative management

1. **Management of fluid administration.** The underlying principle of fluid management following most neurosurgical procedures is the limitation of fluid to the least volume compatible with the preservation of adequate systemic perfusion. Although most data suggest that the rate and composition of maintenance fluid therapy exert minimal effects on ICP and brain water, intravenous fluids customarily are administered at a rate of about one-half to two-thirds of maintenance requirements in both children and adults. This amount will usually maintain adequate intravascular volume and a urinary ouput of 0.5 to 1.0 ml/kg/hr during the first 24 to 48 hours following surgery. If osmotic or loop diuretics have been used, a rapid decline in urinary output to less than 0.5 ml/kg/hr suggests hypovolemia, while a sustained diuresis suggests adequate intravascular volume. Peripheral pulses, skin color, and temperature provide additional, though occasionally misleading, information regarding the adequacy of peripheral perfusion. Neurosurgical patients generally tolerate postoperative fluid restriction well because losses secondary to fluid sequestration are not profound.

Intake and output are carefully measured during the postoperative period, both as a guide to the accumulation of total body sodium and water and to observe for complications of neurologic disease (e.g., diabetes insipidus or SIADH). Accurate daily weight measurements, when compared to preoperative weight, also provide indirect data regarding total body water, although they may not correlate well with intravascular volume.

If empirical fluid management is unsatisfactory, measurement of intracardiac filling pressures and cardiac output may facilitate postoperative volume management. Ideally, CVP and PCWP should be maintained in the low normal range, if that can be achieved while still ensuring adequate systemic perfusion. If intracranial compliance is low, an elevated CVP may increase ICP. If systemic hypoperfusion, manifested by oliguria, peripheral hypoperfusion, or metabolic (lactic) acidosis, occurs at normal filling pressures, cautious additional volume expansion is indicated. If hypoperfusion does not resolve, inotropic support should be considered. Dopamine and dobutamine, the most common choices, will increase cardiac output. However, dopamine will tend to increase CVP and CBF, thereby potentially increasing ICP; dobutamine sometimes causes hypotension, which may further compromise CPP.

An essential component of postoperative fluid management is close monitoring for the development of clinical signs of cerebral edema. Monitoring of ICP, when available, will provide evidence of postoperative edema or hematoma that might compromise neurologic outcome.

2. **Crystalloid versus colloid solutions.** Crystalloid solutions (lactated Ringer's solution or normal saline) are preferred in the intraoperative and postoperative periods. If the blood-brain barrier is intact, both sodium and colloid will remain within the intracranial capillary bed. Some experimental data suggest that rapid volume expansion with colloid solutions will maintain intravascular volume with less risk of precipitating intracranial hypertension [18]. However, if the blood-brain barrier is compromised, colloid-containing solutions will tend to equilibrate with brain interstitial fluid, thereby reducing or abolishing the desired oncotic effect [25,28]. One unresolved question is whether albumin should be administered to chronically ill neurosurgical patients, particularly those with head trauma, who often demonstrate profound hypoalbuminemia [16].

3. **Postoperative fluid mobilization and diuresis.** During the acute phase of surgical management, perioperative fluids must often be given in greater than usual maintenance volumes. As recovery proceeds, often 48 to 72 hours following the insult, third space fluid accumulation will resolve (Fig. 7-5), resulting in an increase in intravascular volume that must then be excreted by the kidneys. Because the mobilization implies an excess of both total body sodium and water, minimal intravenous fluid is necessary during this phase. Usually, spontaneous diuresis is sufficient; however, if the cardiovascular or renal systems cannot compensate for the increased load, loop diuretics may be necessary.

4. **Special considerations in the neurosurgical patient.** Osmotherapy is sometimes necessary in the postoperative period. Circumstances in which mannitol might be useful include intracranial

hypertension secondary to cerebral edema or acute postoperative intracranial hematoma. For postoperative brain edema, doses of 0.25 gm/kg will reduce ICP and can be given repeatedly. Because mannitol given in multiple doses may produce dehydration, hyperosmolality, and electrolyte disturbances, the urine and serum electrolytes and osmolality should be monitored closely. In general, if serum osmolality exceeds 320 mOsm/L, mannitol is withheld. If mannitol is required because of postoperative intracranial bleeding, it is usually given in a large dose of 1.0 to 1.5 gm/kg to rapidly reduce ICP, pending definitive surgical decompression.

Fluid management and cardiovascular support represent particular challenges in patients who receive barbiturates for cerebral protection or elevated ICP in the postoperative period. Barbiturates, when given in doses sufficient to induce coma, depress myocardial contractility and cause systemic vasodilatation. Consequently, the maintenance of hemodynamic stability often requires aggressive intravenous fluid administration to maintain adequate cardiac preload. A pulmonary artery catheter may facilitate systemic hemodynamic support in these patients. Fluid therapy and inotropic-vasopressor support can be titrated using measurements of PCWP and cardiac output to achieve satisfactory peripheral perfusion without aggravating intracranial hypertension. As patients are weaned from barbiturate therapy, they will usually spontaneously diurese, although some may require pharmacologic diuresis.

Patients who develop clinical or angiographic evidence of cerebral vasospasm, either after subarachnoid hemorrhage or craniotomy for aneurysm clip-ligation, present a particular problem of fluid management. Because some brain regions will have "fixed" increases in cerebrovascular resistance, dehydration and/or hypotension may substantially reduce CBF, resulting in a temporary or permanent deterioration in neurologic function. Recent experience suggests that patients who have evidence of vasospasm may improve if intravascular volume is aggressively expanded, usually with blood or colloid [4,10,24]. If there is no risk of rebleeding (i.e., if the aneurysm has been clipped), mean arterial pressure can be maintained in the high-normal range using vasoconstrictor and/or inotropic support as tolerated. Hemodynamic monitoring may be helpful in such patients. Recent evidence suggests that certain calcium entry blocking drugs will reverse vasospasm and improve CBF. To date, the ideal combination of cerebral vasodilatation and systemic hypervolemia and hypertension has not been established and may well vary among individual patients. In other neurologic insults, such as acute stroke, the effects of hemodilution have been less impressive [12,22].

III. Specific fluid and electrolyte problems in the neurosurgical patient

  A. Neurogenic pulmonary edema. Central neurogenic pulmonary edema occasionally complicates life-threatening neurologic disease. Reported in association with severe head trauma, intracranial mass lesions, subarachnoid hemorrhage, intraventricular hemorrhage, stroke, seizures, Guillain-Barré syndrome, and hypothalamic lesions, neurogenic pulmonary edema often occurs despite a previously normal cardiopulmonary system. Although the etiology remains controversial [15], neurogenic pulmonary edema may have elements of both hydrostatic and permeability edema. The hydrostatic component purportedly occurs in relation to the massive, often transient, alpha-adrenergic discharge associated with acute neurologic catastrophe. The resulting systemic and pulmonary hypertension increases the left atrial and pulmonary capillary pressures, producing hydrostatic edema accumulation, and disrupts the pulmonary capillary endothelium, producing capillary leakage of high-protein fluid. In the most severe cases, profuse pulmonary edema may virtually preclude adequate oxygenation and carbon dioxide elimination.

  The most effective treatment of neurogenic pulmonary edema is elimination of the cause (i.e., evacuation of an intracranial hematoma or control of severe intracranial hypertension). Supportive care is similar to the treatment of adult respiratory distress syndrome (ARDS) (see Chap. 5). Carbon dioxide elimination is accomplished with mechanical ventilation, and oxygenation is supported with positive end-expiratory pressure (PEEP). As in any pulmonary capillary leak syndrome, fluid therapy should be limited to the least volume compatible with adequate systemic perfusion because of the aggravation of fluid accumulation associated with increases in pulmonary microvascular pressure. Crystalloid solutions appear to be preferable to colloid-containing solutions in situations where pulmonary capillary integrity may be compromised. Hemodynamic monitoring may help the clinician achieve the difficult balance among intravascular volume, pulmonary gas exchange, systemic perfusion, and cerebral perfusion and may provide useful information regarding the appropriate use of inotropic and systemic vasodilator therapy.

  B. Diabetes insipidus. Acute diabetes insipidus occurs as a consequence of posterior pituitary or pituitary stalk injury. It is an infrequent complication of closed head trauma, skull fractures, and neurosurgical procedures, especially those involving the pituitary gland. Decreased secretion of ADH from the posterior pituitary gland results in water diuresis, progressive dehydration, and hypernatremia. Urinary output may exceed 700 ml/hr; despite serum hyperosmolality, the urine remains dilute.

Diabetes insipidus must be distinguished from solute diuresis induced by vigorous intravenous fluid administration or radiographic contrast media and from diuretic-induced polyuria. The diagnosis depends on the demonstration that the dilute polyuria is nonhomeostatic (i.e., that the patient is unable to concentrate urine or reduce urinary volume even when polyuria leads to hypovolemia or hypernatremia). Characteristically, the excessive urinary output is associated with urinary osmolality that is inappropriately low (60–200 mOsm) relative to serum osmolality and with urinary specific gravity less than 1.005.

The management of diabetes insipidus is both supportive and pharmacologic. Input and output must be carefully monitored because of the rapidity with which hypovolemia and hypernatremia may ensue. Other valuable monitors include serum and urinary electrolytes and osmolality, urinary specific gravity, blood urea nitrogen (BUN), creatinine, and frequent weight determinations. An awake, alert patient who can tolerate oral hydration will usually ingest sufficient water to maintain electrolyte balance and euvolemia. If fluid must be replaced in a patient who cannot regulate fluid intake, solutions containing low concentrations of sodium should be given to replace water losses. However, intravenous administration of large quantities of 5.0% dextrose will produce hyperglycemia that will result in superimposition of glycosuria-induced polyuria on diabetes insipidus. If total losses are modest, 5.0% dextrose in 0.2% saline plus supplemental potassium will replace the hourly urine output plus estimated insensible losses. If the urine output remains excessive (>200–250 ml/hr) or if maintaining fluid balance is difficult, DDAVP (1-desamino-8-D-arginine vasopressin) or aqueous vasopressin will reduce urinary output. DDAVP, considered the drug of choice because of its limited systemic effects, is given in a dose of 1 to 2 μg SC or IV BID. The dose of vasopressin is 5 to 10 IU IM or SC to control excessive urinary output. As output decreases, intravenous or oral fluid intake can be tapered. Since the duration of diabetes insipidus is variable, further pharmacologic treatment is dictated by the recurrence of polyuria. If long-term therapy is required, desmopressin spray can be administered intranasally as needed to control urinary output.

Diabetes insipidus also commonly develops as a manifestation of brain death. If the brain-dead patient is a potential organ donor, careful management of the diabetes insipidus is essential to preserve the viability of the transplantable organs. In combination with vasodilatation, hypovolemia may result in grossly inadequate perfusion of potentially lifesaving organs, particularly in combination with systemic vasodilatation, which occurs with brain death.

C. SIADH. A wide variety of central nervous system disorders, including head trauma, tumor, subarachnoid hemorrhage, and brain abscess, is associated with inappropriate secretion of ADH [3]. Usually self-limited, SIADH most commonly develops 3 to 15 days following trauma or surgery and resolves in fewer than 7 days. The excessive ADH secretion causes continued renal excretion of sodium despite hyponatremia and associated hypo-osmolality. Urine osmolality is therefore high relative to serum osmolality. The patient who has SIADH has no clinical evidence of dehydration; renal and adrenal function are normal. The clinical manifestations of SIADH are variable, depending on the severity of the hyponatremia and the rapidity with which it develops. If the serum sodium falls slowly, even to 120 mEq/L, symptoms are mild. If the hyponatremia occurs more quickly, symptoms include anorexia, nausea, vomiting, irritability, and hyperreflexia, which may progress to seizures, stupor, and coma.

The mainstay of treatment for these water-overloaded, euvolemic patients is water restriction (500 ml/day). If the hyponatremia is severe (serum sodium < than 110 mEq/L), hypertonic (3–5%) saline will return serum sodium toward normal. Because of the rapid increase in extracellular and intravascular volume produced by hypertonic saline, it must be used with caution and patients must be carefully monitored to avoid development of acute pulmonary edema. An alternative treatment regimen for rapid correction of hyponatremia is the administration of 0.9% saline in combination with a loop diuretic. Because the sodium concentration of diuretic-induced urinary losses is usually less than that of 0.9% saline, serum sodium will increase. That approach is sound in patients who have limited cardiac reserve and require rapid partial correction of hyponatremia.

In the absence of severe neurologic complications of hyponatremia, the serum sodium should be gradually corrected. Recently, the syndrome of central pontine myelinolysis has been described in patients who have undergone excessively rapid correction of hyponatremia [5]. When pharmacologic treatment is desirable for more chronic SIADH, demeclocycline is effective [11].

D. Nonketotic hyperglycemic hyperosmolar coma. Nonketotic hyperglycemic hyperosmolar coma (NHHC) [13] complicates a variety of neurosurgical conditions, including intracerebral hemorrhage, head trauma, brain tumor, and cerebral infarction. About two-thirds of patients who have NHHC have no history of diabetes mellitus. Many have concurrent infections, are taking drugs that alter glucose tolerance (e.g., steroids, phenytoin, thiazides), or are dehydrated as a consequence of inadequate fluid intake, hyperosmolar tube feedings, and prolonged osmotherapy.

The diagnostic features of NHHC include hyperglycemia (blood sugar 400–2500 mg/100 ml), glycosuria, and plasma osmolality exceeding 330 mOsm/L in the absence of ketosis. Dehydration and often potassium depletion accompany the osmotic diuresis. Prerenal azotemia, a common finding, can, if untreated, progress to acute renal failure.

Treatment must correct both hypovolemia and hypertonicity. Saline (0.9%) is initially infused to restore the extracellular volume. Although 0.9% saline exceeds normal serum osmolality, it will gradually reduce the even greater osmolality of the patient with NHHC. In patients who have underlying cardiac disease, sufficient volume expansion may require the use of a thermodilution pulmonary artery catheter to measure cardiac filling pressures and cardiac output. After the extracellular volume deficit is corrected with 0.9% saline, the water deficit should be replaced more gradually with 0.2 or 0.45% saline. Excessively rapid reduction of hypertonicity may precipitate cerebral edema.

Hyperglycemia in NHHC is usually sensitive to insulin therapy. Small doses of insulin given as a continuous hourly infusion (1–10 U/hr) will often correct hyperglycemia. Abrupt reduction of the blood sugar may be harmful. The osmotic force exerted by hyperglycemia pulls water from the intracellular space into the PV. Therefore, excessively rapid reduction of blood glucose may result in cerebral edema as water osmotically moves into the brain and may produce hypovolemia as water returns along osmotic gradients from the PV into the intracellular space.

References

1. Albright, A. L., Latchaw, R. E., and Robinson, A. G. Intracranial and systemic effects of osmotic and oncotic therapy in experimental cerebral edema. *J. Neurosurg.* 60:481, 1984.
2. Al-Mufti, H., and Arieff, A. Hyponatremia due to cerebral salt-wasting syndrome: Combined cerebral and distal tubular lesion. *Am. J. Med.* 77:740, 1984.
3. Anderson, R. J., Chung, H.-M., Kluge, R., and Schrier, R. W. Hyponatremia: A prospective analysis of its epidemiology and the pathogenetic role of vasopressin. *Ann. Intern. Med.* 102:164, 1985.
4. Awad, I. A., Carter, L. P., Spetzler, R. F., et al. Clinical vasospasm after subarachnoid hemorrhage: Response to hypervolemic hemodilution and arterial hypertension. *Stroke* 18:365, 1987.
5. Ayus, J. C., Krothapalli, R. K., and Arieff, A. Changing concepts in treatment of severe symptomatic hyponatremia: Rapid correction and possible relation to central pontine myelinolysis. *Am. J. Med.* 78:897, 1985.
6. Chernow, B., Bamberger, S., Stoiko, M., et al. Hypomagnesemia in patients in postoperative intensive care. *Chest* 95:391, 1989.
7. Chung, H.-M., Kluge, R., Schrier, R. W., and Anderson, R. J. Clinical assessment of extracellular fluid volume in hyponatremia. *Am. J. Med.* 83:905, 1987.
8. Cottrell, J. E., Robustelli, A., Post, K., and Turndorf, H. Furosemide- and mannitol-induced changes in intracranial pressure and serum osmolality and electrolytes. *Anesthesiology* 47:28, 1977.
9. Doczi, T., Joo, F., Szerdahelyi, P., and Bodosi, M. Regulation of brain water and electrolyte contents: The possible involvement of central atrial natriuretic factor. *Neurosurgery* 21:454, 1987.

10. Finn, S. S., Stephensen, S. A., Miller, C. A., et al. Observations on the perioperative management of aneurysmal subarachnoid hemorrhage. *J. Neurosurg.* 65:48, 1986.
11. Forrest, J. N., Cox, M., Hong, C., et al. Superiority of demeclocycline over lithium in the treatment of chronic syndrome of inappropriate secretion of antidiuretic hormone. *N. Engl. J. Med.* 298:173, 1978.
12. Hemodilution in Stroke Study Group. Hypervolemic hemodilution treatment of acute stroke: Results of a randomized multicenter trial using pentastarch. *Stroke* 20:317, 1989.
13. Khardori, R., and Soler, N. G. Hyperosmolar hyperglycemic nonketotic syndrome: Report of 22 cases and brief review. *Am. J. Med.* 77:899, 1984.
14. Lanier, W. L., Stangland, K. J., Scheithauer, B. W., et al. The effects of dextrose infusion and head position on neurologic outcome after complete cerebral ischemia in primates: Examination of a model. *Anesthesiology* 66:39, 1987.
15. Malik, A. B. Mechanisms of neurogenic pulmonary edema. *Circ. Res.* 57:1, 1985.
16. McClain, C. J., Hennig, B., Oti, L. G., et al. Mechanisms and implications of hypoalbuminemia in head-injured patients. *J. Neurosurg.* 69:386, 1988.
17. Muizelaar, J. P., Lutz, H. A., III, and Becker, D. P. Effect of mannitol on ICP and CBF and correlation with pressure autoregulation in severely head-injured patients. *J. Neurosurg.* 61:700, 1984.
18. Poole, G. V., Prough, D. S., Johnson, J. C., et al. Effects of resuscitation from hemorrhagic shock on cerebral hemodynamics in the presence of an intracranial mass. *J. Trauma* 27:18, 1987.
19. Prough, D. S., Johnson, J. C., Stump, D. A., et al. Effects of hypertonic saline versus lactated Ringer's solution on cerebral oxygen transport during resuscitation from hemorrhagic shock. *J. Neurosurg.* 64:627, 1986.
20. Roberts, J. L. P., Roberts, J. D., Skinner, C., et al. Extracellular fluid deficit following operation and its correction with Ringer's lactate. *Ann. Surg.* 202:1, 1985.
21. Samson, D., and Beyer, C. W. Furosemide in the intraoperative reduction of intracranial pressure in the patient with subarachnoid hemorrhage. *Neurosurgery* 10:167, 1982.
22. Scandinavian Stroke Study Group. Multicenter trial of hemodilution in acute ischemic stroke. *Stroke* 18:691, 1987.
23. Sieber, F. E., Smith, D. S., Traystman, R. J., and Wollman, H. Glucose: A reevaluation of its intraoperative use. *Anesthesiology* 67:72, 1987.
24. Solomon, R. A., Fink, M. E., and Lennihan, L. Early aneurysm surgery and prophylactic hypervolemic hypertensive therapy for the treatment of aneurysmal subarachnoid hemorrhage. *Neurosurgery* 23:699, 1988.
25. Warner, D. S., and Boehland, L. A. Effects of iso-osmolal intravenous fluid therapy on post-ischemic brain water content in the rat. *Anesthesiology* 68:86, 1988.
26. Worthley, L. I., Cooper, D. J., and Jones, N. Treatment of resistant intracranial hypertension with hypertonic saline. Report of two cases. *J. Neurosurg.* 68:478, 1988.
27. Zaloga, G. P. Interpretation of the serum magnesium level (Editorial). *Chest* 95:257, 1989.
28. Zornow, M. H., Scheller, M. S., Todd, M. M., and Moore, S. S. Acute cerebral effects of isotonic crystalloid and colloid solutions following cryogenic brain injury in the rabbit. *Anesthesiology* 69:180, 1988.

III

Anesthetic Management

8

Intracranial Aneurysms

Neurosurgery

S.J. PEERLESS

Since 1931, when Dott [4] first operated on an intracranial aneurysm, great progress has been made in surgical and anesthetic technique, instrumentation, and results of treatment. Although the application of a clip across the base of an aneurysm remains the procedure of choice, several novel options are available for unclippable lesions. The surgeon may elect to strengthen the wall of the aneurysm through the use of gauze or plastic compounds or to induce intraluminal thrombosis by proximal ligation of feeding vessels. Also, the evolving techniques of interventional radiology hold some promise to obliterate aneurysms by the intravascular insertion of balloons.

The first use of the surgical microscope for aneurysm surgery by Lougheed in 1960 was a turning point in the operative treatment of intracranial aneurysms. The perfect coaxial light and magnification added immensely to the surgeon's precision. The use of the microscope brought with it a new generation of fine instruments and new techniques for exposing the vessels at the base of the brain and dissecting with safety around these complex branching structures.

The details made visible by high magnification have become extremely important for accurate surgical treatment of aneurysms. With the aid of the microscope, the surgeon is able to dissect the neck more precisely and to avoid injury to the tiny branching arteries in the area.

I. **Incidence and classification.** The incidence of subarachnoid hemorrhage (SAH) from ruptured intracranial aneurysms has been estimated to be approximately 15 to 20 per 100,000 population [7]; the incidence of asymptomatic aneurysms is as high as 4%.

In North America, there are approximately 30,000 new cases of SAH secondary to aneurysm rupture each year [7,8]. These figures may actually be underestimated since accurate population studies have been difficult to obtain. Of the 30,000 patients diagnosed as having SAH, 12,000 will die or become significantly disabled: 4000 will be seriously and rapidly brain injured without warning at the time of the first SAH, and 8000 will suffer recurrent hemorrhage after the initial bleed had been ignored or misdiagnosed. Of the remaining 18,000 patients available for treatment, 9000 will die or be disabled as a result of rebleeding, cerebral ischemia secondary to vasospasm, and other medical or surgical complications. Therefore, there will be only 9000 functional survivors. In view of these gloomy figures, contemporary research and therapy of intracranial aneurysms must focus on early, accurate diagnosis of SAH, recognition of aneurysms before they rupture, and elimination of the two most lethal complications: rebleeding and vasospasm.

Aneurysms are most common in the 40- to 60-year age group; 60% of all aneurysms occur in women. Aneurysms are usually classified according to location and size. The location is specified by the vessel of origin and the nearest branch vessel. Aneurysms virtually always arise at a branch or bifurcation and usually at the point where the major vessel makes a turn, changing the axial flow of blood. An aneurysm arising from the carotid artery in the crotch distal to the origin of the posterior communicating artery is called a carotid-posterior communicating aneurysm; the next most distal carotid aneurysm is labeled a carotid-choroidal aneurysm (Fig. 8-1).

After SAH, patients suffering from a ruptured intracranial aneurysm are assigned a clinical grade, depending on the presence of signs of meningeal reaction, level of consciousness, and evidence of focal neurologic dysfunction. Either Botterell's [3] original classification or the modification proposed by Hunt [6] is used by neurosurgeons to provide a means of estimating surgical risk and outcome (Table 8-1). Generally, direct surgical repair of the intracranial aneurysm in a Grade I patient can be accomplished with a low mortality. In contrast, virtually all Grade V patients will perish.

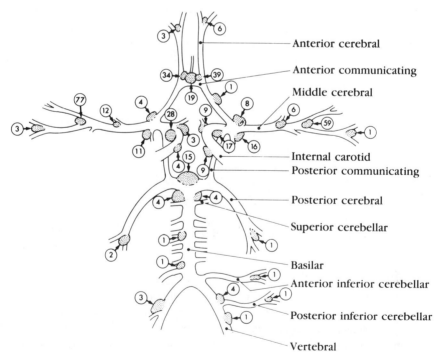

Fig. 8-1. Location of 407 aneurysms in 300 consecutive patients classified by size and location. Numbers in circles reflect the incidence.

Table 8-1. Classification of patients with
intracranial aneurysms according to surgical risk

Grade[a]	Criteria	Perioperative mortality rates (%)[b]
I	Asymptomatic, or minimal headache and slight nuchal rigidity	0–5
II	Moderate to severe headache, nuchal rigidity, no neurologic deficit other than cranial nerve palsy	2–10
III	Drowsiness, confusion, or mild focal deficit	10–15
IV	Stupor, moderate to severe hemiparesis, possibly early decerebrate rigidity and vegetative disturbances	60–70
V	Deep coma, decerebrate rigidity, moribund appearance	70–100

[a] The original classification has been revised to include Grade 0 for patients who have unruptured aneurysms and Grade Ia for patients who have a stable, residual neurologic deficit who are past the period of acute cerebral reaction.
[b] Surgical mortality varies among institutions.
Note: Serious systemic disease such as hypertension, diabetes, severe arteriosclerosis, chronic pulmonary disease, and severe vasospasm seen on arteriography result in placement of the patient in the next less favorable category.

II. Signs and symptoms of SAH

A. Results of initial rupture. The signs and symptoms of SAH result from the eruption of blood into the subarachnoid space under arterial pressure. There is an abrupt, marked rise in the intracranial pressure (ICP), which reaches or momentarily exceeds the systemic arterial pressure. This ICP wave accounts for the acute onset of a severe and excruciating headache with or without loss of consciousness. Minor hemorrhages without coma ("warning leaks") occur in about 50% of patients and may be ignored or misdiagnosed as "flu" or migraine. As the irritant blood floods through the subarachnoid pathways, a meningeal reaction occurs causing photophobia, fever, nuchal rigidity, and persistent headache. After a less severe hemorrhage, normal consciousness is rapidly regained; the patient is usually alert and oriented within 24 hours and has no focal neurologic signs. With more severe bleeds, consciousness may be impaired for days or weeks. Focal or hemispheric signs immediately after the hemorrhage are most often secondary to an intracerebral hematoma. Frequently, the sudden expansion of the aneurysm or the jet of blood will impact on an adjacent cranial nerve, resulting in a focal sign. The most common example is an oculomotor nerve palsy seen in association with a carotid-posterior communicating aneurysm.

B. Focal neurologic dysfunction. Focal neurologic dysfunction most often occurs five to nine days after the hemorrhage owing to cerebral ischemia and infarction secondary to arterial vasospasm. These clinical signs occur in 15 to 20% of patients after a major SAH and frequently may cause permanent hemiparesis, impaired consciousness, intellectual deterioration, or death.

C. Hydrocephalus. Hydrocephalus is also common after SAH owing to impaired cerebrospinal fluid (CSF) circulation through the basal cisterns. Hydrocephalus is best treated after the aneurysm has been secured because reducing the ICP increases the risk of rebleeding significantly. During surgery hydrocephalus is handled by lumbar subarachnoid drainage. The removal of excess fluid provides intracranial relaxation and improves access to the aneurysm. Only rarely is it necessary to insert a permanent shunting device to treat persistent hydrocephalus.

D. Complications of SAH. The sudden rise of ICP in association with aneurysm rupture and the reaction of the meninges and cerebral vasculature to the subarachnoid blood will commonly cause a variety of medical complications. These complications include systemic hypertension, arrhythmias, electrolyte and water disturbances, gastric erosion, and, with coma, aspiration pneumonia.

E. Diagnosis. Positive confirmation of SAH should be made by lumbar puncture, taking care to centrifuge the sample immediately and examine the supernatant for xanthochromia to differentiate between true SAH and traumatic hemorrhage caused by the spinal needle.

The noninvasive computed tomographic (CT) scan may be used in place of or in conjunction with the lumbar puncture. The CT scan may not only provide confirmation of subarachnoid blood but also information about the site and source of bleeding. Aneurysms greater than 1 cm in diameter may be located through CT scanning. Moreover, the early visualization of clot in the subarachnoid cisterns appears to be a reliable way of predicting the subsequent development of vasospasm. After confirmation of SAH, angiography is performed, using a transfemoral catheter approach, selectively injecting both carotid and vertebral arteries, and obtaining lateral, anteroposterior (AP), and often oblique projections. The studies are used to locate the source of bleeding precisely and to rule out other causes of SAH such as arteriovenous malformation (AVM) or neoplasm.

III. Preoperative care after SAH. The goals of preoperative care are to help the brain recover from the effects of SAH and to prevent recurrent hemorrhage. One must strive to maintain normal cerebral perfusion while minimizing the chance of exceeding the bursting pressure of the aneurysm. The patient should be nursed in a quiet, darkened room and given analgesics and sedation to allow sufficient sleep and rest. Phenothiazine derivatives are inadvisable as sedatives because of their variable and uncontrolled hypotensive effect. Analgesic drugs such as codeine or meperidine may be given to alleviate head and neck pain. Phenytoin is used to prevent seizures. One thousand to 1500 calories per day, excluding caffeine, should be given in a soft form to conscious patients at rest in the recumbent position. Cimetidine is used in patients who have impaired consciousness to prevent gastric erosion and hemorrhage. Patients can be fed intravenously for up to three weeks, but after this time a feeding jejunostomy should be used. Straining at stool should be avoided and, therefore, softening agents and suppositories are given routinely. Fluid balance is carefully monitored.

A. Complications

1. Rebleeding. The complications of SAH and surgical treatment of aneurysms include a lengthy list of potential problems that may cause progressive neurologic deterioration (Table 8-2). The most important of these are rebleeding and vasospasm.

Recurrent hemorrhage from an aneurysm is the most devastating complication and carries with it a high morbidity and mortality. Rebleeding from an aneurysm results when the bursting pressure within exceeds the tensile strength of either the clot or the wall of the sac. The bursting pressure is a function of the intra-arterial pressure and the surrounding ICP. Mild elevations in systemic blood pressure are common after SAH and usually respond to bed rest and sedation. If persistent elevation of blood pressure is a problem, it is controlled with loop diuretics (furosemide) and hydralazine as necessary (if the ICP is normal).

The prevention of rebleeding using antifibrinolytic agents (ϵ-aminocaproic acid [Amicar] or tranexamic acid) has been impressive but far from complete. In our experience, the rate of rebleeding has been reduced from about 20% to less than 6%. This dramatic result is not universally accepted and remains controversial. We have found that continuous infusion of ϵ-aminocaproic acid, using a calibrated pump, in a dose of 36 gm/24 hr is necessary to achieve the result.

Table 8-2. Complications of subarachnoid hemorrhage resulting in progressive neurologic deterioration in 420 patients

Complication	%
Vasospasm	33
Hyponatremia (ADH)	19
Hydrocephalus	14
Aseptic meningitis	9
Vascular occlusion	8
Surgery	6
Recurrent hemorrhage	6
Other	9

ADH = antidiuretic hormone.

Smaller doses or oral administration is not as effective in preventing the lysis of clot in the dome of the aneurysm and rebleeding. It is important to maintain the intravenous administration of ε-aminocaproic acid continuously until the patient's aneurysm has been surgically secured in the operating room. We have not noted an increase in hydrocephalus or thrombotic complications with the use of ε-aminocaproic acid. However, ε-aminocaproic acid is hyperosmolar and will produce a net loss of fluid, which should be monitored and replaced. The use of antifibrinolytic agents appears to increase the risk of vasospasm however, and the current trend to operate early, within hours or days of the initial ictus, securing the aneurysm to prevent rebleeding, has resulted in a much reduced use of ε-aminocaproic acid or similar agents [1].

Fundamentally, the goal of the preoperative therapy is to keep the blood pressure within the aneurysm below the bursting pressure of the sac. As noted, carefully controlling the systemic pressure and the ICP and preventing the lysis of the friable clot by sealing the rent in the aneurysm wall are critical in achieving this end. Using this regimen, we have limited the rate of rebleeding to less than 6%. Recurrent rebleeding, when it occurs, is usually attributable to imperfect control of either blood pressure or ICP or to the premature discontinuation of ε-aminocaproic acid.

Should rebleeding occur, the most important initial step is to control the ICP since it is the sudden explosive rise in ICP that is often so damaging. An immediate twist drill ventriculostomy and the rapid intravenous administration of mannitol (1 gm/kg) may be lifesaving. The risk of further hemorrhage is increased after recurrent hemorrhage. A second bleed that occurs during the preoperative period in a patient in less than ideal condition is often considered an indication for immediate surgery.

2. **Vasospasm.** Reactive narrowing of the cerebral arterial tree after SAH occurs in approximately 30% of patients. This narrowing, identifiable angiographically, is associated with neurologic deterioration in about half of these patients. Although the angiogram shows narrowing only in the major conducting vessels at the base of the brain and in the sylvian fissure, it is now clear from cerebral blood flow studies that cerebral perfusion is diminished and cerebral autoregulation is often lost, suggesting that the process extends to the resistance vessels as well. Focal and generalized impairment of perfusion results in cerebral ischemia and, if untreated, may progress to infarction.

Attempts at producing vasodilatation have proven ineffective; no reliable technique or pharmacologic agent appears to exist for reversing the narrowing of arteries and arterioles. This failure may be due to the fact that vasospasm may not be simply a spastic contraction or failure of relaxation of the smooth muscle cells in the media of the vessel, but rather a structural alteration in the vessel wall involving all layers. Moreover, attempts to produce cerebral vasodilatation in the presence of a fixed narrowing of the major conduction vessels may have a paradoxical effect, resulting in decreased blood flow to the ischemic areas. The vessels proximal to the ischemic region are narrowed and cannot dilate, whereas the vessels within the ischemic zone may be already maximally dilated owing to accumulation of acid metabolites. Cerebrovasodilator drugs (aminophylline, isoproterenol, nitroprusside) may dilate arteries in normal areas of the brain, reducing local perfusion pressure and shunting blood from ischemic to normal regions: the intracerebral steal effect. Furthermore, most of the attempts to dilate cerebral vessels run the significant risk of dilating extracerebral vessels and thereby further reducing systemic arterial pressure and cerebral perfusion pressure to below critical levels.

Calcium channel–blocking drugs have been suggested as a method of preventing cerebral arterial vasospasm. These compounds diminish the myoplasmic calcium in smooth and cardiac muscle cells and impede the entry of the slow channel, extracellular calcium that is necessary for the contraction of smooth and cardiac muscle. It is also speculated that these drugs may have a direct effect on the cerebral neuron and supporting glia during the ischemic insult. In experimental animals, calcium channel–blocking agents have been shown to reduce the size of cerebral infarction following ischemia. Several clinical studies have been performed, and randomized trials are ongoing to test the usefulness of the calcium channel–blocking agents in the treatment of cerebral ischemia, both from vasospasm secondary to SAH and after atherosclerotic occlusion of cerebral arteries. To date, the studies have involved a small number of patients and may be considered preliminary. Allen and colleagues [2] noted only 1 of 56 patients treated in a double-blind study using oral nimodipine died or had a persistent neurologic deficit, compared to 8 of 60 patients who received placebo drug. Philippon and coworkers [10] reported a 71% reduction of death and disability due to vasospasm in a controlled study of oral nimodipine in 81 patients, and the Canadian multicentered control study in poor-grade patients reported a 10% reduction of the incidence of delayed neurologic deterioration due to vasospasm. Picard and colleagues [11] have reported a 40% reduction of death and disability related to vasospasm in the largest, and most convincing, control study of 554 patients. Of interest, the incidence, severity, and distribution of angiographically detected vasospasm was not significantly different in the nimodipine and placebo groups, and the overall good outcomes were not significantly improved in the nimodipine-treated patients. In all of these studies, the number of patients were unfortunately too small to exclude with certainty a type-2 error. However, the trends have been encouraging.

The regimen that we have found most effective in dealing with neurologic deterioration secondary to vasospasm consists of rapidly expanding the intravascular volume with colloid and crystalloid infusion to a pulmonary capillary wedge pressure of 18 mmHg or a central venous pressure of 12 mmHg. The vasodepressor response is blocked with atropine, and pitressin is administered to diminish renal diuresis. Administration of digoxin may be necessary to ensure an optimum cardiac output. If the patient does not show signs of immediate improvement on this regimen, the systemic arterial pressure is raised in increments of 10 mmHg using dopamine or dobutamine until the neurologic deficits subside or reverse. It has been found that arterial pressure can be sustained at elevated levels for prolonged intervals using this routine.

Expanding the intravascular volume and elevating systemic arterial pressure in states of cerebrovascular insufficiency secondary to vasospasm have proved to be safe and effective providing meticulous attention is paid to the physiologic, biochemical, and hematologic parameters. Volume expansion and induced hypertension are, however, clearly a hazardous regimen in the presence of an untreated or unruptured aneurysm. In a series of 250 patients, neurologic deterioration was reversed and permanent improvement achieved in 221. Improvement was only transiently maintained in 11 patients; in these 11, the complications of rebleeding from the aneurysm, pulmonary edema, and myocardial infarction necessitated reversing the volume expansion and lowering the blood pressure. In the remaining 18 patients, the vasospasm caused cerebral infarction causing death in 7 and persistent neurologic dysfunction in the remaining 11. These results are superior to any other previously attempted form of vasospasm therapy to date.

IV. Surgery. Hemorrhage from an intracranial aneurysm is a dramatic and often devastating event. If the patient survives the first hemorrhage, then the aim of treatment is to prevent recurrent hemorrhage. There is little doubt now that recurrent hemorrhage is best controlled by surgical obliteration of the sac.

A. Timing of surgery

1. Advantages of delayed surgery. Although surgery within 3 days of SAH was advocated by many surgeons in the past, a delay of 7 to 10 days has become common practice in the United States. Postponing surgery must be balanced, however, by the predictable increase in mortality (40%) from patients who rebleed during this period.

It had been our practice to delay until the patient was in optimum condition and all evidence of vasospasm had disappeared. Delay in surgical approach often allows symptoms secondary to vasospasm to subside and seems to prevent delayed ischemic complications. In addition to antifibrinolytic agents, more precise control of blood pressure and fluid balance has appreciably diminished the wastage from rebleeding and vasospasm during the delay period while providing the surgeon with optimal conditions under which to dissect, isolate, and clip the aneurysm.

An additional advantage to delaying surgery is the almost universal finding of a slack brain that is easy to manipulate during the exposure of the aneurysm. The dissection of the aneurysmal sac also seems easier and safer after much of the blood in the subarachnoid space has been reabsorbed. The aneurysms are firmer, tougher, and less likely to rupture during dissection. Practical reasons for delay include the opportunity to diagnose or treat coexisting cardiopulmonary disease and the ability to obtain detailed and careful preoperative radiologic studies. It is important to have sufficient flexibility in operating room scheduling to provide the surgeon, the anesthetist, and the operating room team with optimal conditions for what is frequently a demanding technical exercise. Finally, our results of an operative morbidity and mortality of less than 8% in more than 2000 aneurysms of all sizes and grades, including 800 arising from the posterior circulation convinced us until 1984 to continue with our practice of delay.

2. **Advantages of early surgery.** Nevertheless, in recent years there has been a growing interest once again in early operation. This interest has come as a result of major technical advances in aneurysm surgery including the microscope, removable clips, the use of the temporary clip, microinstruments, and developments in neurosurgical anesthesia that now almost guarantee a slack brain and the safe induction of controlled hypotension.

Theoretically, the factors in favor of early surgery are attractive. The most impressive, of course, is the prevention of early rebleeding, which is virtually ensured when the neck of the aneurysm is secured. There is also some suggestion that, by operating early and removing blood in the subarachnoid space, the incidence of vasospasm may be reduced. Perhaps a more important consideration is that once the aneurysm is secured, the current treatment of vasospasm (volume expansion and deliberate systemic hypertension to improve cerebral perfusion pressure) can be carried out with relative safety in the knowledge that the aneurysm is clipped and is not likely to rebleed during the manipulations of blood pressure and intravascular volume.

Other factors of possible significance include the reduction of medical complications (e.g., pneumonia, deep vein thrombosis, pulmonary embolus, and fluid and electrolyte abnormalities) as a result of a short stay in bed and a diminished pharmacologic assault. The stress on the patient and family during the tense and anxious period of preoperative delay and the effect of prolonged hospitalization are psychologic and social factors that cannot be ignored.

There have been a few small uncontrolled series from Japan and North America suggesting that early surgery using modern techniques is the optimal method of treatment. These studies, however, lack adequate controls and numbers to be certain of their validity. A larger study from Japan consisting of Grades I and II patients who had surgery within 48 hours of SAH demonstrated a mortality rate of 56.8%, which differs markedly from the more optimistic reports of the smaller series. The controversy regarding early aneurysm surgery was evaluated in an international cooperative study. This study surveyed the results of contemporary surgical and medical management in 3521 patients. At admission, 75% were in good condition and surgery was performed in 83% of the patients. When followed up at six months, 58% had a complete recovery and 26% of the patients were dead. Vasospasm and rebleeding were the leading causes of death and disability, as well as the effect of the initial hemorrhage. There was little significant difference between the outcome of the patients operated on early and those operated on late.

In our own series, we have in the past five years selectively operated early on patients in good condition, and when our schedule and the organization of the operating team made it feasible. About 30% of our patients are now going to the operating room within three days of their hemorrhage and 60% within the first week. During this time, we have operated on more than 1000 patients, with 700 harboring aneurysms arising from the vertebral and basilar arteries. Our results have improved slightly to a combined mortality and morbidity of 6.5%, partly, we believe, from securing the aneurysm early and the more aggressive management of vasospasm.

B. Operative choices

1. Clipping. The best and most effective method of surgical treatment of an aneurysm is complete dissection and clipping of the neck of the sac while sparing the parent vessel and any small perforating arteries or branches in the region. Clipping involves the placement of a removable spring clip across the neck of the aneurysm as close to the feeder artery as possible. If the clip is placed too distally on the neck of the sac, there is a high probability that a new aneurysm will form between the artery and the clip.

Experience, detailed knowledge of the anatomy of the parent vessel, its branches, and the aneurysm, and familiarity with modern microsurgical techniques are all necessary to make the direct operative attack on an aneurysm feasible and safe. It is our opinion that these lesions are best handled by surgeons who operate on many aneurysms a year.

2. **Trapping.** In cases in which the application of a clip is impossible owing to the size of the neck of the aneurysm, consideration can be given to "trapping." Trapping is accomplished by permanently occluding the vessels proximal and distal to the aneurysm and can only be attempted if there is sufficient collateral flow to the affected area of the brain beyond the occluded vessel. Again, trapping is not an alternative if important branch or perforating vessels arise from the segment to be trapped.

3. **Hunterian proximal ligation.** Occasionally, it may be necessary or desirable to ligate the feeder artery to an aneurysm. In some large or otherwise inoperable carotid aneurysms, carotid ligation has been a mainstay of treatment for many years. Reducing the pressure within, or restricting the flow through, the aneurysm decreases the chance of further enlargement and rupture and may induce thrombosis and obliteration of the sac. Such a procedure may be carried out gradually, while the patient is awake, using a graduated screw device such as the Selverstone clamp. Recently, this principle of hunterian ligation has also been applied with some success to middle cerebral, posterior cerebral, and anterior communicating aneurysms, as well as to vertebrobasilar aneurysms. With these more distally located aneurysms, the risk of ischemia and infarction in the territory of the occluded vessel may be reduced by preliminary extracranial to intracranial arterial bypass.

4. **Reinforcement.** In aneurysms in which the aforementioned techniques are impossible because of size or location, reinforcement of the aneurysmal wall using gauze, Gelfoam, or plastic materials may be attempted with the hope of preventing progressive enlargement and rupture of the aneurysm. These techniques are necessarily less than perfect because it is difficult to eradicate the sac completely. Wrapping also does nothing to reduce the bulk of a large or giant aneurysm, which may cause focal deficit by compression.

5. **Embolization.** Some inoperable ophthalmic artery or cavernous sinus aneurysms can be embolized by introducing balloon catheters or embolic material by way of the feeder artery to promote thrombosis. Thrombotic material such as muscle, horsehair, iron filings, acrylic, and silicone have been introduced at surgery as a last resort. Obliteration as a primary technique uses insertion of iron into the aneurysmal sac by stereotactic methods. The balloon techniques are clearly the most promising of these methods, and the technology and skills to accomplish complete obliteration of many intracranial aneurysms is developing rapidly.

V. **Postoperative care.** Immediate reestablishment of normal blood volume and electrolyte balance is necessary postoperatively to compensate for preoperative fluid restriction, negative nitrogen balance, blood loss, and diuresis during surgery. Normal blood pressure, temperature, and cardiopulmonary status should be maintained. Elastic stockings used intraoperatively and postoperatively improve venous circulation and may reduce the incidence of pulmonary embolism. A postoperative angiogram is performed to evaluate the success of the operation. Phenytoin should be continued for three months postoperatively. Corticosteroids are given immediately preoperatively and tapered in the week after the operation. Prophylactic antibiotics are not used.

VI. Operative results. Based on these methods for diagnosing and treating patients who have suffered a ruptured intracranial aneurysm, the operative mortality and morbidity in Grades I and II patients should be less than 5% in the hands of an experienced surgeon.

Treatment of unruptured aneurysms that do not act as mass lesions results in low morbidity and mortality, often reported to be under 1%. As aneurysms increase in size, both mortality and major morbidity increase proportionately.

Anesthesia

PETER S. COLLEY

I. Basic considerations. The major concern in the anesthetic management of patients undergoing craniotomy for surgical treatment of a cerebral aneurysm is the potential for intraoperative rupture of the aneurysm, either during induction of anesthesia or during the surgical procedure itself. Anesthetic management of patients who have cerebral aneurysms is made even more hazardous if cerebral vasospasm and/or raised intracranial pressure (ICP) are present. These complications limit the safety of all anesthetic techniques designed to lessen the risk of aneurysm rupture by lowering systemic blood pressure.

A. Intraoperative aneurysm rupture

1. Aneurysm rupture **during induction** of anesthesia has been reported to occur in less than 1 [49] of 4% [35] of patients undergoing cerebral aneurysm surgery; the mortality rate may be over 50% [49]. When the skull is intact, aneurysmal rupture causes a marked increase in ICP and a decrease in cerebral perfusion pressure (CPP).

2. Incidence of aneurysm rupture **during the surgical period** ranges from 5 [12] to 19% [26], although rates as high as 65% [37] have occasionally been reported. Increased morbidity and mortality in these patients result from greater retraction pressure, the surgical trauma that results from attempts to operate in a restricted and obscured surgical field, and permanent or temporary occlusion of major cerebral vessels to control hemorrhage. Rarely, the ruptured aneurysm may be so difficult to locate that control becomes impossible and the patient exsanguinates. Rupture may occur

    a. When the dura is incised and ICP decreases to atmospheric levels

    b. When excessive brain retraction causes reflex systemic hypertension

    c. During dissection of the aneurysm

    d. As the clip is placed around the neck of the aneurysm

    e. During removal of the clip holder from the aneurysm clip

3. The main goal during induction and maintenance of anesthesia is to **avoid increasing transmural pressure** in the aneurysm. Transmural pressure is defined as the difference between the systemic mean arterial pressure (MAP) and the ICP (Fig. 8-2). The relationship between the transmural pressure and wall stress or tension of the aneurysm is linear [17] (Fig. 8-3). Either an increase in the MAP (e.g., by light anesthesia) or a fall in the ICP (e.g., by ventricular drainage or hyperventilation) will increase the transmural pressure, the wall stress, and the risk of aneurysm rupture.

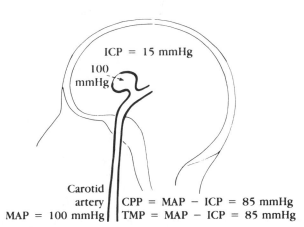

Fig. 8-2. The transmural pressure (TMP) of the aneurysm. TMP is the same as the cerebral perfusion pressure (CPP) and is equal to the difference between mean arterial pressure (MAP) and intracranial pressure (ICP). (Redrawn from [17])

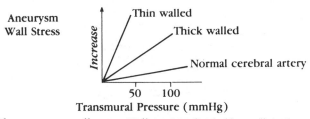

Fig. 8-3. The aneurysm wall stress. Wall tension divided by wall thickness equals aneurysm wall stress. The relationship between transmural pressure (TMP) and wall stress is linear: the thinner the wall, the greater the wall stress at any given pressure. (Redrawn from [17])

4. MAP should be maintained. The CPP also equals the difference between MAP and ICP. If, while attempting to maintain a low aneurysm transmural pressure, the anesthesiologist allows the CPP to fall below the lower limit of autoregulation (i.e., 50 mmHg in the normal brain), a reduction in cerebral blood flow (CBF) will occur (Fig. 8-4). Prolonged reductions in CBF to less than 50% of normal will lead to EEG evidence of cerebral malfunction [48]. MAP, therefore, needs to be maintained within the range of 50 to 90 mmHg. The presence of cerebral vasospasm and raised ICP further narrows this range of "safe" blood pressure.

B. Cerebral vasospasm. After subarachnoid hemorrhage (SAH), a significant number of patients develop vasospasm, which decreases CBF and impairs cerebral autoregulation [16]. CBF thus tends to follow changes in systemic blood pressure passively, increasing the risk of cerebral ischemia after episodes of inadvertent or deliberate hypotension (Fig. 8-4).

When anesthetizing patients who have cerebral vasospasm, it is important to maximize oxygen delivery to the brain by maintaining blood volume, blood oxygenation, and blood pressure (keeping CPP at higher levels than would be necessary in the absence of cerebral vasospasm). Intraoperative hypotension is avoided whenever possible. The anesthesiologist may also reduce cerebral oxygen requirements by the liberal use of barbiturates and low-grade hypothermia.

Calcium entry blockers (i.e., nimodipine) offer promise in preventing cerebral vasospasm [2] and may be used to treat patients in the pre- and postoperative periods. Although these agents decrease peripheral vascular resistance and systolic blood pressure, there are no clinically significant effects on the conduct of anesthesia, especially if the patients are well hydrated [46].

C. Increased intracranial pressure. Most patients coming to surgery for clip ligation of a cerebral aneurysm will have normal ICP but may have decreased intracranial compliance. Patients who have depressed levels of consciousness may have raised ICP owing to the presence of cerebral vasodilatation, cerebral edema, hematoma, or hydrocephalus. About 5% of patients who have a ruptured cerebral aneurysm will have

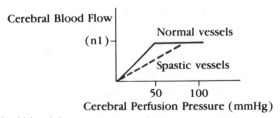

Fig. 8-4. Cerebral blood flow response to changes in cerebral perfusion pressure in the presence of normal autoregulation and impaired autoregulation due to cerebral vasospasm.

severe intracranial hypertension and will require emergency operation for evacuation of an intracranial hematoma [43].

In patients who have intracranial hypertension, it is preferable to avoid inhalation anesthetics until after craniotomy because their vasodilating properties increase the potential for further elevation of ICP. If inhalation agents are required to control systemic blood pressure, moderate hyperventilation should precede their introduction, lowering the $PaCO_2$ to 25 to 30 mmHg, and thereby counteracting their tendency to dilate cerebral vessels. Hypertension, hypercapnia, and coughing are avoided to prevent further increases in ICP.

II. Preoperative evaluation
A. General status
1. A brief neurologic examination should be performed and the patient's **clinical grade** noted. The clinical grade is determined according to the system of Hunt [7] or Botterell [21]. Higher grades (clinically more impaired) tend to be associated with the presence of cerebral vasospasm, increased ICP, and increased surgical mortality. Approximately 55% of patients present in Hunt's Grades I and II, 30% in Grade III, 10% in Grade IV, and 5% in Grade V (see Table 8-1).
2. Any association between a **decrease in blood pressure** and the appearance of **neurologic deterioration** or deficit should be noted. Occasionally a critical level of blood pressure below which neurologic deficits occur may be observed. Blood pressures below this level should be avoided intraoperatively. Previous blood pressure measurements should be reviewed and the preoperative blood pressure determined in both arms to establish a normal value for the patient.
3. Fluid restriction, diuretics, and steroids used in the preoperative management of SAH and intracranial hypertension may cause **dehydration** and **electrolyte abnormalities.** Hyponatremia and hypokalemia occur occasionally and may require correction before surgery.
4. A 1 to 2°C **increase in body temperature** is frequently present in patients who have ruptured aneurysms. This increase is possibly a reaction to blood in the subarachnoid space and should be treated before surgery because an elevated temperature causes an increase in cerebral oxygen requirement.
5. The anesthesiologist should **evaluate** the patient's **CT scan** for the presence of cerebral edema, midline shift, ventricular distortion, hydrocephalus, and hematoma to assess the presence and severity of intracranial hypertension.
6. Note the **location** of the aneurysm; this will determine the surgical approach and the patient's position intraoperatively (see sec. **III.C**).

B. Electrocardiographic abnormalities. Electrocardiographic (ECG) abnormalities occur preoperatively in 60% of patients who have SAH [18]. The ECG alterations are most likely due to increased vagal and sympathetic neural output secondary to SAH. The changes consist most frequently of T-wave inversion or flattening, S–T segment depression or elevation, U waves, and Q–T interval prolongation. Arrhythmias are also common and usually appear within 48 hours of SAH. Sinus bradycardia is present in 66% of patients, and premature ventricular contractions or episodes of ventricular tachycardia appear in 20% of patients [50]. The majority of ECGs return to normal within 10 days of the hemorrhage.

Unless the patient has had ischemic heart disease previously or exhibits pathologic Q waves, these ECG abnormalities are not necessarily indicative of myocardial damage, a contraindication to surgery, or the use of controlled hypotension [18]. In several studies, postmortem examination of hearts in these patients has revealed little evidence of significant coronary artery or myocardial disease [18,44]. Other studies, however, have reported histologic evidence of focal myocardial necrosis [13]. A cardiac consultation, determination of serum myoglobin and CPK isoenzymes [39], serial 12-lead ECGs, and myocardial nuclear scanning [51] may be necessary to evaluate these patients.

C. Informed consent. Some patients can tolerate a fuller appreciation of the risks involved in this operation than can others. A dilemma exists, however, because the physician wishes to avoid causing the patient anxiety and associated increases in blood pressure, but also wishes to comply with laws that protect the patient's right to be informed of the anesthetic risks. It is known that rupture of the aneurysm often occurs during periods of emotional stress. On this basis, we recommend that information, including discussion of extremely remote risks such as the risks of rupture during induction and intubation and of controlled hypotension, that may lead to increased anxiety should not be volunteered to patients who have a history of rupture of a cerebral aneurysm. The family is apprised of all risks and procedures.

Patients, in general, are less anxious if informed of what they may expect on the day of operation. The anesthesiologist should usually give a brief explanation of the anesthetic procedure, the expected duration of operation, and the nature of the anesthetic recovery period.

In all cases, the anesthesiologist should completely explain the procedures and risks to the next of kin in a tactful manner. The risks, including rupture of the aneurysm from intraoperative hypertension and brain damage from induced or unintentional hypotension, should be discussed. Documentation of discussions with the patient and relatives should be entered in the patient's record.

D. Premedication. Patients in grades I and II [21] who appear well tranquilized require little additional preoperative sedation. If tranquilization is less than adequate, an increase in the dose of drugs already in use can be ordered for the 24 hours before surgery. Diazepam, 10 to 15 mg given orally 45 to 60 minutes preoperatively, will usually provide satisfactory sedation. Excessive sedation and narcotics such as morphine or meperidine are best withheld to prevent respiratory depression and the masking of signs of recurrent aneurysmal hemorrhage. Patients who have a decreased level of consciousness (Hunt grades III–V) do not require preoperative sedation.

III. Anesthetic management
A. Preinduction procedures and monitoring
   1. Make available at least four units of **compatible whole blood** before induction of anesthesia.
   2. Place the patient in a 10- to 15-degree head-up position to reduce ICP and minimize venous bleeding.
   3. Insert a large-bore (14–16 gauge) intravenous cannula in a peripheral vein for infusion of lactated Ringer's solution. The intravenous catheter should be equipped with a sidearm attachment with minimal deadspace if infusion of a hypotensive drug is planned. Once an intravenous cannula is inserted, the anesthesiologist can increase sedation (i.e., intravenous diazepam in 2.5- to 5.0-mg increments) if the patient appears anxious. Start a second large intravenous catheter in the opposite arm after the patient is anesthetized. The presence of two venous catheters allows simultaneous administration of a hypotensive drug and blood in the event of intraoperative rupture of the aneurysm.
   4. **Parameters monitored** during induction and maintenance of anesthesia include the following:
      a. **Cardiac rate and rhythm** using an ECG with a V_5 lead.
      b. **Level of neuromuscular blockade** using a peripheral nerve stimulator.
      c. **Arterial pressure and arterial blood gases.** Insert a 20-gauge cannula in the radial artery under local anesthesia prior to induction. Keep the arterial transducer at the level of the head for accurate measurement of CPP.
      d. **Central venous pressure (CVP).** Insert the central venous catheter after the patient is asleep, preferably via a peripheral arm vein [11]. CVP is an especially useful parameter in the event of intraoperative rupture of the aneurysm as it serves as an index of blood volume to monitor blood replacement.
      e. **End-tidal CO_2.** Monitor during both induction and maintenance of anesthesia to ensure adequacy of ventilation. End-tidal CO_2 is typically 0 to 5 mmHg lower than arterial carbon dioxide tension ($PaCO_2$) because of ventilation-perfusion mismatching.
      f. **Heart and lung sounds, body temperature.** Place an esophageal stethoscope and temperature probe in the lower third of the esophagus after induction.

    g. Ventricular CSF pressure (if available). These measurements are needed to diagnose and treat raised ICP.

    h. Urinary output. Insert a urinary catheter after induction.

5. Monitoring brain functions during cerebral aneurysm surgery is a desirable but elusive goal. EEG techniques are limited because of the distance from scalp electrodes to surgical site [23]. Evoked potential monitoring, however, offers promise for the future [14].

6. Prepare a tuberculin syringe containing **sodium nitroprusside, 100 μg,** for use in the event of any hypertensive episodes. Apply 20% benzocaine (Hurricane) for topical anesthesia of the oropharynx and coat the oral airway with lidocaine ointment.

B. Induction technique. To avoid a hypertensive response, it is most important that the patient be smoothly and deeply anesthetized before laryngoscopy and intubation. We recommend thiopental and a narcotic (i.e., fentanyl) as the primary induction drugs. Thiopental rapidly produces unconsciousness and, in patients with normal or moderately elevated ICP (up to 30 mmHg), it reduces the transmural pressure in the aneurysm by decreasing systemic blood pressure more than it decreases ICP [41]. Narcotics provide profound analgesia, blunting the blood pressure response to laryngoscopy and intubation [24,36]. Fentanyl has relatively little effect on ICP and MAP in the presence of controlled ventilation and normal blood volume. Less is known about the effects of sufentanil or alfentanil on ICP, but their use may result in cerebral vasodilatation [30a]. The following sequence has proved to be a satisfactory technique:

1. Initially give the patient **100% oxygen** through a face mask held off to the side of the patient's face to avoid producing anxiety.

2. Administer **narcotic** (i.e., fentanyl, 7–10 μg/kg IV) over one to two minutes while verbally encouraging the patient to breathe. Then give **thiopental,** 1 to 3 mg/kg, to induce anesthesia. As soon as the eyelash reflex disappears, apply the mask to the face and control ventilation manually to keep the end-tidal CO_2 at approximately 30 mmHg. An oral pharyngeal airway is inserted if needed to maintain ventilation.

3. Vecuronium, 0.1 mg/kg, **or metocurine** [40] (formerly called dimethyltubocurarine), 0.3 to 0.4 mg/kg, is given intravenously as soon as possible. Both are good choices having little effect on blood pressure. Pancuronium, 0.1 mg/kg, may be used, but pancuronium occasionally causes an increase in heart rate and blood pressure [27]. Among the choices not recommended are *d*-tubocurarine, which, in intubating doses (0.5–0.6 mg/kg), may cause unpredictable and profound decreases in blood pressure and succinylcholine, which may lead to sympathetic stimulation and hypertension and has also been reported to cause hyperkalemia in patients with cerebral aneurysms [22].

4. If the patient does not have evidence of increased ICP, add a low concentration of **enflurane or isoflurane** (0.5–1.0%). For those few patients who have preoperative evidence of increased ICP, or who develop increased ICP with induction, it is prudent to avoid using nitrous oxide and other inhalation anesthetics during induction because these drugs may cause further increases in ICP.

5. To deepen the level of anesthesia prior to intubation, **fentanyl,** in 25- to 50-μg increments, is administered. A total dose of up to 10 to 15 μg/kg of fentanyl may be used, depending on the response of the blood pressure. Give **lidocaine,** 1.5 mg/kg, intravenously in addition to another 1- to 2-mg/kg bolus of **thiopental** if the blood pressure permits.

6. Three minutes after administration of lidocaine and thiopental, perform **endotracheal intubation** under direct vision as gently and as expeditiously as possible. Use of a stylet is suggested to reduce the time required for intubation and hence the noxious stimulation of laryngoscopy. Fasten the endotracheal tube securely to the patient's face using tincture of benzoin and adhesive tape.

7. Insert the **esophageal stethoscope** with a temperature probe so that the probe will be at the lower third of the esophagus. **Inspect the pupils** for symmetry and carefully cover the eyes.

8. Insert a **urinary catheter** and make sure the legs are wrapped from toes to groin to facilitate venous return and to prevent postoperative venous thrombosis.

C. Positioning. The patient is placed in one of the following positions, depending on the site of the aneurysm [52].

1. Aneurysms arising from the **anterior part of the circle of Willis:** supine position for a frontotemporal approach.

2. Aneurysms arising from the **posterior aspect of the basilic artery:** lateral position for a temporal approach.

3. Aneurysms arising from the **vertebral artery or from the lower basilic artery:** sitting or prone position for a suboccipital approach.

4. Aneurysms arising from the **anterior communicating artery** are frequently approached from the right. Aneurysms arising from the **middle cerebral and posterior communicating arteries** are approached from the side where the aneurysm is located.

D. Maintenance of anesthesia

1. Control ventilation mechanically and adjust it to maintain an appropriate $PaCO_2$. If ICP is normal, maintain $PaCO_2$ at 35 mmHg. This relatively normal $PaCO_2$ is selected to help maintain CBF in the presence of both cerebral vasospasm and controlled hypotension. If intracranial hypertension (above 20 mmHg) is present, the anesthesiologist should lower the $PaCO_2$ to 25 to 30 mmHg by increasing ventilation, thereby reducing ICP. Arterial blood gases and pH should be measured after a stable level of ventilation has been achieved. They are repeated at hourly intervals during the procedure.

2. **Begin surface cooling** shortly after induction if moderate hypothermia is planned (see sec. **IV.C**).

3. **Inject bupivacaine** 0.25% (without epinephrine) subcutaneously and widely along the line of the planned incision to provide excellent prolonged local anesthesia and prevent blood pressure elevations during the early part of the procedure.

4. **Establish a deep plane of anesthesia** before the surgeon makes the scalp incision and turns the bone and dural flaps to avoid a hypertensive response. Depth of anesthesia can be increased by using additional doses of narcotic combined with isoflurane or enflurane, 0.5–1.5%. Isoflurane is perhaps preferable to enflurane or halothane because it appears to have a smaller effect on cerebral blood volume and ICP than enflurane [3], and it markedly decreases the cerebral metabolic rate for oxygen [32]. Isoflurane's low blood-gas solubility also permits rapid elimination at the end of the operative procedure. Isoflurane tends to maintain cardiac output and systemic blood pressure and, unlike enflurane, does not have a tendency to produce spike or seizure patterns on the EEG with increasing concentration. Thiopental infusion (1–3 mg/kg/hr), in place of the volatile agents, is a technique that is also gaining popularity. If marked intracranial hypertension is present, the depth of anesthesia may be increased solely by giving additional increments of narcotic until the skull is opened.

5. **Mannitol** (0.5 gm/kg over 10–15 minutes) may be required to decrease the volume of the brain before opening the dura. Do not give mannitol, however, until after the bone flap is turned to prevent premature shrinkage of the brain and tearing of the bridging veins. Mannitol begins to lower ICP within 4 to 5 minutes of infusion and produces a peak reduction in ICP in about 45 minutes (range 20–120 minutes). It may transiently increase blood volume and blood pressure; if so, the depth of anesthesia should be increased.

6. **Maintain anesthesia** with enflurane or isoflurane (0.5–1.5%) and air-oxygen or nitrous oxide–oxygen. In addition, anesthesia may be supplemented with a continuous infusion of narcotic (i.e., fentanyl, 1–3 μg/kg/hr). The total dose of narcotic should perhaps be limited to minimize the incidence of postoperative respiratory depression unless postoperative controlled ventilation is planned (i.e., in grade III–IV patients).

7. **Begin infusion of the hypotension agent** as the surgeon starts the aneurysm dissection if controlled hypotension is planned (see sec. **IV.B**). Always **consult with the surgeon** prior to inducing hypotension.

8. A unit of whole blood should be immediately available at the beginning of the dissection of the aneurysm for infusion in case of sudden rupture of the aneurysm.

E. **Intraoperative fluid management**

1. **Intravenous fluid therapy.** Ringer's lactate is infused throughout the procedure at a rate of 3 to 4 ml/kg/hr to meet maintenance requirements and to replace fluid losses due to overnight fasting and urine production. If mannitol is used to promote diuresis, then only replace about half the urine volume produced during the period of diuresis with additional Ringer's lactate to avoid overexpanding the intravascular volume with salt solutions. Unlike intraabdominal or intrathoracic surgery, intracranial surgery does not entail significant third-space loss of fluid. Infusion of a large volume of salt solution is thus not needed. Although salt permeates the normal blood-brain barrier poorly, salt solutions may still cause an increase in cerebral edema if intracerebral hemorrhage or ischemia has induced an increase in blood-brain permeability.

2. **Volume loading.** In recent years there has been a trend toward more liberal administration of blood and crystalloid intraoperatively in patients undergoing operation for cerebral aneurysms. This practice evolved from the observation that expansion of blood volume frequently improved cerebral perfusion and reversed neurologic deficits in patients who had vasospasm [38]. The technique of volume loading with whole blood and/or plasma received further support from the observation that patients who had cerebral aneurysms had a blood volume that is approximately 17% below normal values in the preoperative period [30]. We think this decrease in blood volume is due to a combination of supine diuresis, bed rest, decreased erythropoiesis, and negative nitrogen balance. Since craniotomy usually involves a blood loss of 250 to 500 ml, this additional loss, if uncorrected, would result in a 20 to 30% decrease in blood volume.

On the basis of the above observations, at least one unit of blood may be infused immediately after the aneurysm is clipped. A second unit of blood and/or additional Ringer's lactate can be administered if blood loss is greater than 500 ml to maintain the central venous pressure above 5 cm H_2O and a hematocrit of 30 to 35%.

F. **Termination of anesthesia**

1. For patients in grades I and II who had **no intraoperative complications,** the endotracheal tube may be removed in the operating room. The primary goals at the end of surgery are to avoid coughing, straining, hypercapnia, and hypertension, which may occur during placement of the head dressing when head movement causes movement of the endotracheal tube within the trachea and during extu-

bation. These problems may be avoided by maintaining a deep level of anesthesia during placement of the head dressing and tracheal extubation. This must usually be done by increasing the level of inhaled anesthesia concentration as narcotic infusion must be terminated 10 to 45 minutes prior to the end of the procedure to minimize postoperative respiratory depression. Prior to extubation and while still maintaining controlled ventilation, give neostigmine, 2.5 mg, and atropine, 1.2 mg, intravenously to reverse residual muscle relaxation. After return of the muscle twitch to normal (normal train-of-four and lack of fade on tetanic stimulation), suction the oropharynx to remove secretions. Give lidocaine 1.5 mg/kg intravenously; 90 seconds later extubate the trachea. The use of lidocaine in this manner has been shown to reduce hemodynamic responses to extubation.

After extubation, continue controlled ventilation with 100% oxygen by mask for several minutes to eliminate inhalation anesthetics and their respiratory depressant and cerebral vasodilator effects. Gradually decrease ventilation to allow $PaCO_2$ to rise until it stimulates spontaneous ventilation. A delay in the onset of spontaneous ventilation is usually due to the residual depressant effect of narcotic. This may be reversed with naloxone, 0.5–1.0 μg/kg intravenously, and repeated if necessary. Avoid larger doses of naloxone because they cause sudden, violent awakening of the patient and marked increases in systemic blood pressure, which is especially hazardous in the patient with multiple aneurysms.

2. Patients who have **intraoperative complications** such as occlusion of a major vessel, severe blood loss, or excessive surgical trauma and patients in grades III to IV who have depression of consciousness preoperatively retain their endotracheal tubes. The anesthesiologist should plan postoperative mechanical ventilation. Tracheal extubation may be accomplished later when the patient's neurologic status is stable and an unobstructed airway and adequate ventilation can be ensured.

IV. Special techniques

A. **Spinal drainage.** The purpose of spinal drainage is to produce a slack, easily retractable brain and to improve operating conditions for aneurysms situated at the base of the brain. This procedure, however, is not used by all neurosurgeons. If spinal drainage is planned, place the patient in the lateral position in order to insert a subarachnoid catheter through the lumbar 3–4 or 4–5 interspace. For a subarachnoid catheter, our neurosurgeons insert a Cordis lumbar catheter, which has 20 side holes and is 80 cm long.*

* Cordis Corporation, P.O. Box 025700, Miami, FL 33102–5700.

An attempt should be made to avoid excessive loss of cerebrospinal fluid (CSF) when the spinal needle is first placed. Such losses decrease the ICP (increase the aneurysm transmural pressure) and promote further hemorrhage.

During the time prior to beginning CSF drainage, the catheter can be attached to a venous transducer to monitor the lumbar CSF pressure. A normal or moderately elevated lumbar CSF pressure (i.e., 15–30 mmHg) provides some assurance that the aneurysm has not ruptured during induction or the initial period of surgery and provides an assessment of cerebral perfusion pressure (MAP-CSFP). Lumbar CSF pressure measurements are also useful in monitoring effects of the various anesthetic drugs and the level of ventilation.

Initiate spinal drainage only after the dura has been opened to prevent the development of pressure gradients across the brain that could lead to tonsillar herniation. CSF fluid should be removed at a rate no greater than 5 ml/min (approximately 1 drop/sec) to prevent reflex increases in systemic blood pressure [5] (Fig. 8-5). Withdraw 50 to 150 ml of CSF as required for adequate surgical exposure. Spinal drainage is stopped when dural closure begins.

B. Controlled hypotension

   1. General considerations. Although good operative results have been reported when controlled hypotension was not used, controlled hypotension has become an integral part of aneurysm surgery in many institutions. In considering the use of controlled hypotension in aneurysm surgery, one should keep in mind that the blood pressure level below which CBF begins to decrease (i.e., the lower limit of cerebral autoregulation) is elevated in the more clinically ill patients (i.e., the higher clinical grades) [34]. In addition, there is an increasing tendency on the part of the neurosurgeon to manage aneurysm rupture by early placement of **temporary clips** to isolate the aneurysm, in which case normotension should be maintained [6].

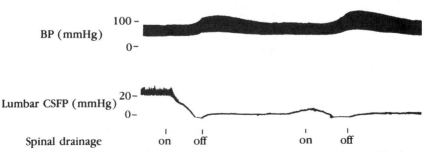

Fig. 8-5. Systemic blood pressure (BP) response to excessively rapid spinal fluid drainage. CSFP = cerebrospinal fluid pressure.

a. Advantages of controlled hypotension

(1) The aneurysm becomes more **mobile,** facilitating dissection and placement of clips.

(2) If the aneurysm ruptures, the **slower rate of blood loss** facilitates control of bleeding.

(3) The incidence of premature rupture is "possibly" decreased by **reducing the transmural pressure.** "Possibly" because no published studies have demonstrated a reduced incidence of intraoperative rupture with the use of hypotension.

b. Choice of hypotensive drug

(1) Nitroprusside, a direct-acting vasodilator, has generally replaced trimethaphan and deep halothane anesthesia and is the authors' recommended agent to produce controlled hypotension during aneurysm surgery. Whether CBF is more effectively maintained during nitroprusside-induced hypotension is controversial [8,19,45]. There is no question, however, that nitroprusside is easier to control in that it has a more rapid onset and briefer duration of action than any other currently used hypotensive agent.

Nitroprusside releases cyanide, which is normally converted to thiocyanate in the presence of endogenous thiosulphate and hepatic rhodanase. Excessive infusion of nitroprusside may overwhelm this metabolic pathway, resulting in increased blood levels of cyanide. Cyanide combines with cytochrome oxidase, which inhibits cellular uptake of oxygen. To avoid cyanide toxicity, it is recommended that infusion rates not exceed 10 μg/kg/min and that the total dose of nitroprusside not exceed 1 mg/kg.

(2) Nitroglycerin, also a direct-acting vasodilator, would appear to have some advantages over nitroprusside. The use of nitroglycerin is associated with a lower incidence of ECG changes characteristic of myocardial ischemia than is nitroprusside [15]. Nitroglycerin is essentially nontoxic and is metabolized to glyceryl dinitrate and nitrite in the presence of glutathione. Large doses (>1 gm), however, may cause small increases in methemoglobin. Nitroglycerin has not replaced nitroprusside because of its somewhat slower onset of action and the belief that more patients are resistant to its hypotensive effect. The drug is adsorbed on many plastics, including polyvinylchloride (PVC), and should be infused using glass bottles and polyethylene tubing.

(3) Trimethaphan, in clinical use as a hypotensive drug for the past 30 years, produces hypotension primarily by ganglionic blockage, although release of histamine and direct relaxation of vascular smooth muscle may also contribute to its hypotensive effect. Its primary advantages, compared to nitroprusside and nitroglycerin, are that fewer patients (especially young adults) are resistant to its hypotensive effect. Trimethaphan produces small increases in ICP [23a], which may be an important consideration in the hypertensive patient before craniotomy. It is used less frequently, however, because of its relatively slow onset of action, because it may cause unreactive, dilated pupils for a variable duration post-operatively, interfering with the neurologic evaluation, and because of evidence of cerebral toxicity when MAP levels are less than 50 mmHg. Trimethaphan undergoes enzymatic hydrolysis in blood and is partly excreted unchanged by the kidney. The drug may prolong the action of succinylcholine by inhibition of plasma pseudocholinesterase [42].

c. Contraindications to controlled hypotension
  (1) Vascular disease of brain, heart, or kidney
  (2) Hypovolemia or anemia
  (3) Narrow angle glaucoma (trimethaphan)
  (4) Leber's optic atrophy*
  (5) Tobacco amblyopia*
  (6) Vitamin B_{12} deficiency*

d. Relative contraindications to controlled hypotension
  (1) Elderly patient
  (2) Chronic hypertension
  (3) Elevated temperature
  (4) Sitting position

e. Doses and characteristics of these hypotensive drugs appear in Table 8-3.

2. Clinical considerations
  a. Discuss the need for and timing of hypotension with the neurosurgeon before starting the procedure.
  b. Use continuous intra-arterial monitoring and oscilloscopic display of blood pressure to increase the safety of controlled hypotension.
  c. Use a volumetric infusion pump for improved control of the rate of infusion.
  d. Calculate the initial dose and set the rate of infusion before hypotension is to be started.
  e. Use lower initial doses for older patients.
  f. Maintain a continuous infusion of Ringer's lactate solution through the intravenous catheter to prevent pooling of the hypotensive agent.

---

* Nitroprusside is contraindicated because of impaired ability to metabolize cyanide.

Table 8-3. Hypotensive drugs

	Nitroprusside	Trimethaphan	Nitroglycerin
Preparation	0.01% 50 mg/500 ml D_5W	0.2% 500 mg/250 ml D_5W	0.04%–0.1% 0.4–1 mg/ml
Concentration	100 μg/ml	2000 μg/ml	400–1000 μg/ml
Initial dose (μg/kg/min)	0.2–0.5	20–50	0.2–0.5
Maintenance (μg/kg/min)	1–3	20–200	5–7
Maximum dose (μg/kg/min)	8–10 or 1 mg/kg total	Unknown	Unknown
Side effects	↑ ICP ↓ PaO_2 Cyanide toxicity	Histamine release Dilated pupils Cerebral toxicity (MAP < 50 mmHg)	↑ ICP ↓ PaO_2

ICP = intracranial pressure, PaO_2 = arterial oxygen tension; MAP = mean arterial pressure.

   g. Although a controversial issue, it is probably best to maintain $PaCO_2$ at levels of more than 25 mmHg to avoid causing brain ischemia during simultaneous hypocapnia and hypotension [4,28,47].

3. Management of controlled hypotension

   a. When the neurosurgeon indicates that he or she is approaching the aneurysm and hypotension is needed, infuse nitroprusside at an initial rate of 0.2 μg/kg/min. Adjust the rate to reduce MAP to 50 mmHg in Grade I patients (i.e., normotensive patients who do not have evidence of cerebral vasospasm). In hypertensive patients, decrease MAP by only 30% of the preoperative value. Treat any inadvertent reduction in blood pressure to less than 50 mmHg by decreasing the infusion rate, by briefly terminating the infusion, or by administering intravenous fluid. If the blood pressure decreases to less than 30 mmHg, give ephedrine in 5-mg increments to raise the blood pressure to desired levels. An infusion of phenylephrine may be used to counteract drug-induced hypotension but, in the author's experience, this is more likely than ephedrine to produce inadvertent hypertension.

   b. Compensatory tachycardia occurring during controlled hypotension can be treated with intravenous propranolol in 0.2-mg increments up to 5.0 mg. Propranolol is contraindicated in patients who have bronchial asthma. Practolol may likewise cause bronchoconstriction but to a lesser extent.

    c. Determine arterial blood gases as soon as hypotension is established. Both nitroprusside and nitroglycerin may decrease PaO_2 by inhibiting hypoxic pulmonary vasoconstriction and increasing blood flow to poorly ventilated or atelectatic areas of the lung [9,10]. An early sign of nitroprusside-induced cyanide toxicity is the appearance of metabolic acidosis. $PaCO_2$ should be maintained at levels of more than 25 mmHg.

    d. Maintain hypotension until after the aneurysm is clipped. Then gradually decrease the infusion rate to avoid rebound hypertension, which, if excessive, may increase cerebral edema and interfere with hemostasis. Return blood pressure to normotensive levels before closure of the dura so the surgeon may detect and coagulate any bleeding sites and make any necessary adjustment in the position of the aneurysm clip.

C. Surgical hypothermia

    1. Moderate hypothermia. Hypothermia reduces the cerebral metabolic requirements for oxygen ($CMRO_2$) by 5% for each degree centigrade decreases in temperature. Moderate hypothermia (i.e., 32°C) is often used during aneurysm surgery in the belief that it will decrease the risk of controlled or inadvertent hypotension and of unanticipated occlusion of a major vessel. Hypothermia in this temperature range decreases $CMRO_2$ by 25% and is not associated with cardiac arrhythmias or other complications. Recently, however, the ability of low-grade hypothermia (32°C) to provide cerebral protection during hypotension has been shown to be absent in animals [25]. The risks of this procedure appear negligible, however, so that hypothermia remains an adjunct to aneurysm surgery in some centers.

    2. Management. After induction of anesthesia, circulate water at a temperature of 4°C through a thermal blanket placed above and beneath the patient until the body temperature begins to fall. Stop cooling as soon as esophageal temperature reaches 33°C; then set the water temperature control to 35 to 40°C. The body temperature will drift downward to 31 to 32°C by the time the aneurysm is clipped. Do not remove the endotracheal tube until the body temperature is 35°C or higher. An in-circuit heated humidifier for inspired gases accelerates rewarming.

    3. Deep hypothermia. More profound levels of hypothermia were used in the late 1950s during operation for cerebral aneurysms in an attempt to provide cerebral protection and reduce the extremely high mortality rates at a time when surgical treatment frequently involved occlusion of major cerebral vessels. The risks of interference with blood clotting mechanisms, increase in operation time, possible increase in the incidence of postoperative vasospasm, cardiac arrhythmias (i.e., ventricular fibrillation), as well as the failure of published reports to show improved results, have gradually led to an avoidance of profound hypothermia in many institutions. The few exceptions have been for treatment of various aneurysms that, by their location or size, are inaccessible to the usual surgical approaches and techniques and require major interruption of CBF. These aneurysms include certain giant aneurysms and aneurysms of the posterior circulation in which cardiac arrest and extracorporeal circulation are required. The development of vascular bypass techniques (i.e., superficial temporal artery to middle cerebral artery anastomosis) has further decreased the need for hypothermia in such situations.

V. Aneurysm rupture

A. Rupture during induction. An abrupt increase in blood pressure during or after induction of anesthesia may be both the result or the cause of aneurysmal rupture. Increases in systemic blood pressure may be treated by administering a bolus of thiopental, 100 to 200 mg, and sodium nitroprusside, 0.5 to 1.0 μg/kg, intravenously to decrease the aneurysm transmural pressure. Marked hypotension is detrimental because a decrease in systemic blood pressure coupled with an increase in ICP may severely impair CPP and reduce CBF.

B. Intraoperative aneurysm rupture

1. Surgical attempts to control hemorrhage from an aneurysm that has ruptured intraoperatively consist initially of placing the tip of the suction catheter over the bleeding site and, if possible, clipping the base of the aneurysm. If this is not possible, control of bleeding is achieved by placing temporary clips on the major cerebral artery proximal to the aneurysm. Some hemorrhage conditions necessitate a trapping procedure (i.e., placement of clips on both proximal and distal arteries).

2. Anesthetic management during rupture of the aneurysm consists of adjusting the infusion rate of nitroprusside to maintain the MAP between 40 and 50 mmHg to decrease the rate of bleeding. If bleeding continues to be excessive and no temporary clips are placed, then the MAP must be lowered to allow the surgeon to remove blood from the field and to see the aneurysm more easily. If temporary clips are placed, normotension should be sought as soon as possible. Blood losses should be continuously replaced with infusions of whole blood to maintain blood volume. Alternatively, one or both carotid arteries may be compressed against the vertebral bodies for up to three minutes. Carotid compression may produce a nearly bloodless field and allow the surgeon to see the aneurysm [7].

C. Barbiturates have been suggested to provide protection against cerebral ischemia when the risk of subsequent neurologic deficit is high. Ischemia may result from prolonged occlusion of a major cerebral artery, cerebral vasospasm, or an episode of severe hypotension. The efficiency of barbiturates in these situations is not yet supported by adequate clinical studies, but perhaps such therapy is worth attempting when the surgical outcome is otherwise likely to be one of severe morbidity or mortality. Some authors have suggested that thiopental, 3 to 5 mg/kg, be given intravenously if temporary occlusion of a major intracranial vessel or deep hypotension is required before aneurysm clipping [31]. If prolonged barbiturate therapy is planned, use pentobarbital 15 to 20 mg/kg as a loading dose followed by pentobarbital 15 mg/kg/24 hr in divided doses for 48 hours postoperatively [20].

VI. Immediate postoperative care

A. In the intensive care unit, place the patient in a 20- to 30-degree head-up position with the head in the midline position to prevent obstruction of the jugular veins. Ensure adequate oxygenation by using supplemental oxygen delivered by face mask and heated nebulizer. Give the nurse caring for the patient a detailed account of the patient's preoperative neurologic state, anesthetic and surgical procedures, intraoperative fluid therapy, and intraoperative and any anticipated complications. Order continuous monitoring of systemic blood pressure and ECG. Maintain MAP at a level above that associated with preoperative neurologic deficits, or no lower than 80 mmHg and no higher than 120 mmHg. Because of the possibility of delayed postoperative respiratory depressant effects of narcotics,[1,29,33], if any deterioration in consciousness or respiration occurs, give naloxone, 0.1 to 0.2 mg, intravenously or instruct the nurse to notify the house staff immediately.

B. Before leaving the intensive care unit, be certain that the vital signs are stable and that the patient is capable of maintaining an unobstructed airway. Carry out a brief neurologic assessment of the patient's level of consciousness, pupillary symmetry and reaction to light, ability to move all extremities, and relative strength of each extremity.

References

ANESTHESIA
1. Adams, A. P., and Pybus, D. A. Delayed respiratory depression after use of fentanyl during anesthesia. *Br. Med. J.* 1:278, 1978.
2. Allen, G. S., Ahn, H. S., Preziosi, T. J., et al. Cerebral arterial spasm — A controlled trial of nimodipine in patients with subarachnoid hemorrhage. *N. Engl. J. Med.* 308:619, 1983.
3. Artru, A. A. A comparison of the effects of isoflurane, enflurane, halothane, and fentanyl on cerebral blood volume and ICP. Abstracts of Scientific Papers. *Anesthesiology* 57:A374, 1982.
4. Artru, A. A., Katz, R. A., and Colley, P. S. Autoregulation of cerebral blood flow during normocapnia and hypocapnia in dogs. *Anesthesiology* 70:288, 1989.
5. Barker, J. An anaesthetic technique for intracranial aneurysms. Correspondence. *Anaesthesia* 30:557, 1982.
6. Batjer, H., and Samson, D. Intraoperative aneurysmal rupture: Incidence, outcome, and suggestions for surgical management. *Neurosurgery* 18:701, 1986.

7. Botterell, E. H., Longhead, W. M., Scott, J. W., et al. Hypothermia and interruption of carotid and vertebral circulation in the surgical management of intracranial aneurysms. *J. Neurosurg.* 13:1, 1956.

8. Brown, F. D., Crockard, H. A., Johns, L. M., et al. The effects of sodium nitroprusside and trimethaphan camsylate on cerebral blood flow in rhesus monkeys. *Neurosurgery* 2:31, 1978.

9. Colley, P. S., Cheney, F. W., and Hlastala, M. P. Ventilation-perfusion and gas exchange effects of sodium nitroprusside in dogs with normal and edematous lungs. *Anesthesiology* 50:489, 1979.

10. Colley, P. S., Cheney, F. W., and Hlastala, M. P. Pulmonary gas exchange effects of nitroglycerin in canine edematous lungs. *Anesthesiology* 55:114, 1981.

11. Cucchiara, R. F., Messick, J. M., Gronert, G. G., et al. Time required and success rate of percutaneous right atrial catheterization: Description of a technique. *Can. Anaesth. Soc. J.* 27:572, 1980.

12. Dahlgren, B. E., Gordon, E., and Steiner, L. Evaluation of controlled hypotension during surgery for intracranial arterial aneurysms. In *Prog. Anaesthesiology,* Excerpta Medica, 1970. P. 1232.

13. Doshi, R., and Neil-Dwyer, G. Hypothalamic and myocardial lesions after subarachnoid haemorrhage. *J. Neurol. Neurosurg. Psychiatry* 40:821, 1977.

14. Ducati, A., Landi, A., Cenzato, M., et al. Monitoring of brain function by means of evoked potentials in cerebral aneurysm surgery. *Acta. Neurochir. Suppl. (Wien),* 1988. Pp. 8–13.

15. Fahmy, N. R. Nitroglycerin as a hypotensive drug during general anesthesia. *Anesthesiology* 49:17, 1978.

16. Farrar, J. K., Gamache, F. W., Ferguson, G. G., et al. Effects of profound hypotension on cerebral blood flow during surgery for intracranial aneurysms. *J. Neurosurg.* 55:857, 1981.

17. Ferguson, G. Physical factors in the initiation, growth and rupture of human intracranial aneurysms. *J. Neurosurg.* 37:666, 1972.

18. Galloon, S., Rees, G. A. O., Briscoe, L. E., et al. Prospective study of electrocardiographic changes associated with subarachnoid haemorrhage. *Br. J. Anaesth.* 44:511, 1972.

19. Grubb, R. L., and Raichle, M. E. Effects of hemorrhage and pharmacologic hypotension on cerebral oxygen utilization and blood flow. *Anesthesiology* 56:3, 1982.

20. Hoff, J. T., Pitts, L. H., and Spetzler, R. Barbiturates for protection from cerebral ischemia in aneurysm surgery. *Acta Neurol. Scand.* (Suppl. 64) 56:158, 1977.

21. Hunt, W. E., and Hess, R. M. Surgical risk as related to time of intervention in the repair of intracranial aneurysms. *J. Neurosurg.* 28:14, 1968.

22. Iwatsuki, N., Kuroda, N., Amaha, K., and Iwatsuki, K. Succinylcholine-induced hyperkalemia in patients with ruptured cerebral aneurysms. *Anesthesiology* 53:64, 1980.

23. Jones, T. H., Chiappa, K. H., Young, R. R., et al. EEG monitoring for induced hypotension for surgery of intracranial aneurysms. *Stroke* 10:292, 1979.

23a. Karlin, A., Hartung, J., and Cottrell, J. E. Rate of induction of hypotension with trimetaphan modifies the intracranial pressure response in cats. *Brit. J. Anaesth.* 60(2):161, 1988.

24. Kautto, U-M. Attenuation of the circulatory response to laryngoscopy and intubation of fentanyl. *Acta Anaesthesiol. Scand.* 26:217, 1982.

25. Keykhah, M. M., Welsh, F. A., Hagerdal, M., et al. Reduction of the cerebral protective effect of hypothermia by oligemic hypotension during hypoxia and the protective effect of hypothermia by oligemic hypotension during hypoxia in the rat. *Stroke* 13:171, 1982.

26. Krayenbühl, H., Yasargil, G., Flamm, E. S., et al. Microsurgical treatment of intracranial saccular aneurysms. *J. Neurosurg.* 37:678, 1972.

27. Lebowitz, P. W., Ramsey, F. M., Savarese, J. J., et al. Combination of pancuronium and metacurine. Neuromuscular and hemodynamic advantages over pancuronium alone. *Anesth. Analg.* 60:12, 1981.
28. Levin, R. M., Zadigian, M. E., and Hall, S. C. The combined effect of hyperventilation and hypotension on cerebral oxygenation in anaesthetized dogs. *Can. Anaesth. Soc. J.* 27:264, 1980.
29. Mahla, M. E., White, S. E., and Moneta, M. D. Delayed respiratory depression after alfentanil. *Anesthesiology* 69:593, 1988.
30. Maroon, J. B., and Nelson, P. B. Hypovolemia in patients with subarachnoid hemorrhage: Therapeutic implications. *Neurosurgery* 4:223, 1979.
30a. Marx, W., Shah, N., Long, C., et al. Sufentanil, Alfentanil, and Fentanyl: Impact on Cerebrospinal Fluid Pressure in Patients with Brain Tumors. *J. Neurosurg. Anesth.* 1(1):3, 1989.
31. Michenfelder, J. D. Physiology and pharmacology of brain protection. Annual ASA Refresher Course Lectures, 1982, P. 242.
32. Newberg, L. A., Milde, J. H., and Michenfelder, J. D. Cerebral metabolic effects of isoflurane at and above concentrations which suppress the EEG. *Anesthesiology* 57:A334, 1982.
33. Nilsson, C., and Rosberg, B. Recurrence of respiratory depression following neurolept analgesia. *Acta Anaesthesiol. Scand.* 26:240, 1982.
34. Nornes, H., Knutzen, H. B., and Wikeby, P. Cerebral arterial blood flow and aneurysm surgery. *J. Neurosurg.* 47:819, 1977.
35. Nornes, H., and Wikeby, P. Results of microsurgical management of intracranial aneurysms. *J. Neurosurg.* 51:608, 1979.
36. Payne, K. A., Murray, W. B., and Oosthuizen, J. H. Obtunding the sympathetic response to intubation. Experience at 2 minutes after administration of the test agent in patients with cerebral aneurysms. *S. Afr. Med. J.* 73:584, 1988.
37. Pertuiset, B., Van Effenterre, R., Goutorbe, J., et al. Management of aneurysmal rupture during surgery, using bipolar coagulation, deep hypotension, and the operating microscope. *Acta Neurochir.* 30:195, 1974.
38. Pritz, M. B., Giannotta, S. L., Kindt, G. W., et al. Treatment of patients with neurological deficits associated with cerebral vasospasm by intravascular volume expansion. *Neurosurgery* 3:364, 1978.
39. Rudehill, A., Gordon, E., Sundqvist, K., et al. A study of ECG abnormalities and myocardial specific enzymes in patients with subarachnoid haemorrhage. *Acta Anaesthesiol. Scand.* 26:344, 1982.
40. Savarese, J. J., Hassan, H. A., and Antonio, R. P. The clinical pharmacology of metacurine. *Anesthesiology* 47:277, 1977.
41. Shapiro, H. M., Galindo, A., Wyte, S. R., et al. Rapid intraoperative reduction of intracranial pressure with thiopentone. *Br. J. Anaesth.* 45:1057, 1973.
42. Sklar, G. S., and Lanks, K. W. Effects of trimethaphan and sodium nitroprusside on hydrolysis of succinylcholine in vitro. *Anesthesiology* 47:31, 1977.
43. Skultety, F. M., and Nishioka, H. The results of intracranial surgery in the treatment of aneurysms. *J. Neurosurg.* 25:683, 1966.
44. Srivastava, S. C., and Robson, A. O. Electrocardiographic abnormalities associated with subarachnoid haemorrhage. *Lancet* 2:431, 1964.
45. Stoyka, W. W., and Schultz, H. The cerebral response to sodium nitroprusside and trimethaphan controlled hypotension. *Can. Anaesth. Soc. J.* 22:275, 1975.
46. Stullken, E. H., Jr., Balestrieri, F. J., Prough, D. S., et al. The hemodynamic effects of nimodipine in patients anesthetized for cerebral aneurysm clipping (1984).
47. Sullivan, K. H., Keenan, R. L., Isrow, L., et al. The critical importance of $PaCO_2$ during intracranial aneurysm surgery. *J. Neurosurg.* 52:426, 1980.
48. Trojaborg, W., and Boysen, G. Relation between EEG, regional cerebral blood flow and internal carotid artery pressure during carotid endarterectomy. *Electroencephalogr. Clin. Neurophysiol.* 34:61, 1973.

49. Tsementzis, S. A., and Hitchcock, E. R. Outcome from "rescue clipping" of ruptured intracranial "aneurysms" during induction anaesthesia and endotracheal intubation. *J. Neurol. Neurosurg. Psychiatry* 48:160, 1985.
50. Vidal, B. E., Dergal, E. G., Cesarman, E., et al. Cardiac arrhythmias associated with subarachnoid hemorrhage: Prospective study. *Neurosurgery* 5:675, 1979.
51. White, J. C., Parker, S. D., and Rogers, M. D. Pre-anesthetic evaluation of a patient with pathologic Q waves following subarachnoid hemorrhage. *Anesthesiology* 62:351, 1985.
52. Yasargil, M. G., and Fox, J. L. The microsurgical approach to intracranial aneurysms. *Surg. Neurol.* 3:7, 1975.

NEUROSURGERY

1. Adams, H. P., Kassell, N. F., Torner, J. C., et al. Predicting cerebral ischemia after aneurysmal subarachnoid hemorrhage: Influences of clinical condition, CT results, and antifibrinolytic therapy. A report of the Cooperative Aneurysm Study. *Neurology* 37:1586, 1987.
2. Allen G. S., Ahn, H. S., Preziosi T. J., et al. Cerebral arterial spasm — A controlled trial of nimodipine in patients with subarachnoid hemorrhage. *N. Engl. J. Med.* 308:619, 1983.
3. Botterell, E. H., Longhead, W. M., Scott, J. W., and Vandewater, S. L. Hypothermia and interruption of carotid or carotid and vertebral circulation in the surgical management of intracranial aneurysms. *J. Neurosurg.* 13:1, 1956.
4. Dott, N. W. Intracranial Aneurysm: Cerebral Arterioradiography: Surgical Treatment. *Transcripts of the Medical Chirurgical Society,* Edinburgh, 1932–1933. Pp. 219–234.
5. Henry, P. D. Clinical pharmacology of calcium antagonist: Effects on muscle and normuscle cells. In R. Battye (Ed.), *Calcium Antagonists: Possible Therapeutic Use in Neurosurgery.* New York: Raven Health Care Communications, 1983.
6. Hunt, W. E., and Hess, R. M. Surgical risk as related to time of intervention in the repair of intracranial aneurysms. *J. Neurosurg.* 28:14, 1968.
7. Kurtzke, J. F. *Epidemiology of Cerebrovascular Disease.* New York: Springer, 1969. P. 195.
8. Locksley, H. B. Report on the cooperative study of intracranial aneurysms and subarachnoid hemorrhage: Natural history of subarachnoid hemorrhage, intracranial aneurysms and arteriovenous malformations. Based on 6368 cases in the Cooperative Study. *J. Neurosurg.* 22:219, 1965.
9. Petruk, K. C., West, M., Mohr, G., et al. Nimodipine treatment in poor-grade aneurysm patients. Results of a multicenter double-blind placebo-controlled trial. *J. Neurosurg.* 68:505, 1988.
10. Philippon, J., Grob, R., Dagreou, F., et al. Prevention of vasospasm in subarachnoid haemorrhage. A controlled study with nimodipine. *Acta Neurochir. (Wien)* 82:110, 1982.
11. Picard, J. D., Murray, G. D., Illingworth, R., et al. Effect of oral nimodipine on cerebral infarction and outcome after subarachnoid haemorrhage: British aneurysm nimodipine trial. *Br. Med. J.* 298:636, 1989.
12. White, B. C., Wiegenstein, J. G., and Winegar, C. G. Brain ischemic anoxia. *J.A.M.A.* 251:1586, 1984.

9

Ischemic Cerebrovascular Disease

ELIZABETH A. M. FROST

All anesthetic drugs and techniques influence cerebral circulation and metabolism. In patients who have cerebral ischemic disease, these changes may prove inappropriate to the brain's nutritional needs, and the consequences may be devastating. Thus, anesthetic effects must be carefully controlled to provide optimal protection and improved conditions.

I. Basic considerations of cerebral circulation
A. Anatomy
1. **Cerebral arterial supply** is provided by the carotid and vertebral circulations. Normally 90% of the cerebral blood flow (CBF) is supplied through the carotid arteries and 10% through the vertebral arteries.
   a. **Carotid arteries.** The left carotid and left subclavian arteries are direct branches of the aortic arch. The right carotid and right subclavian arteries arise from the innominate branch of the aorta. Each common carotid artery divides at the level of the fourth cervical vertebra (C4) into the internal and external carotid arteries. The external carotid artery supplies the glands, muscles, and bones of the head and face, and the dura mater. The internal carotid artery enters the skull through the foramen lacerum and carotid canal and crosses the cavernous sinus. Ophthalmic, posterior communicating, and anterior choroidal branches are given off before the internal carotid artery terminates on the basal surface of the brain by dividing into the anterior and middle cerebral arteries.
   b. **Vertebral arteries.** The vertebral arteries are given off by the subclavian arteries. The larger left vertebral and the smaller right vertebral arteries enter the foramen transversarium of C6 on either side and ascend through the neck to C1 where they cross the dura to the anterolateral surface of the upper cervical spinal cord.

   The vertebral arteries give origin to (1) the posterior inferior cerebellar arteries and (2) the rami for the common midline anterior spinal artery that supplies the anterior two-thirds of the spinal cord before joining at the midline to form the basilar artery. Paired branches of the basilar artery include the anterior inferior cerebellar arteries, the segmental perforating branches, the superior cerebellar arteries, and the terminal posterior cerebral arteries.

2. Venous drainage is through superficial and deep systems. Cortical veins drain into the veins of Trolard and Labbé laterally and inferiorly and into the superior sagittal sinus medially and superiorly. Drainage from the deep gray nuclei passes along periependymal veins to the basal veins of Rosenthal and the vein of Galen, to the straight sinus and torcular, and thence to the superior sagittal sinus. Lateral sinuses carry venous blood to the sigmoid sinus and to internal jugular veins that empty into the superior vena cava. From the posterior fossa, drainage is through cerebellar and basilar plexi into the sigmoid sinus.

3. Anastomotic pathways between the arterial systems, of which there are several, exist to maintain flow in cases of cerebral ischemic disease. The circle of Willis connects the left and right carotid circulations and the carotid and vertebrobasilar circulations. Retrograde flow from maxillary ophthalmic arteries can fill the internal carotid artery. Emissary channels connect scalp, bony, and dural arteries through petrotympanic branches to the internal carotid artery.

B. Physiology

1. The brain's lack of phosphorylase and glycogen means that it requires a continuous supply of glucose and oxygen to function. A relatively high blood flow is therefore mandatory and is maintained as long as autoregulatory mechanisms remain intact. The normal value for global CBF is 44 ml/100 gm/min. However, this figure may vary regionally from 20 to 80 ml/100 gm/min, the faster flows generally occurring through gray matter and the slower rates calculated from white matter. Values for metabolic rates for consumption of cerebral nutrients are given in Table 9-1.

2. Physiologic control of the cerebral circulation is maintained by a precise interaction of myogenic, metabolic, chemical, and neurogenic vascular responses (Table 9-2).

    a. Autoregulation, or myogenic control, maintains CBF near a constant value even though the mean arterial pressure (MAP) may range between 50 and 150 mmHg [14]. The exact mechanism for this control is not completely understood, although it is known to be dependent on changing cerebrovascular resistance. Autoregulation is not an instantaneous effect, as several minutes are required for equilibration. This myogenic response is impaired by trauma, hypoxia, anesthetic agents, seizures, chronic hypertension, diabetes, and vasospasm [1].

    b. Metabolic control of CBF refers to the close association between flow and the level of oxidative metabolism in brain tissue. As the metabolic rate increases or the relative supply of oxygen within small areas of the brain decreases, release of local metabolites results in vasodilatation. An increase in hydrogen ion (H^+) concentration rather than a decrease in oxygen is considered the

Table 9-1. Normal values for metabolic rates of consumption of cerebral nutrients

Full name	Abbreviation	Normal values and units
Cerebral blood flow	CBF	44 ml/100 gm/min
Regional cerebral blood flow	rCBF	20–80 ml/100 gm/min
Cerebral perfusion pressure*	CPP	80 mmHg
Cerebrovascular resistance	CVR	1.8 mmHg/ml/100 gm/min
Arteriovenous oxygen content difference	$(A-V)O_2$	6.8 ml/100 ml
Cerebral metabolic rate for oxygen	$CMRO_2$	3.0 ml/100 gm/min
Cerebral metabolic rate for glucose	CMR glucose	4.5 mg/100 gm/min
Cerebral metabolic rate for lactate	CMR lactate	2.3 mg/100 gm/min
Cerebral venous oxygen tension	PvO_2	35–40 mmHg
Oxygen glucose index	OGI	90–100%
Lactate glucose index	LGI	0–10%
Cerebral blood flow equivalent	$CBF/CMRO_2$	14–15 ml blood/ml O_2

* Defined as mean arterial pressure minus mean cerebral venous pressure or mean arterial pressure minus intracranial pressure.

Table 9-2. Physiologic control of the cerebral circulation

Autoregulation (myogenic)
    SABP ↑ or ↓ → CVR ↑ or ↓ → flow constant
Metabolic
    H^+ ↑
    CMR lactate ↑
    K^+ ↑   → vasodilatation
    $CMRO_2$ ↑
Chemical
    $PaCO_2$ ↑ or ↓ → CBF ↑ or ↓
    PaO_2 <50 mmHg → CBF ↑
Neurogenic
    Adrenergic
    Cholinergic

SABP = systemic arterial blood pressure; CVR = cerebrovascular resistance; H^+ = hydrogen ion; CMR = cerebral metabolic rate; K^+ = serum potassium; $CMRO_2$ = cerebral metabolic rate of oxygen consumption; $PaCO_2$ = arterial carbon dioxide tension; CBF = cerebral blood flow; PaO_2 = arterial oxygen tension.

major metabolic factor coupling flow and metabolism. Alteration of serum calcium (Ca^{2+}) and potassium (K^+) levels and changes in carbonic anhydrase activity, and adenosine diphosphate concentrations influence local flow.

   c. **Chemical control** is mediated by alteration of arterial carbon dioxide tension ($PaCO_2$)[11]. A linear relationship exists between CBF and $PaCO_2$: there is a 4% rise in CBF for each 1 mmHg increase in $PaCO_2$ between $PaCO_2$ levels of 30 to 60 mmHg. Within the same range, $PaCO_2$ has no apparent effect on cerebral metabolic rate of oxygen consumption ($CMRO_2$). Alteration of CBF by changing $PaCO_2$ occurs almost immediately as carbon dioxide (CO_2) diffuses rapidly from blood vessels to affect the pH of extracellular fluid. If $PaCO_2$ is kept constant and only arterial H^+ or bicarbonate (HCO_3^-) is altered, little immediate change is seen in CBF, since these ions enter the extracellular fluid space more slowly.

   The decrease in CBF with hypocapnia is limited, and minimal flow is reached at about 15 to 20 mmHg, when cerebral tissue hypoxia may prevent further reduction in flow. Lowering arterial oxygen tension (PaO_2) when the $PaCO_2$ is normal does not affect CBF until PaO_2 falls below 50 mmHg, at which point cerebral vasodilatation occurs and CBF increases.

   d. The precise role of **neurogenic control** is still debated. Both adrenergic and cholinergic nerves innervate extracranial and intracranial blood vessels. Stimulation of nerves can markedly affect the caliber of pial vessels. However, the response of these pial vessels — to hypoxia, hypercapnia, and hypertension — appears to be similar whether the nervous pathways are intact or not. The nerve plexuses on cerebral vessels are identical to those in other vascular beds, but the nerve actions are minimal or nonexistent. Neurogenic control is probably not of major significance under normal circumstances but becomes important during stress states such as hypovolemic shock.

3. Noninvasive **quantitative assessment** of CBF and metabolism may be made by monitoring washout of xenon-133 (^{133}Xe) from small areas of the brain after the patient inhales the isotope. CBF can also be measured externally by using up to 250 scintillation counters, each of which looks at a small cylinder of brain tissue [15]. In centers with access to a cyclotron, it is possible to measure the metabolic rates for CO_2 generation, ammonia turnover, oxygen consumption, and local cerebral blood volume in small regions of cerebral tissue using tomographic scanners that image positron-emitting radioisotopes. The new techniques of nuclear magnetic resonance (NMR) have provided much information about the metabolic requirements and patterns of the brain.

C. Pathophysiology. Anesthetic management of patients who have ischemic cerebrovascular disease must be aimed at institution of conditions that will favor resolution of ischemia, protection against the development of ischemic infarction, and maintenance of normal intracranial dynamics.

1. Development of cerebral infarction is governed by the degree to which the metabolic needs of the brain are met by the cerebral circulation. Factors that decrease substrate supply or increase metabolic demand increase the risk of infarction. Factors that augment blood flow or lower metabolism decrease the chance of infarction. How much ischemia produces a clinical deficit is unknown, but slowing of the electroencephalogram (EEG) is seen when CBF is less than 20 ml/100 gm/min.

2. CBF is decreased by systemic hypotension and focal vascular occlusion; also sickle cell anemia and paraproteinemias increase cerebrovascular resistance and decrease CBF. Cerebral edema and hydrocephalus increase critical closing pressures and reduce CBF. Hematomas cause a mass effect and decrease perfusion pressure at the point of focal compression; reactive edema and hyperemia are present in the surrounding brain.

3. Hypoxic ischemia from respiratory or central neurogenic disorders causes a relative shift from oxidative metabolism within mitochondria to anaerobic, largely extra-mitochondrial glycolysis with conversion of pyruvate to lactate. As lactate concentration increases, there is a decrease in the rate of production of adenosine triphosphate by oxidative phosphorylation. The blood-brain barrier, which restricts permeability, breaks down, and injury to the endothelial cells of the capillaries occurs. Edema aggravates ischemia by increasing critical closing pressure. A vicious cycle of ischemia and edema may then lead to irreversible infarction.

4. Therapy can interrupt this sequence of events at several points and must be directed toward increasing CBF, reducing edema formation, or decreasing metabolic demand. Anesthetic techniques and drugs may be used to maintain or decrease CBF or to exert a protective effect on the brain by reducing the metabolic rate of oxygen utilization.

II. Major cerebrovascular ischemic disease entities

A. Thromboembolism accounts for approximately 78% of new "strokes" [21]. Sources of emboli include obstructive lesions in the arterial circulation from atheromas, cardiac emboli, or ulceration of atheromatous plaques. Other causes of stroke include vasculitis and hematologic disorders.

B. Classification of ischemic disease reflects duration and severity of the clinical deficit. *Transient ischemic attacks* (TIAs) are characterized by deficits that persist for less than 24 hours and resolve completely. *Reversible ischemic neurologic deficits* (RINDs) persist for longer than 24 hours but resolve within a week. *Progressive stroke* (PS) is the most unstable condition and is characterized by serial worsening of the deficit. *Completed stroke* (CS) describes a persistent deficit that may range from minor to disabling.

C. **Noninvasive tests** to evaluate the extent of the ischemic disease include ophthalmodynamometry, assessment of flow reversal in ophthalmic-facial collaterals with directional Doppler equipment, thermography, and oculoplethysmography. Plain skull and cervical x-rays may show calcification, and computed tomographic (CT) scan with contrast enhancement may show the extent of infarction. Noninvasive arteriographic methods, including digital subtraction (or intravenous) angiography, permit visualization of arterial channels. Arterial angiography is often reserved either for symptomatic patients or for visualization of intracranial vessels [4].

D. Decision to **operate** is determined by the site of the lesion. Severe stenosis or ulcerative plaques near the carotid bifurcation are best treated by carotid endarterectomy. Complete occlusion or inaccessible stenosis of the internal carotid or middle cerebral arteries were previously treated by microvascular anastomosis of an extracranial to an intracranial artery. However, results of an international randomized trial failed to confirm that extracranial-intracranial anastomosis is effective in preventing cerebral ischemia in patients with artherosclerotic arterial disease in the carotid and middle cerebral arteries [3]. Nonfatal and fatal stroke occurred more frequently and earlier in operated patients. Medical therapy involves decreasing the risk factors (i.e., control of hypertension, diabetes, and obesity, and discontinuing smoking). Acetylsalicylic acid (325 mg 4 times daily) is administered unless contraindicated or not tolerated.

III. Preoperative anesthetic evaluation
A. Multisystem disease
1. **Hypertension.** The majority of patients who have cerebrovascular disease are hypertensive and pose a number of problems for the anesthetist [5].
   a. The hypertensive patient undergoing general anesthesia is at increased risk of **myocardial infarction.**
   b. Hypertensive patients may be particularly **unstable during the anesthetic period,** becoming hypotensive intraoperatively and further compromising an ischemic area of the brain [9].
   c. **Postoperatively, hypertension** may develop, putting atheromatous cerebral vessels at risk of rupture.
   d. **Control.** Since patients who have untreated or inadequately treated hypertension are at greater risk during anesthesia of ar-

terial hypotension and of associated myocardial and cerebral ischemia, it has been recommended that the arterial pressures be brought under control *before* the patient undergoes anesthesia. The risk of anesthesia can be reduced when the diastolic pressure is stable and not higher than 110 mmHg, and when close monitoring and prompt therapy avoid intraoperative and postoperative episodes of hypotension or hypertension [10].

2. **Carotid artery disease.** Cerebral ischemia usually does not cause neurologic deficit until carotid artery stenosis reaches about 80% or embolization of an atheromatous plaque occurs. The disease is bilateral in about 50% of cases. Abnormalities of the circle of Willis (usually hypoplastic communicating vessels) are found in the majority of cases and further decrease the ability to augment collateral flow. Thus, the margin of safety is greatly reduced, and relatively small decreases in systemic blood pressure or cerebral vessel diameter may precipitate a catastrophic situation. Preoperative evaluation of patients who have carotid artery disease should include a test of neck motion to ascertain that consciousness is maintained with lateral and extension movements.

3. **Myocardial infarction.** A history of previous myocardial infarction is obtained from 25% of patients and has been shown to correlate closely with postoperative cardiac complications regardless of the age or the severity of the infarction. If patients also have ischemic cardiac disease and require coronary artery bypass, their cerebral ischemia should be relieved before they undergo heart surgery. About 20% of patients have also had previous major vascular surgery.

4. **Diabetes mellitus** occurs in about 20% of patients who have cerebrovascular disease, and they usually require insulin for control. Coincidental use of corticosteroids in neurosurgical management to decrease cerebral edema may aggravate hyperglycemia and increase insulin needs.

5. About 40% of patients have smoked one or two packs of **cigarettes** per day for more than 20 years. Consequently, bronchitis, emphysema, chronic hypoxia, or even carcinoma are frequently complicating factors.

6. Stroke victims also have altered muscular function [20]. **Hyperkalemia** is a recognized danger in patients who have central nervous system lesions and skeletal muscle paralysis. The phenomenon may occur in patients who have both upper and lower motor neuron abnormalities. Elevated serum potassium levels persist in the venous blood returning from all paralyzed muscles for several weeks after injury, indicating that the source of the potassium is the abnormal muscle distal to the neural lesion. Therefore, administration of succinylcholine to these patients may increase serum potassium levels and cause cardiac dysrrhythmias or even arrest. It is imperative that

preoperative serum potassium levels be within normal limits. Adequate muscle relaxation for intubation and intraoperatively is provided by drugs with moderate duration of action such as atracurium or vecuronium.

B. Multiple pharmacologic regimens

  1. Approximately 85% of patients who have cerebrovascular insufficiency take a combination of several drugs. Most commonly, these medications include digitalis, diuretic, antihypertensive, antiarrhythmic, anticoagulant, insulin, and corticosteroid preparations.

  2. Antihypertensive and antiarrhythmic drugs should be continued until the morning of surgery to minimize the risk of postoperative rebound hypertension. Rebound hypertension is most commonly seen after withdrawal from clonidine. It is important to restart hypertensive drugs as soon as possible in the postoperative period.

  3. Diuretics may cause fluid and electrolyte imbalance that can result in critical intraoperative hypotension and arrhythmias. Serum electrolytes must be measured immediately before surgery. Input-output charts should be carefully balanced for 24 to 48 hours preoperatively to assess fluid status.

  4. Patients receiving long-acting insulin preparations should be stabilized preoperatively on soluble compounds.

  5. Aspirin, usually given for several weeks before surgery to reduce platelet adhesives, may decrease the effectiveness of other essential coagulation factors. In addition, patients who have suffered TIAs often take coumadin preparations. These drugs must be discontinued for up to one week to allow clotting to revert to normal. Emergency therapy with large doses of vitamin K may prove relatively ineffective in returning prothrombin times to standard levels. A clotting profile is essential on the day of surgery.

C. Preanesthetic medication. The use of atropine is best avoided because of its unpleasant drying and tachycardic effects. Small doses of tranquilizers such as diazepam (5–10 mg orally) may be given about one hour before surgery. If the patient exhibits bradycardia after succinylcholine is given or after intubation, atropine may be given intravenously.

IV. Intraoperative anesthetic management

A. Carotid endarterectomy (Table 9-3)

  1. Cerebral perfusion pressure (CPP) must be maintained. Normotension or slight hypertension is essential since autoregulatory mechanisms are frequently altered regionally if not globally. The long-term use of antihypertensive medications makes patients susceptible to hypotensive episodes initially. These changes may be detected immediately if an arterial line has been established before or during induction. Stabilization of blood pressure is achieved by

Table 9-3. Anesthetic management of the
patient undergoing carotid endarterectomy

Careful preoperative history
    Assessment of multisystem disease
    Optimal medical condition
    Continue cardiovascular therapeutic regimen
Maintain cerebral perfusion pressure
    Avoid hypotension and bradycardia
    Normocapnia
    Surgical shunt
Select anesthetic agent to lower $CMRO_2$ and maintain cerebral blood flow
Monitoring
    ECG
    Intra-arterial BP
    Cerebral function
    Stump pressure
    CBF
Close postoperative observation
    Maintain normotension or slight hypertension
    Resume antihypertensive drugs
    Clear airway
    Neurologic assessment

$CMRO_2$ = cerebral metabolic rate of oxygen consumption; ECG = electrocardiogram;
BP = blood pressure; CBF = cerebral blood flow.

increasing fluid administration, infusing a 0.02% phenylephrine hydrochloride solution, and using light planes of anesthesia [7].

2. $PaCO_2$ should be kept in the normocapnic range (35–40 mmHg), since CBF increases linearly with increase in $PaCO_2$.

    a. In cases of carotid artery stenosis, establishment of **hypercapnia** will increase collateral flow and might be beneficial. However, ischemic areas of the brain are probably already maximally dilated owing to regional autoregulation, and a reduction in resistance in nonischemic areas may cause blood to flow from ischemic to normal areas of the brain, resulting in the **intracerebral steal phenomenon.** Retained CO_2 increases systemic blood pressure (which is beneficial) but causes a higher incidence of arrhythmias, especially in patients who already have generalized vascular disease. In addition, hypercapnia decreases stump pressure and increases cerebral venous pressure, both of which lower CPP.

    b. Hypocapnia has the opposite effect: it increases resistance in nonischemic areas and may direct flow to ischemic areas. However, this effect may jeopardize healthy brain tissue and increase resistance in collateral vessels supplying ischemic areas. A shift of the oxygen dissociation curve to the left in respiratory alkalosis also makes oxygen less available to tissues.

3. Precise, continuous **monitoring** is essential. Monitoring should include electrocardiogram, direct arterial blood pressure and gases (from an arterial line), and temperature. The Cerebral Function Monitor, an electroencephalographic processor giving information essentially from a single pair of parietal electrodes, provides only a gross indication of activity (see Chap. 3). Continuous, full EEG recording or power spectral analyses are preferable, especially during the period of carotid clamping. Although stump pressures above 50 mmHg are said to indicate adequate flow, the EEG may be abnormal at values even higher than this. Therefore, stump pressures are an indication of global flow at best and afford no information as to regional conditions.

4. **Assessing the adequacy of cerebral circulation**
   a. Assessment is most accurate when **local anesthesia** allows the patient to respond verbally. Even though carotid endarterectomy is performed successfully in many centers under cervical plexus block, local anesthesia is not always possible because of either lack of patient acceptance or surgical difficulties. In addition, this technique may cause the patient anxiety and some pain, resulting in tachycardia, hypertension, hypercapnia (from rebreathing under the drapes), and increased myocardial and brain oxygen consumption. Finally, neurologic damage does not always occur immediately after carotid artery clamping and may even be delayed for up to 30 minutes, a time when surgical attention may be directed elsewhere.
   b. Under general anesthesia, means of assessing cerebral circulation include jugular bulb oxygen tension (an indicator of global flow), EEG monitoring (regional and global flow), stump pressure (indicating the pressure of back flow from the opposite carotid artery and vertebral arteries), and the Cerebral Function Monitor [17,19]. The use of collimated scintillation crystals and measurement of ^{133}Xe washout rates after inhalation is an accurate, if not readily available, means of measuring regional flow intraoperatively. Recently transcranial Doppler monitoring gives visual and auditory assessment of CBF, most usually over the middle cerebral artery.

5. An **anesthetic agent** should be used that will lower cerebral metabolic oxygen requirements but maintain flow without myocardial depression.
   a. **Barbiturates** decrease $CMRO_2$ but they also decrease CBF. In addition, blood pressure may be difficult to maintain, and emergence is frequently delayed. A cerebral protective effect of barbi-

turate has been suggested but is still under considerable question (see Chap. 4).

b. An **inhalation agent** such as isoflurane also decreases cerebral metabolic rate, but will increase total CBF (which may result in some, but not total, intracerebral steal effect). Although blood pressure may decrease initially, emergence from anesthesia is usually prompt and complete. Isoflurane may also confer some protective effect. Thus, low-dose inhalational techniques are probably preferable to barbiturates [8].

c. The effects of **narcotics** on $CMRO_2$ and CBF, especially clinically, are less well defined [2,18]. Intravenous fentanyl (100 μg/kg) produced depression of $CMRO_2$ and CBF by 35 and 50% respectively [2]. Smaller doses of fentanyl (5 μg/kg or less) may have no effect on $CMRO_2$ [2]. In animal studies, fentanyl given prior to an hypoxic insult did not provide cerebral protection [13]. High-dose sufentanil has also been shown to reduce CBF and $CMRO_2$, with maximum decreases of 53 and 40% respectively, occurring at a dose of 80 μg/kg. Higher doses caused no further significant changes [12].

d. The effect of **nitrous oxide** on cerebral dynamics has been the subject of much controversy. In summary, nitrous oxide 70% causes cerebral vasodilatation and increases $CMRO_2$. No cerebral protective effect is obtained [6].

e. Reliance on the mechanical effect of a **surgical shunt** to maintain flow during clamping is preferable to the assumption that the metabolic requirements of the brain have been adequately reduced pharmacologically.

6. Sudden episodes of **bradycardia and hypotension** intraoperatively are caused by surgical manipulation at the carotid bifurcation. The reflex may be blocked by intravenous atropine 0.4 mg, repeated twice, as necessary, or by local instillation of 1% lidocaine. The surgeon should be advised immediately of the response.

B. Extracranial-intracranial (EC-IC) anastomosis. The technique of microvascular EC-IC anastomosis was developed to increase collateral blood flow in patients who have cerebrovascular insufficiency from atheromatous disease that is inaccessible by carotid surgery.

As already stated, this procedure has not been proven beneficial in preventing strokes. However, EC-IC anastomosis is still used to increase intracranial flow prior to carotid clamping in the treatment of a giant or other inaccessible aneurysm or as therapy for Moya-Moya disease — a pathologic condition characterized by decreased CBF at a young age. Although not strictly ischemic cerebrovascular disease, some notes on anesthetic considerations are important.

1. Surgical considerations. Anastomosis may be performed in the anterior circulation between the superficial temporal artery and the middle cerebral artery or in the posterior circulation between the occipital artery and the posterior inferior cerebellar artery. If the occipital artery is used, surgery is performed in a sitting position and all precautions necessitated by this position must be observed (see Chap. 11).

2. **Anesthetic considerations.** The main anesthetic considerations are to maintain cerebral perfusion pressure (CPP), maintain normo-capnia, decrease $CMRO_2$, reduce brain movement, and administer low-molecular—weight dextran.

   a. **Maintenance of adequate CPP** is essential. An arterial line must be established immediately, and systemic arterial pressure must be held as close to the patient's customary levels as possible with the use of 0.02% phenylephrine hydrochloride solution intravenously, if necessary, to avoid thrombosis in newly anasto-mosed vessels.

   b. **Routine monitoring** should include all vital signs, pulse oxime input-output charting, temperature recording, and frequent blood gas determinations. The inspired oxygen concentration may require adjustment if significant lung disease exists. Blood transfusion is rarely necessary although blood should be available in the event of profuse scalp bleeding or accidental displacement of the arterial clamp.

   c. **Reduction of brain movement.** The operation is performed under high magnification through a narrow exposure. Respira-tory and cardiac pulsations are magnified and cause a distracting brain bounce, which may be attenuated by a head-up position, minimal head turning, lower tidal volumes with increased respi-ratory rate, removal of small amounts of cerebrospinal fluid, and use of small doses of furosemide. Although not yet clinically employed, a modification of jet ventilation may lend itself to these situations. Anesthesia should then be maintained by intravenous means.

   d. **Anesthetic drugs**

      (1) The surgical technique necessitates clamping a branch of the middle cerebral artery for approximately one hour. There-fore, a drug that may afford ischemic protection, such as a barbiturate, may seem to be preferable for anesthesia. However, barbiturates cause marked cerebral vasoconstric-tion, which could impair collateral flow.

      (2) Alternatively, low-dose inhalational drugs in combination with efforts to maintain normocapnia cause some cerebral vasodilatation and decrease $CMRO_2$.

   e. **Low-molecular—weight dextran** infused at a rate of 50 to 100 ml/hr has been shown to maintain flow through freshly anastomosed vessels. In about 50% of patients, however, persistent oozing of blood or increasing blood pressure results, at which point this therapy should be discontinued.

f. The surgery essentially does not invade the brain. Thus, **extremely light planes of anesthesia** can be tolerated and the patient should be awake at the end of the operation. Intravenous administration of lidocaine, 50 to 100 mg, as the head dressing is applied will prevent or greatly decrease the coughing that not only puts strain on newly anastomosed vessels but possibly causes considerable tissue damage if the pin headholder has not been removed.

V. Postoperative care
A. Carotid endarterectomy
1. **Careful monitoring** and trend recording in an intensive care unit setting are essential. Frequent evaluation of neurologic status is important to detect obstruction of the carotid artery, hematoma, or embolization that may require additional surgical exploration.
2. **Blood pressure** must be kept at or slightly above normal to prevent thrombosis. Both hypotensive and hypertensive episodes may occur in the immediate postoperative period because of reduced baroreflex function. Hypotension reduces perfusion of both the brain and the heart; hypertension increases the work and the oxygen demand of the myocardium. In both instances the end result is likely to be myocardial ischemia. The major cause of serious postoperative morbidity in patients undergoing carotid endarterectomy is myocardial infarction. In addition, hypertension may increase capillary hydrostatic pressure, especially in ischemic areas of the brain, and lead to protein leakage, edema, or hemorrhagic infarction.

   a. Hypotension is treated with fluid replacement, ventilation, and infusion of 0.02% phenylephrine hydrochloride solution as necessary.

   b. For **hypertensive episodes,** which occur more commonly, preoperative antihypertensive medications should be restarted as soon as possible. When MAP rises more than 15 to 20% above baseline recordings, aggressive therapy is required. However, rapid reduction of arterial pressure by more than 25% may in itself cause cerebral ischemia. Therefore, therapy must be instituted with care, and extremely close observation of continuous arterial pressure recordings is mandatory. Useful drugs for parenteral therapy include sodium nitroprusside by slow infusion (70 μg/kg/hr), hydralazine (5–20 mg IM or IV), or diazoxide in a bolus injection of 50 mg that may be repeated twice. Propranolol 0.5 to 1.0 mg given slowly may augment the effects of hydralazine. There is some evidence to suggest that intraoperative use of propranolol (0.5–1.0 mg/hr slowly) may attenuate hypertensive responses in the postoperative period.

3. The **airway must be easily accessible;** close monitoring is necessary to detect intrinsic or extrinsic obstruction from laryngeal edema or hematoma formation. Patients frequently complain of throat pain probably related to introperative retraction on the trachea or esophagus. Treatment consists of reassurance and topical anesthetic lozenges.

B. EC-IC anastomosis

1. Because these anastomoses involve only the superficial cortex of the brain, patients should be awake and their tracheas should be extubated before entry to the recovery room.

2. Close observation in the intensive care unit of all vital signs for 48 to 72 hours is necessary. Blood pressure should be maintained as close to preoperative levels as possible (see sec. **V.A.2**). Careful, frequent neurologic assessment must be performed and charted. Alteration of CBF may increase the risk of rupture of an aneurysm.

3. All previous medications (with the exception of ϵ-aminocaproic acid that is used as an antifibrinolytic agent) should be restarted as quickly as possible. Patients who had been taking barbiturate preparations to control seizures should not receive full doses in the immediate postoperative period since this will interfere with emergence from anesthesia.

4. Necrosis of the flap may occur in the area of the scalp supplied by the diverted superficial temporal artery and may cause postoperative fever or sepsis.

References

1. Bentsen, N., Larsen, B., and Lassen, N. A. Chronically impaired autoregulation of cerebral blood flow in long term diabetics. *Stroke* 6:497, 1975.
2. Carlsson, C., Smith, D. S., Keykhah, M. M., et al. The effects of high dose fentanyl in cerebral circulation and metabolism in rats. *Anesthesiology* 57:375, 1982.
3. EC/IC Bypass Study Group. Failure of extracranial-intracranial arterial bypass to reduce the risk of ischemic stroke: Results of an international randomized trial. *N. Engl. J. Med.* 313:19, 1191, 1985.
4. Fein, J. M. Contemporary Techniques of Cerebral Revascularization. In J. M. Fein and O. H. Reichman (Eds.), *Microvascular Anastomoses for Cerebral Ischemia.* New York: Springer Verlag, 1978. Pp. 161–177.
5. Foex, P., and Prys-Roberts, C. Anesthesia and the hypertensive patient. *Br. J. Anaesth.* 46:575, 1974.
6. Frost, E. Central Nervous System Effects of Nitrous Oxide. In E. I. Eger (Ed.), *Nitrous Oxide N₂O.* New York: Elsevier, 1985. Pp. 157–176.
7. Frost, E. A. M. Anaesthetic management of cerebrovascular disease. *Br. J. Anaesth.* 53:745, 1981.
8. Frost, E. A. M. Inhalation anaesthetic agents in neurosurgery. *Br. J. Anaesth.* 56:47S, 1984.
9. Goldman, L., and Caldera, D. L. Risks of general anesthesia and elective operation in the hypertensive patient. *Anesthesiology* 50:25, 1979.

10. Goldman, L., Caldera, D. L., Southwick, F. S., et al. Cardiac risk factors and complications in noncardiac surgery. *Medicine* 57:357, 1978.
11. Harper, A. M. The inter-relationship between $PaCO_2$ and blood pressure in the regulation of blood flow through the cerebral cortex. *Acta Neurol. Scand.* 41 (Suppl 14):95, 1965.
12. Keykhah, M. M., Smith, D. S., Carlsson, C., et al. Influence of sufentanil on cerebral metabolism and circulation in the rat. *Anesthesiology* 63:274, 1985.
13. Keykhah, M. M., Smith, D. S., Englebach, I, et al. Effects of high dose fentanyl on cerebral high energy metabolites during hypoxia. *Anesthesiology* 61:A368, 1984.
14. Lassen, N. Cerebral blood flow and oxygen consumption in man. *Physiologie* 39:183, 1959.
15. Lassen, N. A., Ingvar, D. H., and Skinhoj, E. Brain function and blood flow. *Sci. Am.* 239:62, 1978.
16. Malley, R. A., and Frost, E. A. M. Moya-moya disease: Pathophysiology and anesthetic management. *J. Neurosurg. Anesthesiol.* 1:2, 1989.
17. McKay, R. D., Sundt, T. M., Michenfelder, J. E., et al. Internal carotid artery stump pressure and cerebral blood flow during carotid endarterectomy. Modification by halothane, enflurane and Innovar. *Anesthesiology* 45:390, 1976.
18. Michenfelder, J. D. The Cerebral Circulation. In C. Prys-Roberts (Ed.), *The Circulation in Anaesthesia, Applied Physiology and Pharmacology.* Oxford: Blackwell Scientific Publications, 1980. Pp. 209–225.
19. Sharbrough, F. W., Messick, J. M., Jr., and Sundt, T. M., Jr. Correlation of continuous electroencephalograms with cerebral blood flow measurements during carotid endarterectomy. *Stroke* 4:674, 1973.
20. Tobey, R. E., Jacobsen, P. M., Kahle, C. T., et al. The serum potassium response to muscle relaxants in neural injury. *Anesthesiology* 37:332, 1972.
21. Wylie, E. J., and Ehrenfeld, W. K. Extracranial occlusive cerebrovascular disease. Philadelphia: Saunders, 1970. P. 231.

10

Cerebrovascular Lesions and Tumors in the Pregnant Patient

MARK A. ROSEN

Maternal mortality has declined during the past 35 years owing to better management of the major obstetric problems of hemorrhage, infection, and toxemia. As a result, there has been an increase in the incidence of maternal deaths from nonobstetric causes. Prominent among nonobstetric causes of maternal mortality are neurosurgical disorders, of which the most commonly encountered during pregnancy are subarachnoid hemorrhage (SAH) and intracranial tumor. SAH secondary to rupture of either a saccular aneurysm [3,11,18,22,35,37,39,42,54] or an arteriovenous malformation (AVM) [8,15,16,27,46] now ranks high as a cause of maternal mortality. As documented by angiography, surgery, or autopsy, SAH is reported to cause 12 to 24% of maternal deaths [6,22,35]. Primary and metastatic intracranial tumors are uncommon during the childbearing years, but their clinical course may be aggravated by pregnancy, and surgery may be necessary before it is possible to deliver a viable infant.

This chapter will review the pathophysiology of SAH and intracranial tumors during pregnancy, and discuss an approach to the anesthetic management of these clinical situations. Although other neurosurgical disorders such as pseudotumor cerebri, cerebral cysts or abscesses, sinus thrombosis, and spinal cord diseases occur less frequently, the principles of anesthetic management discussed in this chapter are applicable to them as well.

Regardless of the neuropathology, the anesthesiologist will be involved in providing anesthesia for either the neurosurgical procedure or the vaginal or abdominal delivery. The objectives in the neuroanesthetic management of pregnant women are (1) ensuring maternal safety, (2) avoiding teratogenic drugs, (3) avoiding fetal asphyxia, and (4) preventing preterm labor. The goal of anesthesia for labor and delivery is to provide analgesia without either endangering the fetus or aggravating the maternal neurologic disorder.

I. **Intracranial tumors during pregnancy.** Although the incidence of brain tumors is not greater in pregnant women than in nonpregnant women, a tumor's clinical course is often aggravated by pregnancy [17,28,34]. The mechanism for the exacerbation of tumor progression in pregnancy is probably the generalized water retention that occurs, which causes tumor swelling [13,51]. There is no evidence that mitotic activity increases. Clinical presentation, signs, symptoms, indications for diagnostic workup, and decisions regarding radiation therapy are not altered by pregnancy. Consideration should be given to postponing elective surgical resection until after delivery, when the maternal physiologic changes of pregnancy have returned toward normal and there is no chance to adversely affect the fetus. Craniotomy may be necessary during pregnancy, however, if the patient's clinical condition deteriorates.

II. SAH during pregnancy

A. Etiology and incidence. SAH during pregnancy is most commonly related to congenital saccular (berry) aneurysms or cerebral AVMs with approximately equal frequency. Although the precise incidence is not known, estimates from different series vary from less than 1 per 10,000 to 1 per 2500 pregnancies [11,33].

B. Pathology

1. Saccular aneurysms are caused by congenital defects in the muscularis of arterial walls that occur at bifurcation or branching sites at or near the circle of Willis. These aneurysms are usually less than 1 cm in diameter but can be as large as 5 cm. Autopsy specimens from women of reproductive age reveal an incidence of unruptured saccular aneurysms of 0.5 to 1.0%. With continued overstretching by the forces of blood pressure, the internal elastica undergoes degeneration.

2. AVMS are a network of tangled, interconnected thin-walled vessels in which arterial blood passes directly to venous drainage without intervening capillaries. The network is usually supplied by more than one artery and ranges in size from microscopic to massive. AVMs commonly extend from the surface of the brain into the parenchyma and can occur in the spinal cord.

C. Etiology of rupture. Although distention leading to rupture of an AVM or saccular aneurysm often occurs at rest, the most clearly related predisposing factor appears to be an episode of increased blood pressure, which may occur with coughing, straining, coitus, defecation, lifting, or emotional stress.

D. Relation of pregnancy to rupture. A clear correlation between pregnancy and rupture of saccular aneurysms or AVMs has not been established. Although some conclude that the association is merely coincidental [3,11,18,37], there is an increased incidence of rupture of saccular aneurysms in the thirtieth to fortieth gestational week and of AVMs during the second trimester, shortly before labor, during delivery, and in the early puerperium [41]. Rupture of either aneurysms or AVMs can occur, however, at any time during gestation, labor, or delivery. Several physiologic factors may cause rupture during pregnancy. The cardiovascular stresses of increased cardiac output and increased blood volume and the hormonal changes affecting the connective tissue integrity of the vessel walls may all play contributory roles, but none has been proven or directly implicated.

E. Pathophysiology. With rupture of AVMs or aneurysms, the sudden high-pressure leakage of blood raises the intracranial pressure (ICP) and can cause rapid brain displacement and death, coma, drowsiness, or merely headache, depending on the severity of the hemorrhage. The hemorrhage may remain subarachnoid or blood may dissect into brain parenchyma, resulting in focal neurologic deficits. Parenchymal involvement is more common with AVMs than aneurysms. The blood and its breakdown products are irritants to meninges, blood vessels, and brain parenchyma. Meningeal irritation causes headache and sterile meningitis, which can lead to subacute or chronic communicating hydrocephalus. Brain irritation can evoke adverse descending autonomic discharges, causing hypertension or cardiac arrhythmias. Vasospasm, at least partially caused by the breakdown products of extravasated blood, can lead to ischemia or infarction with resulting neurologic deficits five to seven days after the initial hemorrhage.

F. Prognosis. The prognosis after rupture of either a saccular aneurysm or AVM in pregnancy is comparable to nonpregnant patients. There is a high incidence of recurrent hemorrhage within the first few weeks, especially within the first 48 hours after the initial bleed. The overall mortality is higher in hemorrhages from saccular aneurysms than from AVMs, although there is increased neurologic disability among survivors of AVMs because of their location and tendency to bleed into brain tissue.

G. Diagnosis. The diagnosis of AVM (more often than aneurysm) can sometimes be made before rupture by history of severe headaches, seizures, bruits, cranial nerve palsies, or focal neurologic deficits. The presentation, however, is almost invariably SAH. The initial symptoms are abrupt onset of severe headache (usually described as bursting or explosive), photophobia, nuchal rigidity, diplopia, nausea, vomiting, disturbance of consciousness ranging from drowsiness or confusion to coma, seizures, migraines, bruits, and possibly focal or lateralizing neurologic signs.

The diagnosis of SAH is made by history and physical examination and confirmed by computed tomographic (CT) scanning and grossly bloody or xanthochromic cerebrospinal fluid (CSF) (if sufficient time has elapsed for the blood to hemolyze after the rupture) at lumbar puncture. If there are lateralizing neurologic deficits or suspicion of increased ICP, the lumbar puncture should be deferred. The specific etiology is confirmed by angiography. Protective radiographic shielding for the fetus is important and should be used.

H. Differential diagnosis. The principal differential diagnosis is either fulminant toxemia of pregnancy, with or without intracerebral hemorrhage, or a cerebrovascular accident secondary to chronic hypertension. In fact, many patients with SAH are erroneously diagnosed and treated as toxemics. Hypertension, proteinuria, and earlier convulsions or coma can occur with both toxemia and SAH. Severe hypertension, generalized edema, and severe proteinuria are more often associated with toxemia, however. The headache of toxemia is usually frontal and boring or throbbing rather than explosive, and the epigastric pain sometimes seen with toxemia is not a symptom of SAH. Although unusually high blood pressure occurs more frequently with toxemia, the hemorrhage of a ruptured aneurysm or AVM may raise ICP, causing a reflex increase in blood pressure. Because of these similarities, early neurosurgical consultation is advised whenever toxemics present with unusual findings.

I. Treatment. Successful outcome requires aggressive and prompt investigation and treatment. The neurologic management of SAH in pregnancy is the same as that for the nonpregnant patient. The goals of treatment are (1) to preserve life, (2) to reduce disability, (3) to prevent recurrent hemorrhage, and (4) for the pregnant patient [18], to preserve fetal life.

  1. Medical treatment. The initial treatment is conservative.

   a. Avoid increase in blood pressure by the following measures:

   (1) Antihypertensives for hypertension caused by preexisting disease or secondary to the irritation from subarachnoid blood

   (2) Absolute bed rest in a dark, quiet room to avoid emotional excitement

   (3) Cautious use of sedatives to prevent excitement

   (4) Cautious use of analgesics

   (5) Stool softeners to avoid straining and Valsalva maneuver

   b. Administer steroids to reduce edema.

   c. Administer antifibrinolytic agents (ϵ-aminocaproic acid) to inhibit lysis of the clot formed at the bleeding site to prevent rebleeding (see Chap. 8).

   d. Treat vasospasm. Abortion or cesarean section are performed only for obstetric indications. However, when massive hemorrhage occurs late in pregnancy and the mother is deeply comatose and moribund, cesarean section is necessary to save a viable baby, and the staff must be prepared to perform an agonal cesearean section [24,25].

  2. Surgical treatment. The decision to operate, as well as the timing of operation, are based on the site and surgical accessibility of the lesion, the patient's clinical condition, and the presence of vasospasm. These decisions should rarely, if ever, be influenced by pregnancy. Surgery reduces the mortality and incidence of recurrent hemorrhage from saccular aneurysms. The advantages of surgical resection and ligation of the feeding arteries of AVMs depend on the size and location. Alternative interventional therapy includes particulate embolization, obliteration with intravascular glue, and proton-beam irradiation.

III. Physiologic changes of pregnancy and their anesthetic implications. The particular hazards of anesthesia during pregnancy are related to the physiologic changes in the mother and to the possible adverse effects on the fetus. Hormonal secretions from the corpus luteum and the placenta and mechanical effects of the gravid uterus induce major changes in practically every organ system. Familiarity with these alterations and their implications for anesthetic management is essential for the safest possible administration of anesthesia to the pregnant woman.

A. Pulmonary changes

1. **Decreased functional residual capacity (FRC).** FRC is decreased 10% at 16 weeks' gestation and 20% at term, owing to an increase in tidal volume and a decrease in expiratory reserve volume in the face of unchanged total lung capacity.

2. **Increased ventilation.** Alveolar ventilation is increased 25% at 16 weeks' gestation and 70% at term because of an increase in tidal volume with only small increases in respiratory rate. With this increased ventilation, normal arterial carbon dioxide tension ($PaCO_2$) is decreased to 32 mmHg. Compensatory metabolic acidosis (bicarbonate reduced to 22 mEq/L) keeps maternal pH close to 7.4 units.

3. **Increased oxygen consumption.** Oxygen consumption increases 20% from the development of the fetus, placenta, and uterus.

B. Anesthetic implications of pulmonary changes

1. **Rapid inhalation induction.** With a decreased FRC and increased alveolar ventilation, the rapidity of induction with inhalation anesthetics is increased. This effect is partially balanced by an increase in cardiac output.

2. **Decreased oxygen reserve.** A decreased FRC combined with increased oxygen consumption makes pregnant women more likely to become hypoxic in the face of respiratory obstruction or difficult intubation during the period of apnea. Rapid development of hypoxia is avoided by administering 100% oxygen before induction and intubation. Even during rapid intubation with only 30 seconds of apnea, arterial oxygen tension (PaO_2) can fall to 50 mmHg if preoxygenation is not performed.

C. Cardiovascular changes

1. **Increased cardiac output.** Cardiac output increases 30 to 40% during the first trimester and remains elevated throughout gestation. It increases even more during labor with painful uterine contractions and reaches its greatest increase (80% elevation) immediately after delivery. Despite this increase in cardiac output, there is normally no increase in blood pressure, indicating a decrease in peripheral vascular resistance.

2. **Increased blood volume.** Increases in maternal blood volume begin in the first trimester. The increase in plasma volume is greater than the increase in red blood cell (RBC) volume. This accounts for

the relative anemia of pregnancy. At term, the RBC volume is increased about 20% and the plasma volume is increased about 40%.

3. Supine hypotension. When lying supine, pregnant women in the second and third trimesters may develop hypotension from aortocaval compression by the gravid uterus. Caval compression impedes venous return to the heart, which decreases cardiac output. Uterine blood flow decreases both from increased uterine venous pressure and, occasionally (in 10% of parturients), from uterine arterial hypotension. Direct compression of the aorta by the gravid uterus will directly decrease uterine blood flow. Anesthesia may augment these detrimental changes by mechanisms such as the vasodilatation produced by halothane and thiopental or the sympathectomy from regional epidural anesthesia, both of which reduce venous return to the heart. Therefore, it is important to avoid the supine position. For uterine displacement off the great vessels to prevent supine hypotension and uterine hypoperfusion, left lateral tilt should be employed during all anesthetic procedures.

D. Gastrointestinal changes

1. Increased gastric acid production. The hormone gastrin is produced by the placenta. Gastrin levels are elevated throughout pregnancy, with especially high levels occurring in the second and third trimesters. This hormone stimulates gastric acid and enzyme production.

2. Gastroesophageal sphincter incompetence. During pregnancy there is a shift in the position of the stomach due to the enlarging uterus, which changes the angle of the gastroesophageal junction and may permit passive regurgitation.

E. Anesthetic implications of gastrointestinal changes. With increased gastric acid production and compromise of the cardiac sphincter, the pregnant woman, when anesthetized, is more susceptible than her nonpregnant counterpart to regurgitation and aspiration of acidic gastric contents. Although the precise time in gestation when she is at greater risk is unknown, the gastric emptying time is significantly increased in pregnant women beyond 34 weeks' gestation.

All pregnant women should receive 15 ml of 0.3 M sodium citrate before undergoing anesthesia. The safety and effectiveness of other drugs, such as metoclopramide and cimetidine, for reducing gastric volume and acidity are currently being investigated.

Airway protection using cuffed endotracheal tubes and rapid intubation with preoxygenation and cricoid pressure should be employed for women in the second half of pregnancy or anytime during pregnancy if the woman has symptoms of reflux esophagitis.

F. Neurologic changes

1. Decreased inhalation anesthetic requirement. The minimum alveolar concentration (MAC) of pregnant women is reduced 25 to 40%, which is possibly related to elevated endorphin levels.

      2. Decreased size of epidural and subarachnoid spaces. With the increase in femoral venous and intra-abdominal pressures, the epidural veins are enlarged, decreasing the epidural space. This increased epidural pressure is transmitted to the subarachnoid space, decreasing the volume of CSF in the vertebral column. The CSF pressure is not elevated.

   G. Anesthetic implications of neurologic changes

      1. Increased likelihood of inhalation anesthesia overdose. With the decreased MAC, pregnant women are more sensitive to inhalation anesthetics. Concentrations that would otherwise be safe may produce overdose and cardiovascular depression.

      2. Decrease in epidural anesthetic requirements. With the decrease in epidural space and CSF volume, there is a 30% decrease in the amount of local anesthetic required to produce a given level of epidural or subarachnoid block in parturients during the period from midpregnancy to term as compared to the nonpregnant patient.

  H. Renal and hepatic changes. During pregnancy there is an increase in the renal plasma flow, glomerular filtration rate, and tubular reabsorption of water and electrolytes, with an increased creatinine clearance. Therefore, the normal blood urea nitrogen (BUN) is 8 to 9 mg/100 ml, and the normal creatine is 0.6 mg/100 ml, but electrolytes are unchanged.

     Many liver enzymes are normally elevated during pregnancy, including serum glutamic-oxaloacetic transaminase (SGOT) lactic dehydrogenase (LDH), and alkaline phosphatase, although bilirubin levels and hepatic blood flow remain unchanged. There is a decrease in total protein and the albumin-globulin ratio. Serum cholinesterase is also decreased, which is usually clinically insignificant but may prolong the neuromuscular blockade of succinylcholine.

  I. Uterine blood flow. Uterine blood flow at term is about 700 ml/min, which is 10% of the maternal cardiac output. About 70 to 90% of the uterine blood flow perfuses the placenta and the rest supplies the myometrium. The uterine vascular bed, almost maximally dilated under normal conditions, has little capacity to dilate further. It is not autoregulated, so the uterine blood flow is proportional to the mean perfusion pressure. The uterine vessels are, however, capable of marked vasoconstriction.

  J. Anesthetic implications of uterine blood flow. Reductions in uterine blood flow can cause serious fetal hypoxia with disastrous results. Uterine blood flow is significantly decreased by several factors relevant to the anesthesiologist.

     1. Hypotension

        a. Sympathetic blockade

        b. Hypovolemic shock

    c. Supine-hypotension syndrome

    d. Iatrogenic: nitroprusside-induced hypotension or deep halothane anesthesia

  2. Vasoconstriction (increased uterine vascular resistance)

    a. Endogenous sympathetic discharge

    b. Essential hypertension

    c. Toxemia

    d. Exogenous alpha-adrenergic drugs (e.g., phenylephrine)

  3. Uterine contractions or hypertonus

  4. Excessive positive pressure ventilation (by decreasing venous return and cardiac output)

IV. Anesthesia for craniotomy during pregnancy. Anesthetic management of patients undergoing neurosurgical procedures is modified during pregnancy to protect the fetus (by avoiding asphyxia, teratogenicity, and preterm labor) and the mother.

A. Fetal considerations

  1. Avoidance of fetal asphyxia. Fetal oxygenation is dependent on maternal arterial oxygen content and placental blood flow. Induced hypotension and hypocapnia are commonly employed during neurosurgery, but these techniques may affect the fetus adversely. Intrauterine fetal asphyxia is avoided by maintaining normal maternal PaO_2, $PaCO_2$, and uterine blood flow.

    The causes of maternal hypoxia during general anesthesia do not differ from those for any ventilated patient. Elevated maternal oxygen tensions that commonly occur during anesthesia are safe for the fetus. A rise of maternal PaO_2 even to 600 mmHg seldom produces a fetal PaO_2 above 45 mmHg and never above 60 mmHg. Thus, premature closure of the ductus arteriosus or retrolental fibroplasia cannot be produced in utero with normobaric maternal hyperoxia.

    Fetal $PaCO_2$ is directly related to maternal $PaCO_2$. Maternal hypercapnia will cause fetal respiratory acidosis. Maternal hypocapnia produced by excessive positive pressure ventilation may increase mean intrathoracic pressure, decrease venous return, and hence decrease cardiac output. This causes a fall in the uterine blood flow, which is deleterious to the fetus. Also, maternal alkalosis reduces umbilical blood flow by direct vasoconstriction, and shifts the oxyhemoglobin dissociation curve to the left. This shift increases the affinity of maternal hemoglobin for oxygen and decreases the release of oxygen to the fetus at the placenta. Thus, fetal hypoxia and acidosis can result from maternal hyperventilation.

    As uterine arterial blood flow is directly dependent on maternal blood pressure, maternal hypotension will cause a fall in uterine blood flow and may lead to asphyxia. A small fall in blood pressure with low concentrations of halothane is not associated with significant reduction of uterine blood flow because of concomitant decrease in uterine vascular resistance. Deep halothane anesthesia that results in maternal hypotension (30% decrease from control) will, however, produce fetal asphyxia. Significant maternal hypotension should therefore be avoided or corrected promptly by administering fluids, reducing anesthetic concentration or, if necessary, administering an appropriate vasopressor (ephedrine).

2. **Avoidance of teratogenic drugs.** Teratogenicity may be induced at any stage of gestation by exogenous agents and detected at birth, or later. To produce a defect, the teratogenic agent must be given in an appropriate dose, during a particular developmental stage of the embryo or fetus, in a species or individual who has a particular genetic susceptibility. Each organ and each system undergoes a critical stage of differentiation during which vulnerability to teratogens is greatest and specific malformations can be produced. In humans, the first trimester appears to be the most vulnerable period.

   Almost all commonly used anesthetic and premedicant drugs have been shown to be teratogenic in some animal species. Also, in the experimental animal, hyperbaric oxygenation, hypoxia, and hypercapnia may be teratogenic. In several surveys of women who received anesthesia for operations during pregnancy, including the vulnerable first trimester, no drug has been shown to be safer than another, and no specific agent has been implicated as a teratogen [44,45]. These studies in humans are too small, however, to support a categorical statement that anesthetic drugs are *not* teratogenic. At this time, the choice of specific anesthetic agents for pregnant women undergoing neurosurgical procedures is not influenced by concerns of teratogenicity.

3. **Prevention of preterm labor.** There have been suggestions that abdominal operations during pregnancy may cause preterm labor during the postoperative period, and that anesthesia and surgery during pregnancy are associated with an increased risk of first and second trimester spontaneous abortions. Despite this, there is no association between neurosurgical procedures and preterm labor. It is unknown whether anesthetics can stimulate or inhibit preterm labor, but it is unlikely that preterm labor would begin during the neurosurgical intraoperative period. Patients should be monitored for uterine contractions intraoperatively and postoperatively for at least 24 hours. Early detection of preterm labor is important because effective drugs are available to inhibit labor and avoid premature delivery.

   Drugs that increase uterine tone such as alpha-adrenergic vasopressors should be avoided as should rapid intravenous administration of anticholinesterase drugs.

4. **Possible fetal complications of adjuvants to lower ICP.** Osmotic diuresis, controlled hypotension, hypothermia, and hypocapnia are commonly employed during neurosurgery. These adjuvants may, however, have adverse effects on the fetus. Special consideration must be given to the fetus in relation to the use of these techniques and adjuncts during the anesthetic course. Their use depends on the seriousness of the maternal impairment, and whether that impairment will result in more severe fetal morbidity than the morbidity associated with the therapy.

   a. **Osmotic diuretics.** Osmotic diuretics (mannitol, urea) used to reduce cerebral water content, have been shown to traverse the placenta, raise the fetal plasma osmotic pressure, and cause a net flow of water from the fetus to the mother [7,10]. This decreases fetal blood volume, total body water, and extracellular fluid volume. Such fluid exchange can cause severe fetal dehydration. Therefore, these drugs should only be used when absolutely necessary during pregnancy.

   b. **Induced hypotension.** Induced hypotension reduces cerebral bleeding and the likelihood of rupture of a saccular aneurysm during surgical manipulation, but it can cause fetal asphyxia with disastrous effects on the newborn. Although there have been several successful cases reported using hypotensive techniques for craniotomies during pregnancy [11,35,53], there have also been reports of fetal demise or distress (based on fetal heart rate monitoring) [2,38,42]. Further, the "success" reported has often been a living fetus or live birth with neither follow-up nor assessment of neurologic status.

      (1) **Fetal asphyxia.** The hazard to the fetus depends on the severity and duration of maternal hypotension. Fetal risk is directly related to uterine blood flow, which varies directly with maternal blood pressure. When uterine blood flow is reduced sufficiently, fetal asphyxia results. Fetal asphyxia is most damaging to the central nervous system, heart, and lungs. In experimental fetal monkeys who sustained fetal asphyxia of intermediate severity and duration with consequent acidosis, permanent brain injury occurred, with lesions similar to those of human cerebral palsy [9]. Severe asphyxia produces fetal death from myocardial failure.

      (2) **Hypotensive drugs.** The drugs commonly used to induce hypotension are halogenated inhalational anesthetics, nitroprusside, nitroglycerin, and trimethaphan. Regardless of which drugs are used, the reduced maternal blood pressure may lead to fetal asphyxia.

         (a) **Halogenated anesthetics.** Light halothane anesthesia is not associated with significant reductions in uterine blood flow because of concomitant decreases in uterine vascular resistance. High concentrations of halothane anesthesia that depress myocardial contractility and produce significant hypotension cause a fall in uterine blood flow and, consequently, fetal asphyxia.

(b) Nitroprusside. Nitroprusside, the most widely used drug for inducing hypotension, carries the potential hazard of fetal toxicity. The placenta is readily permeable to nitroprusside. It is degraded to cyanogen, which is transformed to thiocyanate by the liver enzyme rhodonase. In experimental animals, peak fetal arterial cyanide levels have been shown to be significantly higher than maternal levels [26,36]. This may be due to either more rapid formation of cyanide or a slower rate of detoxification and excretion by the fetus. Although several patients have received nitroprusside for acute treatment of systemic and pulmonary hypertension without adverse effects on the fetus [14,40], nitroprusside administration should be limited to small doses for short periods of time.

(c) Nitroglycerin. To date, the use of nitroglycerin during pregnancy has demonstrated no adverse fetal or neonatal effects. Nitroglycerin has been shown to be effective in reducing norepinephrine-induced hypertension in gravid ewes [52] and has been used successfully in humans [21,47]. It is essentially nontoxic and metabolizes to glyceryl dinitrate and nitrite in the presence of glutathione. Onset of action is slower than that of nitroprusside, and more patients are resistant to its hypotensive effect. Since nitroglycerin is adsorbed on many plastics, it should be infused using glass bottles and polyethylene tubing.

(d)Trimethaphan. Pregnant women have a greater reaction to ganglionic blockade, as with trimethaphan, than nonpregnant women. The hypotensive effect of autonomic blockade in supine pregnant women depends mainly on venous pooling of blood with decreased return to the heart and a consequent diminution of cardiac output. Autonomic blockade prevents the increased neurogenic tone of the capacitance vessels that ordinarily compensates for the interference with venous return from uterine compression.

(3) Monitoring. When it is necessary to induce hypotension, blood pressure reduction should be limited in depth and duration to the minimum required, based on clinical judgment, and fetal heart rate should be closely monitored. Fetal tolerance will depend on fetoplacental reserve. Maternal arterial pH should be measured frequently to avoid potentially severe fetal toxicity.

c. **Hypocapnia.** Extreme maternal hyperventilation may result in a reduction of uterine blood flow, a fall in placental oxygen transfer, a fall in fetal oxygen partial pressure (PO_2), anaerobic metabolism, and fetal metabolic acidosis. In theory, hyperventilation should therefore be avoided. Mild hyperventilation is probably safe, however, especially if the fetal heart rate is monitored for adverse effects. Some fetuses that have good reserve will not become acidotic because of anaerobic metabolism. Fetuses in borderline or in precarious situations, however, may react adversely to even mild degrees of maternal hyperventilation. The normal $PaCO_2$ in pregnant women is 32 mmHg, with a pH of 7.4 units. Hyperventilation to decrease $PaCO_2$ to 20 mmHg is most likely safe and easily reversible if fetal tachycardia or bradycardia indicates fetal intolerance. As with induced hypotension, the use of hyperventilation should be limited in extent and duration to the minimum required, based on clinical judgment.

d. **Hypothermia.** Moderate hypothermia (temperatures of 28–32°C), properly used, decreases cerebral oxygen demand and reduces blood flow to the brain. If maternal respiratory acidosis is prevented, the gas and acid-base contents of fetal blood will parallel those of the mother [50]. Although uterine vascular resistance increases and uteroplacental blood flow falls during hypothermia, oxygen transfer is unaffected. Since the fetus also becomes hypothermic, its metabolic needs are proportionately decreased [4]. Hypothermia as an ancillary aid to intracranial surgery does not increase fetal morbidity, which is substantiated by many case reports [8,11,15,19,23,30,38,39,42,46,48,53]. Fetal heart rate will decrease in parallel when maternal heart rate decreases, then increase again when rewarming occurs [20,48].

5. **Monitoring during craniotomy.** Besides the usual monitors for major neurosurgical procedures (intra-arterial catheter, Doppler air-embolism monitor, and right atrial catheter), the fetus and uterus should be monitored when a pregnant woman undergoes craniotomy. After the sixteenth week of pregnancy, the external Doppler fetal heart rate monitor should be employed. Monitoring fetal heart rate provides an indication of abnormalities in maternal ventilation or uterine perfusion, as well as fetal well-being. Careful observation of the maternal blood pressure and prompt correction of hypotension and hypoxia are mandatory if the fetus is to have the best chance of survival with an intact nervous system.

Anesthetics that readily traverse the placenta diminish the normal beat-to-beat variability of the fetal heart rate. During induced hypothermia, the fall in fetal heart rate parallels the decrease in maternal heart rate. Patterns of bradycardia are, however, associated predominantly with maternal hypotension or hypoxia and, as such, are valuable for diagnosis. The relationship between maternal hypotension and fetal bradycardia is well known in obstetrics. A maternal systolic blood pressure of less than 100 mmHg may be associated with pathologic fetal bradycardia, which begins a few minutes after the onset of the hypotension, and is sometimes preceded by mild fetal tachycardia. Fetal tachycardia has also been recognized as an early sign of maternal hypoxia in the third trimester of pregnancy and of fetal distress in the full-term infant.

Additionally, an external tocodynamometer to monitor uterine tone is indicated if the uterine fundus is above the level of the umbilicus.

B. Preanesthetic visit. The preanesthetic visit, an essential part of each patient's preparation and assessment before operation, includes attention to physical examination, history, laboratory findings, and consultants' reports. Special efforts should be made to decrease the patient's apprehension by providing reassurance and emotional support. Maternal stress and anxiety are associated with increased release of endogenous catecholamines, which decreases uterine blood flow. These women are concerned not only for their own welfare, but for that of their unborn child. The anesthesiologist should convey optimism about both maternal and fetal prognosis and reassure the mother that the welfare of the baby will be considered at all times.

C. Premedication. Heavy sedation is contraindicated because of possible respiratory depression, potential exacerbation of depressed consciousness, and delayed postoperative recovery of consciousness. Preoperative sedation may be omitted in most cases with increased safety for the patient. If some sedation is necessary, pentobarbital, 50 to 100 mg IM, is preferred to benzodiazepines, phenothiazines, or narcotics. All patients should receive an oral antacid 30 to 60 minutes before induction to reduce gastric acidity.

D. Transport and positioning. Beginning in the second trimester, women must not be transported or positioned on the surgical table in a supine or prone position. They should either be placed in a sitting or lateral decubitus position. Proper positioning will minimize the risk of obstruction of the vena cava by displacing the gravid uterus off the great vessels. The legs should be wrapped in elastic bandages and placed at the level of the heart to facilitate venous return from the lower extremities. The eyes should be protected with a small amount of protective eye ointment, tape, and patches.

E. Induction and intubation. Induction of anesthesia with intravenous drugs, followed by immediate endotracheal intubation, is performed with standard rapid-sequence technique to establish an airway and protect the patient from possible regurgitation and aspiration. This is important for pregnant women whose gestation is greater than 20 weeks and for all women who have a history of gastric reflux.

The rapid-sequence intravenous induction and endotracheal intubation, commonly performed for women undergoing cesarean section, is acceptable for the neurosurgical patient provided she is adequately anesthetized before laryngoscopy. The conscious patient can be asked to voluntarily hyperventilate just before induction of anesthesia. Succinylcholine after pretreatment with a nondepolarizing drug will not itself raise the ICP. Alternatively, a priming dose of a short-acting, nondepolarizing drug can be given before the intubating dose [32,43,49]. Laryngoscopy and intubation in a lightly anesthetized patient will cause hypertension, but a large dose of thiopental ameliorates this response. Additionally, the use of nitroprusside to achieve a stable, modest blood pressure reduction (15–20%) during the few minutes prior to induction will blunt the hypertensive response from the rapid-sequence intravenous induction. The technique is as follows.

1. Induce a stable, modest blood pressure reduction (15–20%) with nitroprusside, using an infusion pump and direct arterial pressure monitoring.
2. Administer 100% oxygen for at least three minutes to avoid maternal hypoxia during intubation, asking the patient to hyperventilate.
3. Administer *d*-tubocurarine, 3 mg IV. Reassure the patient that she and the fetus are both doing well. Wait three to five minutes, continuing preoxygenation.
4. Apply pressure over cricoid cartilage to occlude the esophagus and prevent passive regurgitation (Sellick maneuver). This pressure should be applied by an assistant until the trachea is successfully intubated and the endotracheal tube cuff is inflated.
5. Administer thiopental, 4 to 5 mg/kg IV, to conscious patients (less thiopental required for patients with altered states of consciousness) *and* administer succinylcholine, 1.5–2.0 mg/kg IV, followed by a 60- to 90-second pause, during which positive pressure ventilation by mask is avoided.
6. Intubate the trachea with a cuffed endotracheal tube, using a stylet.
7. Inflate the cuff immediately after the trachea is intubated.
8. Control the ventilation, and undertake maneuvers to ensure correct endotracheal tube placement.
9. Stop the nitroprusside infusion.
10. Administer narcotics to deepen anesthesia.

F. **Maintenance of anesthesia.** Fifty percent nitrous oxide with 50% oxygen supplemented by intravenous thiopental, narcotics, and neuromuscular blocking drugs will be adequate for positioning and placement of the pin headholder. Once adequate hyperventilation has been ensured by blood gas determination, anesthesia can be supplemented by the addition of low concentrations of halogenated anesthetic agents.

    G. Postoperative management. The posoperative management of a pregnant woman after craniotomy involves only a few modifications from that of her nonpregnant counterpart.

        1. Extubation. Although smooth emergence and extubation are ideal, extubation should be delayed until the patient is sufficiently awake to protect her airway from regurgitation and aspiration of gastric contents.

        2. Position. Maintenance of left uterine displacement is important to avoid supine hypotension from compression of the great vessels by the gravid uterus. The patient should be maintained in a lateral position, with the head slightly elevated, during the entire postoperative period (including transport from the operating room to the recovery area).

        3. Monitoring. The fetal heart rate and uterine tone should be monitored for at least 24 hours, or until the mother's condition is stable. Maternal hypotension, hypertension, or respiratory depression may have adverse effects on the fetus as well as the mother. Efforts should be made to avoid these complications. If they do occur, they should be promptly investigated, diagnosed, and aggressively treated.

V. Obstetric management and anesthesia for vaginal delivery or cesarean section. For the patient who has a documented saccular aneurysm or AVM, whether ruptured or unruptured, surgically or conservatively treated, elective cesarean section is not necessarily warranted since it affords no advantage over vaginal delivery in protecting against intracerebral hemorrhage [3,5,12,22,35,37,39,42]. Cesarean section should be performed only for accepted obstetric indications. If labor supervenes after SAH, vaginal or even abdominal delivery should be considered before neurosurgical intervention [42,54]. This decision is affected by the severity of the maternal clinical condition, the feasibility of stopping preterm labor, and the maturity of the fetus.

    Management of labor and delivery in women who have documented aneurysms, AVMs, or intracranial tumors (especially tumors that have not been surgically treated) includes avoidance of hypertension and increased ICP. The second stage of labor should be shortened and maternal straining should be avoided. Maternal straining with the Valsalva maneuver raises both ICP and CSF pressure [22,29,31]. After the Valsalva maneuver, there is an immediate reduction in CSF pressure but an increase in cardiac output and blood pressure owing to increased venous return to the heart. The net effect on transmural pressure of cerebral vessels from the Valsalva maneuver is not precisely known. Until cerebral hemodynamics during labor are better understood, it is best to avoid Valsalva maneuvers in women who have increased ICP or cerebrovascular disease to reduce the possibility of herniation of the brain or rupture of tenuous cerebral vessels.

Shortening the second stage of labor and avoiding maternal straining can be best achieved by segmental lumbar epidural or caudal anesthesia and the elective application of outlet forceps for delivery. For the first stage of labor, a properly administered epidural block for labor will (1) decrease pain and prevent the increased blood pressure and cardiac output from painful contractions and (2) avoid the Valsalva maneuver by blocking the reflex urge to bear down. There is an obvious risk of lumbar epidural techniques in these women because of inadvertent dural puncture. A sudden leakage of CSF can result in cerebral herniation. There is a somewhat reduced likelihood of dural puncture with the caudal approach to the epidural space. However, neurologic sequelae have resulted from caudal anesthesia in patients with increased ICP [1].

Alternate forms of analgesia include paracervical and pudendal blocks, inhalation analgesia, and systemic narcotics. These techniques are not as effective as epidural anesthesia, but paracervical and pudendal blocks may be satisfactory alternatives for women with increased ICP. Administration of narcotics and inhalation agents during spontaneous ventilation may raise $PaCO_2$, increase cerebral blood flow, raise ICP, and induce maternal respiratory acidosis. If general anesthesia is necessary for either vaginal delivery or manual removal of the placenta, the anesthetic considerations and techniques for induction and intubation discussed in this section **V** should be employed.

Low spinal anesthesia may be contraindicated in patients who have intracranial hypertension in the presence of an aneurysm or AVM. A reduction in CSF pressure might increase the transmural pressure (MAP-ICP) in the aneurysm and the risk of aneurysm rupture (see Chap. 8).

Should a cesarean section be required, epidural anesthesia with a sensory level of T4 is recommended. However, if general anesthesia is indicated, the considerations and techniques discussed here are applicable.

After successful surgical occlusion of an aneurysm or AVM, there appears to be no need for specialized management of labor and delivery. Even elective induction of labor employing an oxytocic agent is not contraindicated. Considering that the reported incidence of aneurysms is 0.5 to 1.0%, a large number of women who have this vascular anomaly must go through labor and delivery without undue difficulty.

References

1. Abouleish, E. Caudal analgesia. In E. Abouleish (Ed.). *Pain Control in Obstetrics.* Philadelphia: Lippincott, 1977. Pp. 225–256.
2. Aitken, R. R., and Drake, C. G. A technique of anesthesia with induced hypotension for surgical correction of intracranial hemorrhages. *Clin. Neurosurg.* 21:107, 1974.
3. Amias, A. G. Cerebral vascular disease in pregnancy. I. Haemorrhage. *J. Obstet. Gynaecol. Br. Commonw.* 77:100, 1970.
4. Assali, N. S., and Westin, B. Effects of hypothermia on uterine circulation and on the fetus. *Proc. Soc. Exper. Biol. Med.* 109:485, 1962.

5. Baker, J. W. Subarachnoid haemmorrhage associated with pregnancy. *Aust. N.Z. J. Obstet. Gynaecol.* 9:12, 1969.
6. Barno, A., and Freeman, D. W. Maternal deaths due to spontaneous subarachnoid hemorrhage. *Am. J. Obstet. Gynecol.* 125:384, 1976.
7. Battaglia, F., Prystowsky, H., Smisson, C., et al. Fetal blood studies XIII. The effect of the administration of fluids intravenously to mothers upon the concentrations of water and electrolytes in plasma of human fetuses. *Pediatrics* 25:2, 1960.
8. Boba, A. Hypothermia: Appraisal of risk in 110 consecutive patients. *J. Neurosurg.* 19:924, 1962.
9. Brann, A. W., Jr., and Myers, R. E. Central nervous system findings in the newborn monkey following severe in utero partial asphyxia. *Neurology* 25:327, 1975.
10. Bruns, P. D., Linder, R. O., Drose, V. E., and Battaglia, F. The placental transfer of water from fetus to mother following the intravenous infusion of hypertonic mannitol to the maternal rabbit. *Am. J. Obstet. Gynecol.* 86:160, 1963.
11. Cannell, D. E., and Botterell, E. H. Subarachnoid hemorrhage and pregnancy. *Am. J. Obstet. Gynecol.* 72:844, 1956.
12. Daane, T. A., and Tandy, R. W. Rupture of congenital intracranial aneurysms in pregnancy. *Obstet. Gynecol.* 15:305, 1960.
13. Donaldson, J. O. Tumours. In *Neurology of Pregnancy.* Philadelphia: Saunders, 1978. P. 158.
14. Donchin, Y., Amiray, B., Sahar, A., and Yarkoni, S. Sodium nitroprusside for aneurysm surgery in pregnancy. *Br. J. Anaesth.* 50:849, 1978.
15. Dunn, J. M., and Raskind, R. Rupture of a cerebral arteriovenous malformation during pregnancy. *Obstet. Gynecol.* 30:423, 1967.
16. Dunn, J. M., Weiss, S. R., and Raskind, R. Rupture of intracranial arteriovenous malformation in pregnancy. *Int. Surg.* 49:241, 1968.
17. Ehlers, N., and Malmros, R. The suprasellar meningiomas. *Acta Ophthalmol.* 121(Suppl):1, 1973.
18. Fliegner, J. R. H., Hooper, R. S., and Kloss, M. Subarachnoid haemorrhage and pregnancy. *J. Obstet. Gynecol. Brit. Commonw.* 76:912, 1969.
19. Hehre, F. W. Hypothermia for operations during pregnancy. *Anesth. Analg. Curr. Res.* 44:424, 1965.
20. Hess, O. W., and Davis, C. D. Electronic evaluation of the fetal and maternal heart rate during hypothermia in a pregnant woman. *Am. J. Obstet. Gynecol.* 89:801, 1964.
21. Hood, D. D., Dewan, D. M., James, F. M., III, et al. The use of nitroglycerin in preventing the hypertensive response to tracheal intubation on severe preeclamptics. *Anesthesiology* 59:A423, 1983.
22. Hunt, H. B., Schifrin, B. S., and Suzuki, K. Ruptured berry aneurysms and pregnancy. *Obstet. Gynecol.* 43:827, 1974.
23. Kamrin, R. P., and Masland, W. Intracranial surgery under hypothermia during pregnancy. *Arch. Neurol.* 13:70, 1965.
24. Kofke, W. A., Wuest, H. P., and McGinnis, L. A. Cesarean section following ruptured cerebral aneurysm and neuroresuscitation. *Anesthesiology* 60:242, 1984.
25. Lennon, R. L., Sundt, T. M., Jr., and Gronert, G. A. Combined cesarean section and clipping of intracerebral aneurysm. *Anesthesiology* 60:240, 1984.
26. Lewis, P. E., Cefalo, R. C., Naulty, J. S., and Rodkey, F. L. Placental transfer and fetal toxicity of sodium nitroprusside. *Gynecol. Invest.* 8:46, 1977.
27. Locksley, H. B. Report on the cooperative study of intracranial aneurysms and subarachnoid hemorrhage: Section V, Part II. Natural history of subarachnoid hemorrhage, intracranial aneurysms and arteriovenous malformations. Based on 6368 cases in the cooperative study. *J. Neurosurg.* 25:321, 1966.
28. Magyar, D. M., and Marshall, J. R. Pituitary tumors and pregnancy. *Am. J. Obstet. Gynecol.* 132:739, 1978.

29. Marx, G. F., Zemaitis, M. T., and Orkin, L. R. Cerebrospinal fluid pressures during labor and obstetrical anesthesia. *Anesthesiology* 22:348, 1961.
30. Matsuki, A., and Oyama, T. Operation under hypothermia in a pregnant woman with an intracranial arteriovenous malformation. *Can. Anaesth. Soc. J.* 19:184, 1972.
31. McCausland, A. M., and Holmes, F. Spinal fluid pressures during labor: Preliminary report. *West. J. Surg. Obstet. Gynecol.* 65:220, 1957.
32. Mehta, M. P., Choi, W. W., Gergis, S. D., et al. Facilitation of rapid endotracheal intubations with divided doses of nondepolarizing neuromuscular blocking drugs. *Anesthesiology* 62:392, 1985.
33. Miller, H. J., and Hinkley, C. M. Berry aneurysms in pregnancy: A ten year report. *South Med. J.* 63:279, 1970.
34. Mills, R. P., Harris, A. B., Heinrichs, L., and Burry, K. A. Pituitary tumor made symptomatic during hormone therapy and induced pregnancy. *Ann. Ophthalmol.* 11:1672, 1979.
35. Minielly, R., Yuzpe, A. A., and Drake, C. G. Subarachnoid hemorrhage secondary to ruptured cerebral aneurysm in pregnancy. *Obstet. Gynecol.* 53:64, 1979.
36. Naulty, J., Cephalo, R. C., and Lewis, P. E. Fetal toxicity of nitroprusside in the pregnant ewe. *Am. J. Obstet. Gynecol.* 139:708, 1981.
37. Pedowitz, P., and Perell, A. Aneurysms complicated by pregnancy. Part II. Aneurysms of the cerebral vessels. *Am. J. Obstet. Gynecol.* 73:736, 1957.
38. Pevehouse, B. C., and Boldrey, E. Hypothermia and hypotension for intracranial surgery during pregnancy. *Am. J. Surg.* 100:633, 1960.
39. Pool, J. L. Treatment of intracranial aneurysms during pregnancy. *J.A.M.A.* 192:209, 1965.
40. Rigg, D., and McDonogh, A. Use of sodium nitroprusside for deliberate hypotension during pregnancy. *Br. J. Anaesth.* 53:985, 1981.
41. Rish, B. L. Treatment of intracranial aneurysms associated with other entities. *South Med. J.* 71:553, 1978.
42. Robinson, J. L., Chir, B., Hall, C. J., and Sedzimir, C. B. Subarachnoid hemorrhage in pregnancy. *J. Neurosurg.* 37:27, 1972.
43. Schwarz, S., Ilias, W., Lackner, F., et al. Rapid tracheal intubation with vecuronium: The priming principle. *Anesthesiology* 62:388, 1985.
44. Shnider, S. M., and Webster, G. M. Maternal and fetal hazards of surgery during pregnancy. *Am. J. Obstet. Gynecol.* 92:891, 1965.
45. Smith, B. E. Fetal prognosis after anesthesia during gestation. *Anesth. Analg. Curr. Res.* 42:521, 1963.
46. Smolik, E. A., Nash, F. P., and Clawson, J. W. Neurological and neurosurgical complications associated with pregnancy and the puerperium. *South. Med. J.* 50:561, 1957.
47. Snyder, S. W., Wheeler, A. S., and James, F. M., III. The use of nitroglycerin to control severe hypertension of pregnancy during cesarean section. *Anesthesiology* 51:563, 1979.
48. Stange, K., and Halldin, M. Hypothermia in pregnancy. *Anesthesiology* 58:460, 461, 1983.
49. Taboada, J. A., Rupp, S. M., and Miller, R. D. Redefining the priming principle for vecuronium during rapid sequence induction of anesthesia. *Anesthesiology* 63:A573, 1985.
50. Vandewater, S. L., and Paul, W. M. Observations on the foetus during experimental hypothermia. *Can. Anaesth. Soc. J.* 7:44, 1960.
51. Weyand, R. D., MacCarty, C., and Wilson, R. B. The effect of pregnancy on intracranial meningiomas occurring about the optic chiasm. *Surg. Clin. North Am.* 31:1225, 1951.
52. Wheeler, A. S., James, F. M., III, Meis, P. J., et al. Effects of nitroglycerin and

nitroprusside on the uterine vasculature of gravid ewes. *Anesthesiology* 52:390, 1980.

53. Wilson, F., and Sedzimir, C. B. Hypothermia and hypotension during craniotomy in a pregnant woman. *Lancet* 2:947, 1959.

54. Young, D. C., Leveno, K. J., and Whalley, P. J. Induced delivery prior to surgery for ruptured cerebral aneurysm. *Obstet. Gynecol.* 61:749, 1983.

11

Posterior Fossa Procedures

ROBERT F. BEDFORD

I. Physiologic considerations
A. Brainstem considerations
1. Within the posterior fossa, the pons and medulla contain the major motor and sensory pathways, the primary respiratory and cardiovascular centers, and the lower cranial nerve nuclei. Because of the posterior fossa's small size, a localized lesion or a small amount of edema may have profound neurologic effects.
2. Patients who have posterior fossa lesions have decreased levels of consciousness, increased sensitivity to sedative medications, depressed respiration, and impaired airway protective reflexes, all of which must be carefully considered throughout the perioperative period [4].
3. Posterior fossa operations are complicated by fluctuations in heart rate and blood pressure [1]. Meticulous cardiovascular monitoring is therefore required during operation and in the postoperative period [5].
B. Obstructive hydrocephalus and increased intracranial pressure. Exploration of the posterior fossa is frequently performed in the presence of obstruction of cerebrospinal fluid (CSF) outflow at the level of the fourth ventricle from compression by tumor or cyst. Continued production of CSF by the choroid plexus of the lateral ventricles causes intracranial hypertension. When intracranial pressure (ICP) is increased further by volatile anesthetics or arterial hypertension, herniation of brain contents may result, causing potentially fatal brainstem compression [24]. Signs of increased ICP must be sought constantly and techniques for prompt decompression must be available.

II. Preoperative evaluation
A. Patient history
1. Headache, vomiting, and lethargy are indicative of **intracranial hypertension** and often subside after corticosteroid therapy. If signs of intracranial hypertension persist, a ventriculostomy drainage tube or ICP monitor should be placed preoperatively under local anesthesia before general anesthesia is induced [2].
2. A history of a recent preoperative **air-contrast study** should be sought since residual air may take up to a week to reabsorb. Nitrous oxide (N_2O) inhalation will expand the volume of residual intracranial air and thus increase ICP [21].

3. The patient's **sensitivity to general anesthetics** can be estimated from his or her response to sedative medications if they were used for preoperative neuroradiologic procedures. Prolonged somnolence after sedatives usually indicates a decrease in intraoperative anesthetic requirement.

B. Physical examination

1. Intravascular volume depletion often occurs during an extensive period of neurologic diagnosis. Somnolence may limit fluid intake, bed rest causes supine diuresis, and these patients often develop vomiting. Flat neck veins and poor tissue turgor indicate the need for vigorous preoperative volume replacement.

2. Vascular sites for monitoring catheters require evaluation. Allen's test for ulnar-artery collateral blood flow to the hand should be performed before radial artery cannulation, and suitable sites for peripheral and central venous catheters must be sought. Increased ICP from head-down positioning and decreased cerebral venous outflow can be avoided if antecubital veins are used instead of the jugular or subclavian route [25].

3. Preoperative papilledema confirms the diagnosis of increased ICP and limited intracranial compliance. If papilledema disappears after corticosteroid therapy, improved intracranial compliance can be anticipated.

4. Preoperative **pulmonary function** should be evaluated. Impaired consciousness and protective reflexes may have allowed "silent" aspiration to occur. Previously undiagnosed pulmonary dysfunction may present as intraoperative hypoxia and may be life-threatening if combined with uncontrolled hemorrhage during surgery.

5. Evaluation of **concurrent cardiovascular disease** is important. Patients who have limited myocardial reserve or cerebrovascular insufficiency should be considered for operation in the prone or lateral decubitus position rather than risking cardiovascular instability in the seated position [18].

C. Medications.
High-potency corticosteroids reduce edema around brain tumors [13] and frequently cause marked preoperative neurologic improvement. The potential complications of hyperglycemia and electrolyte disturbances must be evaluated, and plans for continued perioperative steroid and diuretic therapy should be formulated.

III. Intraoperative considerations
A. Choice of anesthetic

1. The use of **N_2O and oxygen in combination with narcotic and muscle relaxant** usually has minimal effect on cerebral blood flow and ICP, yet it allows maximal cardiovascular stability during postural changes [18]. This technique is preferred for positioning patients who have space-occupying lesions undergoing operations in the seated position. Once surgery has begun, many neuroanesthetists choose to discontinue N_2O to reduce the risks of air embolism [20] and tension pneumocephalus [3].

2. **Volatile drugs** may be used in patients who have normal intracranial dynamics for nerve root section, microvascular decompression, or electrode implantation. Patients who have obstructive pulmonary disease or coronary artery disease may require volatile anesthetics. An ICP monitor facilitates titration of inhalational agents against their effect on ICP [15]; cerebral perfusion pressure (CPP) can be maintained through hyperventilation and other measures to control ICP.

B. Monitoring

1. **Direct arterial pressure monitoring** is extremely useful during posterior fossa exploration in the seated position. An estimate of CPP can be obtained by placing the pressure transducer at head level, and sudden cardiovascular changes can be observed on a beat-to-beat basis. Furthermore, correlation of pulse-pressure waveforms with electrocardiogram (ECG) patterns allows instant recognition of the hemodynamic impact of arrhythmias caused by brainstem or cranial nerve stimulation [1,4].

2. **Right atrial and pulmonary artery pressure monitoring** afford means for diagnosis and recovery of intravenous air and also reflect cardiac preload. Furthermore, by measuring right atrial and pulmonary capillary wedge pressures, it is possible to identify patients who may sustain paradoxical air embolism via a probe-patent foramen ovale [23]. Although insertion of flow-directed balloon-tipped catheters requires added time and effort, several centers now use them routinely. However, most institutions still prefer right atrial catheterization with ECG or x-ray confirmation of the position of the tip.

3. **Precordial Doppler monitoring** is virtually mandatory. The probe is affixed along the right sternal border between the third and sixth intercostal spaces. Proper positioning over the right atrium is confirmed by eliciting a change in Doppler signal when a 10-ml bolus of saline is injected rapidly into the right atrial catheter [26].

4. **End-tidal CO_2 analysis** complements the capabilities of the Doppler device, since small, hemodynamically insignificant air emboli heard with the Doppler device can be differentiated from emboli that may produce arterial hypotension. Capnography is virtually as sensitive as pulmonary artery pressure monitoring [5] but has the added advantage of being noninvasive. Initial cost, however, ranges from $2000 to $7000.

5. **Intraoperative monitoring** of anesthetic gases using mass spectroscopy permits the accurate diagnosis of air embolism by indicating an increase in exhaled nitrogen concentration as air reaching

the pulmonary circulation crosses the alveolar-capillary membrane and is exhaled. For all practical purposes the changes in **end-tidal nitrogen concentration** during air embolism parallel the changes in **end-tidal CO_2 concentration and pulmonary artery pressure** during air embolism [11,19]. A disadvantage of relying on mass spectroscopy, however, is that the instrument must be shared by several operating rooms, thus delaying observation of an increase in end-tidal nitrogen concentration by as much as a minute.

6. **Transesophageal echocardiography** (TEE) is the most sensitive method for air embolism detection [9] but is also the most expensive (currently about $75,000). It is possible to observe both cardiac contractility and air bubbles as they pass through the heart.

7. **Brainstem auditory evoked potential (BAEP) monitoring** has also achieved widespread use for detection of untoward surgical dissection near the brainstem and eighth cranial nerve. This is particularly true for acoustic tumor excision, but is also applicable to other procedures. Usually, abnormalities in BAEPs develop just at the time that cardiovascular changes occur during brainstem manipulation, thus verifying that the heart rate and blood pressure alterations are neurogenic in origin.

8. **Neuromuscular transmission** requires monitoring during posterior fossa surgery, particularly if there is a possibility that the patient will cough or strain during the light levels of anesthesia occasionally required for the seated position to prevent cardiovascular instability.

9. Knowledge of **urinary output** is necessary as an indicator of perioperative fluid balance. During craniotomy the initial diuresis is frequently augmented by osmotic or loop diuretics. Urine output, however, may be reduced by either hypovolemia or release of antidiuretic hormone (ADH).

C. Position

1. **The seated position** affords access to the apex of the posterior fossa and facilitates exploration and dissection because blood and CSF drain away from the surgical site. In addition, it is possible to observe the airway and to note the response to cranial nerve stimulation.

2. **Cardiovascular instability** is the primary disadvantage of the seated position. General anesthesia and positive pressure breathing reduce blood pressure mainly by reducing cardiac output. These effects are augmented as patients are placed in the seated position since venous return is impeded. Vigorous volume replacement with balanced salt solutions, wrapping the legs with ace bandages, and keeping the knees flexed at heart level are all techniques that promote venous return and maintain cardiac output (Fig. 11-1). Although blood pressure at the level of the heart may be normal, it is

crucial to remember that mean arterial pressure (MAP) at the level of the head is approximately 20 mmHg lower in the seated position.

3. Positional complications

    a. Hyperflexion of the neck causes **jugular venous obstruction,** which can result in increased ICP and a "tight" posterior fossa. Swelling of the face and tongue may also occur [12]. Excessive neck flexion may cause **quadriplegia** from ischemia of the cervical spine [17]. Placing two fingers between the chin and suprasternal notch while the patient's head is being fixed in position in the headholder is a simple method for preventing neck hyperflexion and its attendant complications.

    b. Ulnar nerve compression may occur at the elbow if the ulnar groove is in contact with either the edge of the operating table or the arm boards. The ulnar grooves can remain free of pressure if the forearms are crossed over the abdomen and affixed with 4-inch–wide tape running from one elbow to the other. Padding the elbows also minimizes compression.

    c. Sciatic nerve damage may be induced by severe flexion of the hips while the knees are held straight. Although optimal venous

Fig. 11-1. Diagrammatic representation of patient properly positioned for seated posterior fossa operation with knees at heart level and neck not hyperflexed. Monitoring devices are discussed in text. ECG = electrocardiogram; SAP = systemic arterial pressure; PAP = pulmonary artery pressure; CVP = central venous pressure.

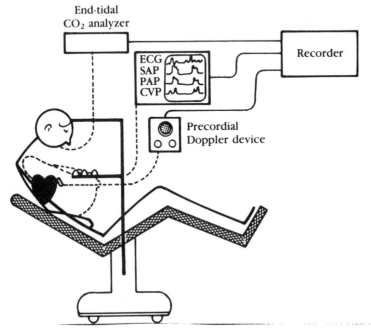

return to the heart occurs with the knees at heart level, it is best to flex the knees in order to reduce tension on the sciatic nerve.

d. Lateral peroneal nerve compression may occur from pressure from the headrest brackets near the lateral aspect of the knees. Liberal padding should be applied at this point to avoid contact with metal supports.

D. Air embolism

1. Pathophysiology. Whenever the operative site is higher than the level of the heart, venous blood falls freely past the incision. In this situation, room air may be entrained into the circulation through surgical openings in the veins. During posterior fossa operations, there is a high incidence (30–50%) of air embolism because of the large hydrostatic pressure gradient between the occiput and the heart and because dural tacking to bony structures tends to hold the veins open [1,5]. Air then enters the circulation as a fine stream of bubbles, passes through the right side of the heart, and subsequently lodges in the pulmonary arterioles. Intensive vasoconstriction occurs, resulting in ventilation-perfusion mismatch, interstitial pulmonary edema, and reduced cardiac output as pulmonary vascular resistance increases. Small amounts of air can be excreted through the lungs, but as the capacity of the pulmonary vasculature is exceeded, air bubbles back up into the right side of the heart and prevent cardiac ejection by causing an "air lock" effect.

Paradoxical air embolism is a particular concern in the sitting position because air bubbles that enter the systemic circulation tend to travel preferentially to the cerebral vasculature where cerebral ischemic injury may result [14]. As demonstrated in Figure 11-2, paradoxical air embolism usually occurs when venous air bubbles traverse a probe-patent foramen ovale and enter the left atrium. Thirty percent of patients have a probe-patent foramen ovale [16] and air bubbles may pass through whenever right atrial pressure exceeds left atrial pressure. This occurs during moderately large episodes of air embolism when pulmonary vascular resistance increases markedly, but also may occur if air embolism develops at a time when left atrial pressure has fallen below right atrial pressure as a result of fluid restriction in the sitting position [8].

During posterior fossa procedures, air embolism develops frequently when the posterior neck muscles are dissected free from the subocciput, when bone is excised, and when a vascular tumor bed is entered. Particular vigilance is necessary at these times so that the surgeon can be alerted to the presence of air embolism and can take appropriate measures to stop entrainment of air.

2. Diagnosis

a. The simplest method for detecting air embolism is by monitoring the signal of a 2-Hz precordial **Doppler ultrasound probe** placed over the right atrium. Air bubbles as small as 0.1 ml elicit a

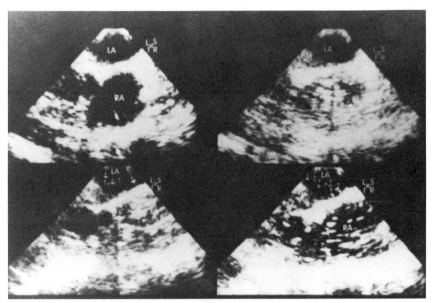

Fig. 11-2. Two-dimensional echocardiographic record of air embolism developing during a posterior fossa operation in the sitting position. Air bubbles appear as a "snowstorm" in the right atrium (RA) and then progress into the left atrium (LA) through the foramen ovale (see arrows) when right atrial pressure increases above left atrial pressure. Note change of interatrial septum from concave to convex configuration as interatrial pressure gradient changes. (From R. F. Cucchiara, M. Nugent, J. B. Seward, and J. M. Messick. Air embolism in upright neurosurgical patients: Detection and localization by two-dimensional echocardiography. *Anesthesiology* 60:353–355, 1984. With permission.)

distinctive change in Doppler frequency since they reflect the ultrasound beam more effectively than erythrocytes when they pass through the right side of the heart. The Doppler device is not foolproof, however, since it cannot accurately quantitate the volume of air passing through the heart. Conversely, the Doppler may fail to detect a very fine stream of air bubbles or its position may shift during a long operation. It is most effective when used in conjunction with at least one other modality for detection of air embolism.

b. Infrared end-tidal CO_2 analysis is less sensitive than is Doppler monitoring, but does permit quantification of the severity of an air embolus. When enough air has entered the circulation to produce pulmonary vasoconstriction, wasted ventilation increases and end-tidal CO_2 concentration promptly decreases in proportion. False-positive diagnoses are possible, however, since an abrupt decrease in cardiac output (as caused by an arrhythmia or brainstem compression) will also decrease end-tidal CO_2 and may be misinterpreted as an air embolus (Fig. 11-3).

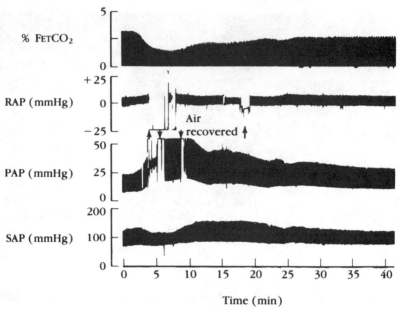

Fig. 11-3. Record of air embolism occurring during posterior fossa exploration. Concomitant with a modest reduction in systemic arterial pressure (SAP) is a marked increase in pulmonary artery pressure (PAP), a fall in end-tidal CO_2 fraction (FETCO$_2$), and a slight increase in right atrial pressure (RAP). Breaks in RAP and PAP traces indicate where a small volume of air (5–10 ml total) was recovered from both the right atrium and pulmonary artery.

    c. Pulmonary artery pressure monitoring affords positive diagnosis of air embolism and also quantifies its severity since pulmonary artery pressure increases proportionally with the volume of air embolized. Pulmonary artery pressure is not readily affected by sudden changes in cardiac output unless associated with acute left ventricular failure. Pulmonary artery catheters may allow recovery of air from both the pulmonary artery and right atrium, although recovery has not been as successful as with multiorifice central venous catheters [6]. Late signs of air embolism, such as premature ventricular beats, a mill-wheel murmur, or systemic hypotension, are of little diagnostic value because they reflect ongoing cardiovascular decompensation from large volumes of air.

    Pulmonary artery pressure monitoring also affords an estimate of left atrial pressure when pulmonary capillary wedge pressure is measured. Frequent determination of pulmonary capillary wedge pressure can thus indicate when left atrial pressure is falling below right atrial pressure and when measures that will elevate left atrial pressure should be undertaken (e.g., volume loading or gradual lowering of the head of the operating table) [8].

d. End-tidal nitrogen concentration changes in concert with end-tidal CO_2 concentrations and pulmonary artery pressure during air embolism. It is available in all operating rooms equipped with mass spectroscopy, but is currently of limited value for early diagnosis of air embolism because one unit is shared among several operating rooms. Thus, from a clinical standpoint, there is a crucial delay between when an air embolus occurs and when the end-tidal nitrogen concentration is observed by the anesthesiologist. If single-use mass specs become available, however, they will be of considerable value in making a positive diagnosis of air embolism, since no other intraoperative pathologic condition causes an increase in end-tidal nitrogen concentration.

e. Two-dimensional echocardiography (2-D echo) has been shown to be more sensitive than precordial Doppler monitoring for venous air embolism, and the appearance of air bubbles on the screen is unmistakable (see Fig. 11-2). Furthermore, the 2-D echo not only allows a visual estimation of ventricular contractility but also permits identification of a probe-patent foramen ovale if it is present. By forcibly injecting saline solution through a central venous catheter, one can observe the flow of saline passing through a foramen ovale, particularly if a Valsalva maneuver is performed simultaneously so that right atrial pressure is elevated above left atrial pressure [10]. If a patent foramen ovale is detected, one would be particularly loath to use the sitting position for surgery with a high risk of air embolism.

Disadvantages of the 2-D echo are its expense (approximately $250,000) and the necessity of watching an oscilloscope screen. Because of these problems it is unlikely it will achieve much use outside of busy neurosurgical centers.

3. Treatment. Treatment of air embolism must be directed first at stopping further entrainment of air. The incision should be packed with soaked sponges and the bone edges should be waxed. Compression of the neck veins may be performed to increase venous pressure, temporarily slow air entry, and demonstrate the bleeding site. N_2O must be discontinued promptly so that embolized air bubbles do not expand [20]. Recovery of air from the right side of the heart or pulmonary artery is accomplished by aspirating the mixture of blood and air from the right atrial or pulmonary artery catheter. Systemic hypotension responds readily to ephedrine, 10 to 15 mg IV, but is rarely needed if a prompt diagnosis is made and appropriate surgical intervention is conducted. If arterial hypotension persists, the head of the operating table should be lowered. With increased venous pressure, not only does entrainment of air stop, but active bleeding can indicate where air is entering the circulation and these sites can be cauterized and sealed. The use of 10 cm of positive end-expiratory pressure (PEEP) is not effective in the acute treatment of air embolism and may serve to promote paradoxical air embolism by raising right atrial pressure acutely [22].

E. **Cardiovascular changes.** Surgical manipulation near the brainstem and cranial nerves often causes abrupt fluctuations in blood pressure and heart rate. Stimulation of the fifth cranial nerve, the periventricular gray area, the medullary reticular formation, or the nucleus of the tractus solitarius may produce arterial hypertension, whereas stimulation of the vagus nerve causes bradycardia [1,4]. Compression of the medulla and pons results in sudden arterial hypotension. Differentiating arterial hypotension from an air embolus not heard with a Doppler may be difficult without confirmatory monitors such as a pulmonary artery catheter, end-tidal nitrogen analyzer, or 2-D–echo device.

F. **Fluid management.** Since formation of edema at the operative site is potentially fatal, patients should receive balanced salt solution replacement only in volumes compatible with hemodynamic stability. Blood loss is replaced with 5% albumin solution, blood, or both, depending on the hematocrit. Since blood loss may be massive and temporarily uncontrollable, routine use of two large-bore peripheral intravenous routes is recommended.

IV. **Anesthetic management**
A. **Induction sequence**
   1. General anesthesia is induced with thiopental (2–4 mg/kg IV), and airway patency is assured by positive pressure ventilation with oxygen by a bag and mask. A paralyzing dose of nondepolarizing muscle relaxant is given and N_2O (50–70% in oxygen) is added if no recent air-contrast study has been done [21]. If N_2O cannot be used, then low concentrations of volatile anesthetic and oxygen are employed. Controlled hyperventilation is maintained until total neuromuscular blockade is observed.
   2. Before endotracheal intubation, lidocaine, 1.5 mg/kg IV, and additional thiopental, 2 to 3 mg/kg IV, are given. Laryngoscopy is begun just as arterial pressure begins to decrease in response to these drugs. This, in turn, minimizes the increase that often occurs in both arterial and intracranial pressures after endotracheal intubation.
   3. After endotracheal intubation, an esophageal stethoscope and themistor are introduced, the eyes are taped closed, and the endotracheal tube is secured with liberal amounts of adhesive tape. If 2-D–echo monitoring is used, the probe should be placed at this time and presence of a foramen ovale is sought by injection of 10 ml of saline solution. [10].

B. The seated position

1. Before positioning, the legs are wrapped from toes to groin with ace bandages, and a urinary catheter is inserted. The operating table is slowly maneuvered into a semiseated position with the patient's hips and knees flexed, legs elevated, and knees at heart level. Both arterial and ICP transducers are secured at head level to verify adequate CPP. The forearms are crossed over the abdomen and secured with tape.

2. If a **pin headholder** is to be used, additional thiopental and lidocaine should first be given intravenously, or a local anesthetic should be used to infiltrate the scalp [7] to prevent intracranial hypertension as the pins are secured in the skull. As the head is positioned, care must be taken to avoid hyperflexion of the neck [12,17], and the eyes must be checked to ensure that there is no external pressure being applied from the headrest. Once the headrest is in place, the endotracheal tube and circle absorber hoses can be suspended from the headrest bracket to avoid traction on the airway.

3. After the patient has been placed in the seated position, the precordial Doppler can be placed over the right atrium and the capnograph line inserted into the endotracheal tube. Care must be taken to avoid skin burns from patient contact with the capnography head, which becomes quite hot with prolonged use.

4. Once cardiovascular stability has been achieved in the seated position, the level of anesthesia may be deepened with judicious doses of narcotics or volatile agents (ideally with an ICP monitor in use) before the skin incision. Many prefer to discontinue N_2O immediately before the skin incision is made in an effort to prevent an increase in size of any air emboli that may occur [20]. Intravenous drugs, such as barbiturates, diazepam, and droperidol should be used with caution, however, since prolonged somnolence may make postoperative neurologic assessment more difficult.

C. Ventilation

1. Ventilation is controlled throughout posterior fossa procedures to maintain modest hypocapnia. Changes in blood pressure, heart rate, or both are used as an indication of brainstem ischemia or harmful manipulation [4]. A minority of clinicians believe that changes in depth, pattern, or frequency of respiration during spontaneous ventilation are a more sensitive indicator of brainstem involvement than are cardiovascular changes. The risks of hypercapnia or coughing during operation, however, contraindicate this technique. Brainstem, auditory, and somatosensory evoked potential monitoring has largely eliminated previous concerns relating to brainstem function during posterior fossa surgery.

2. The patient's requirement for **postoperative mechanical ventilation** should be assessed before the end of the procedure. In general, with patients who have had minimally traumatic procedures, such as microvascular nerve-root decompression, the trachea can be extubated at the conclusion of the operation. Conversely, patients who have had extensive posterior fossa exploration and possible damage to respiratory centers or protective reflex pathways should be observed until they are fully awake. Extubation is then performed only when they are able to breathe and cough adequately.

D. Fluid and medication management

  1. Maintenance **IV fluid requirements** during operation are met with balanced salt solutions without dextrose. If cardiovascular instability is associated with either low cardiac filling pressures or poor urinary output, then 5% albumin, whole blood, or both are used for intravascular volume expansion.

  2. Patients who are receiving **corticosteroids** preoperatively receive a constant infusion of dexmethasone, 4 mg/kg, throughout the procedure. Mannitol, 0.25 to 0.5 gm/kg, or furosemide, 20 to 40 mg, is given if needed to reduce brain bulk once the craniectomy has been performed.

  3. Serum electrolytes and glucose are determined every few hours during operation, since hyperventilation and diuretics can profoundly alter sodium and potassium levels and steroid therapy may cause severe hyperglycemia. Arterial blood gases and pH are checked frequently to document the adequacy of ventilation and oxygenation.

V. Postoperative care

  A. Ventilation

  1. A patent airway and adequate alveolar ventilation are prerequisites for accurate assessment of neurologic status. Since respiratory centers or airway protective reflexes may be compromised during extensive posterior fossa dissection [4], some patients may require intubation postoperatively. Ventilation is assisted or controlled to maintain arterial carbon dioxide tension ($PaCO_2$) at approximately 35 mmHg.

  2. Intraoperative **air embolism** may result in interstitial pulmonary edema. Patients who have sustained air embolism should have serial blood gas analyses and chest x-rays postoperatively. The use of oxygen therapy, ventilatory support, or PEEP is dictated by the results of these studies.

  3. Choosing the proper time for **extubation** is difficult. Coughing and straining on an endotracheal tube are hazardous because they may precipitate intracranial bleeding. Conversely, aspiration and pneumonitis may result from premature extubation if patients are not alert and able to cough and swallow effectively. Occasionally, patients may require intubation for several days before airway protective reflexes return. Usually these patients can be identified early because they do not react vigorously to prolonged intubation and they require minimal sedation during the postoperative period.

B. Neurologic care

1. Patients are nursed in the 30-degree head-up position to reduce formation of edema around the brainstem and cranial nerves. **Level of consciousness** is the most reliable sign of early brainstem compromise, and for this reason long-acting, nonreversible sedatives, such as diazepam and droperidol, should be avoided. Sudden postoperative deterioration of consciousness may indicate obstructive hydrocephalus or brainstem encroachment by hematoma.

2. **Tension pneumocephalus** is recognized as a potential cause of serious postoperative neurologic dysfunction [3]. As CSF leaks out of the subarachnoid space during posterior fossa operations in the seated position, the cerebral hemispheres can collapse and allow air to enter through the craniectomy and accumulate over the cortex. This effect is probably enhanced further in patients who have functioning lateral ventricular shunts where the hydrostatic pressure gradient between the head and the chest tends to promote loss of CSF. After the incision has been closed, CSF accumulates faster than the air can be absorbed, producing a tension pneumocephalus. If suspected, the diagnosis can be made easily with skull x-ray, and the intracranial air can be released through a small twist drill burr hole placed after local anesthetic infiltration of the area.

3. **ICP monitoring and computed tomography (CT)** capability are mutually complementary in the postoperative assessment of patients who are slow to awaken. Increased ICP may result from brain edema, obstructive hydrocephalus, or tension pneumocephalus. CT scanning can rapidly identify causes of elevated ICP and indicate which patients require prompt surgical intervention. Patients who remain somnolent despite the absence of a surgically correctable lesion and the reversal of sedatives usually have developed brain edema or vasospasm and require prolonged supportive care until consciousness returns. Often, evoked potential monitoring can play an important role in detecting postoperative brainstem dysfunction.

C. Cardiovascular control

1. Continuous direct arterial and venous pressure and ECG **monitoring** are necessary for the first 24 to 48 hours postoperatively.

2. **Arterial hypertension** frequently occurs after posterior fossa exploration and should be treated aggressively with sympathetic blocking drugs such as labetalol before brain edema or hematoma formation occurs. Since arterial hypotension may lead to cerebral

vasospasm, meticulous maintenance of normal cardiac filling pressures and arterial blood pressure is mandatory.

D. Fluid and electrolyte management. Corticosteroid therapy is continued into the postoperative period at doses equivalent to those used preoperatively. Immediately after operation, serum electrolyte concentrations are determined and appropriate fluid replacement with sodium- and potassium-containing solutions is begun. Insulin is given to treat high blood glucose levels. In general, fluid restriction is continued to prevent both brain edema and dilutional hyponatremia secondary to high postoperative ADH levels.

References

1. Albin, M. S., Babinski, M., Maroon, J. C., et al. Anesthetic management of posterior fossa surgery in the sitting position. *Acta Anaesth. Scand.* 20:117, 1976.
2. Albright, L., and Reigel, D. M. Management of hydrocephalus secondary to posterior fossa tumors. *J. Neurosurg.* 46:52, 1977.
3. Artru, A. A. Nitrous oxide plays a direct role in the development of tension pneumocephalus intraoperatively. *Anesthesiology* 57:59, 1982.
4. Artru, A. A., Cucchiara, R. F., and Messick, J. M. Cardiorespiratory and cranial nerve sequellae of surgical procedures involving the posterior fossa. *Anesthesiology* 52:83, 1980.
5. Bedford, R. F., Marshall, W. K., Butler, A., et al. Cardiac catheters for diagnosis and treatment of venous air embolism. *J. Neurosurg.* 55:610, 1981.
6. Bunegin, L., Albin, M. S., Helsel, P. E., et al. Positioning the right atrial catheter: A model for reappraisal. *Anesthesiology* 55:343, 1981.
7. Colley, P. S. Prevention of blood pressure response to skull pin head holder by local anesthesia. *Anesth. Analg.* 58:241, 1979.
8. Colohan, A. R. T., Perkins, N. A. K., Bedford, R. F., et al. Intravenous fluid loading as prophylaxis for paradoxical air embolism. *J. Neurosurg.* 62:839, 1985.
9. Cucchiara, R. F., Nugent, M., Seward, J. B., et al. Air embolism in upright neurosurgical patients: Detection and localization by two-dimensional echocardiography. *Anesthesiology* 60:353, 1984.
10. Cucchiara, R. F., Seward, J. B., Nishimura, R. A., et al. Identification of patent foramen ovale during sitting position craniotomy by transesophageal echocardiography with positive airway pressure. *Anesthesiology* 63:107, 1985.
11. Drummond, J. C., Prutow, R. J., and Scheller, M. S. A comparison of the sensitivity of pulmonary artery pressure, end-tidal carbon dioxide, and end-tidal nitrogen in the detection of venous air embolism in the dog. *Anesth. Analg.* 64:688, 1985.
12. Ellis, S. C., Bryan-Brown, C. W., and Hyderally, H. Massive swelling of the head and neck. *Anesthesiology* 42:102, 1975.
13. Galicich, J. H., and French, L. A. Use of dexamethasone in the treatment of brain tumors and brain surgery. *Am. Prac.* 12:169, 1961.
14. Gronert, J. A., Messick, J. M., Cucchiara, R. F., et al. Paradoxical air embolism from a patent foramen ovale. *Anesthesiology* 50:548, 1979.
15. Grosslight, K., Foster, R., Colohan, A. R., et al. Isoflurane for neuroanesthesia: Risk factors for increases in ICP. *Anesthesiology* 63:533, 1985.
16. Hagen, P. T., Scholz, D. G., and Edwards, W. D. Incidence and size of patent foramen ovale during the first 10 decades of life: An autopsy study of 965 normal hearts. *Mayo Clin. Proc.* 59:17, 1984.
17. Hitselberger, W. E., and House, W. S. A. Warning regarding the sitting position for acoustic tumor surgery. *Arch. Otolaryngol.* 106:69, 1980.

18. Marshall, W. K., Bedford, R. F., and Miller, E. D. Cardiovascular responses in the seated position — Impact of four anesthetic techniques. *Anesth. Analg.* 62:648, 1983.
19. Matjasko, J., Petrozza, P., and Mackenzie, C. F. Sensitivity of end-tidal nitrogen in venous air embolism detection in dogs. *Anesthesiology* 63:418, 1985.
20. Munson, E. S., and Merrick, H. C. Effect of nitrous oxide on venous air embolism. *Anesthesiology* 27:783, 1966.
21. Paul, W. L., Munson, E. S., and Maniscalo, J. E. Cerebrospinal fluid pressure during O_2 encephalography and N_2O inhalation. *Anesth. Analg.* 55:849, 1976.
22. Perkins, N. A. K., and Bedford, R. F. Hemodynamic consequences of PEEP in seated neurosurgical patients: Implications for paradoxical air embolism. *Anesth. Analg.* 63:429, 1984.
23. Perkins-Pearson, N. A. K., Marshall, W. K., and Bedford, R. F. Atrial pressures in the seated position: Implications for paradoxical air embolism. *Anesthesiology* 57:493, 1982.
24. Shapiro, H. M. Intracranial hypertension. *Anesthesiology* 43:445, 1975.
25. Smith, S. L., Albin, M. S., Ritter, R. R., et al. CVP catheter placement from the antecubital veins using a J-wire catheter guide. *Anesthesiology* 60:238, 1984.
26. Tinker, J. H. Detection of air embolism: A test for positioning of right atrial catheter and Doppler probe. *Anesthesiology* 43:104, 1975.

12

Transsphenoidal Procedures

KALMON D. POST

PHILIPPA NEWFIELD

I. General principles. Although the transsphenoidal operation dates back
to 1907, and Cushing [6] performed over 200 such operations for resection
of pituitary tumors, it was not until 1959 that Guiot and Thibaut [4]
popularized the operation using image-intensified fluoroscopy. Hardy [5]
further modernized the procedure by introducing the operating microscope, which had the advantages of both magnifying and significantly
improving focal illumination. With these advances, the transsphenoidal
approach to sellar lesions has become increasingly popular and successful.
   A. Advantages of the transsphenoidal approach
      1. Morbidity and mortality are extremely low.
      2. Trauma to the brain is minimized.
      3. Operation is tolerated extremely well by acutely ill and aged pa-
      tients.
      4. Approach allows visual differentiation of small tumors within the
      gland.
      5. Anesthetic and convalescent times are short.
      6. Incidence of diabetes insipidus is low.
      7. Blood loss is minimal.
   B. Disadvantages of the transsphenoidal approach
      1. Neural structures adjacent to a large tumor cannot be visualized.
      2. Approach is through a nonsterile field (although meningitis is ex-
      tremely rare).
      3. Capabilities are limited if the diagnosis is questionable.
      4. Suprasellar extension of the tumor into frontal fossa, middle fossa,
      or retroclival area that is asymmetric cannot be removed.

II. Indications for transsphenoidal approach to the sellar region. The
indications for the transsphenoidal approach are most often limited to
sellar and suprasellar lesions such as pituitary tumors, intrasellar and
cystic craniopharyngiomas, cerebrospinal fluid (CSF) leaks, and intrasellar
masses of uncertain types. The transsphenoidal approach is also used for
hypophysectomy performed for breast or prostatic cancer as well as for
intrasinus lesions such as tumors or mucoceles. Experience is increasing
in the utilization of this approach for clival lesions such as chordomas.
   A. Pituitary tumors. Pituitary tumors can be divided into two broad
   categories, nonfunctional and hypersecreting. In the past, radiation was
   the treatment of choice for small tumors when diagnosis was reason-

264

ably certain on visual, endocrinologic, and radiologic bases. Craniotomy and primary decompression were reserved for (1) large tumors that compromised vision to 20/200 or worse, (2) cystic adenomas, (3) pituitary apoplexy, or (4) uncertain diagnosis.

1. Nonfunctional tumors (Fig. 12-1)

   a. Diagnosis. Unless they either appear as incidental findings on skull film or cause headaches or mild endocrinopathies, nonfunctional tumors are usually diagnosed when they become large enough to produce a mass effect with visual changes and hypopituitarism secondary to compression of the optic chiasm and pituitary gland, respectively.

   b. Indications for surgery. The size of the nonfunctional tumor may mandate surgical intervention. Any cranial nerve deficit (e.g., intraocular muscle abnormalities from dysfunction of cranial nerves III, IV, VI) other than that of the optic nerve also demands surgical treatment. Progressive visual loss in acuity or fields and other mass effects, such as CSF obstruction with hydrocephalus, a generalized increase in intracranial pressure (ICP) from a large tumor in either the frontal or middle fossa, and specific neuroendocrine deficits because of hypothalamic dysfunction, also mandate sugical removal and decompression. Additional indications include pituitary apoplexy, uncertain diagnosis, tumor recurrence after radiation treatment, and CSF leak.

   In autopsies performed on patients who did not have evidence of pituitary dysfunction, as many as 23% had pituitary adenomas

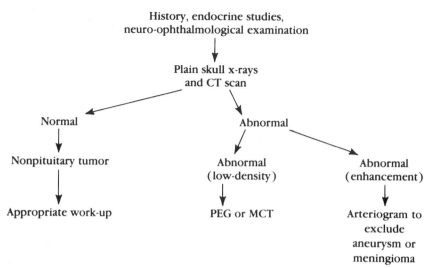

Fig. 12-1. Suggested tests for nonsecretory tumors. CT = computed tomography; MCT = metrizamide computed tomography; PEG = pneumoencephalography.

[2], presumably nonfunctional and requiring no treatment. (Although they had no signs of Cushing's disease or acromegaly, prolactin secretion could have been present.) Undoubtedly, then, a large proportion of small nonfunctional or prolactin-secreting tumors may have a benign natural history. Therefore, the incidental nonfunctional tumor that produces neither neurologic nor endocrinologic deficit can either be followed conservatively with the use of computed tomography (CT) until evidence of growth is present or it may be treated with radiation therapy to arrest growth; surgery is not usually performed. Occasionally, for psychological reasons, a patient will desire the removal of even a small tumor, and this is done.

2. Hypersecreting tumors (Fig. 12-2)

   a. Presentation. Hypersecreting tumors may produce adrenocorticotropic hormone (ACTH), growth hormone (GH), thyroid-stimulating hormone (TSH), and prolactin, singly or in combination. Because of the effects of the excessive hormone secretion, patients usually seek treatment while the tumors are small, and therefore mass effect with compression of the neural structures is less common as an early manifestation.

   b. Indications for surgery include all the indications for nonfunctional tumors and the following.

   (1) Cushing's disease. Cushing's disease is almost always secondary to a pituitary microadenoma, but x-ray studies of the sella are more often normal than abnormal. In a series of 86 patients who had Cushing's disease, only 20 were noted to have abnormalities on sella tomograms or plain skull films. Tyrrell and colleagues [18] explored the sella in 20 consecutive cases of Cushing's disease, 8 of whom had normal sellae by x-ray study. In 2, there were technical difficulties that precluded intrasellar exploration, but in 17 of the other 18, a microadenoma was found and removed. In the other patient, a hypophysectomy was performed and 1.5-mm adenoma was seen in the specimen. Hypercortisolism was corrected in all but one of these patients.

   We recommend sellar exploration of all patients who have Cushing's disease since the systemic effects of excessive ACTH and cortisol, such as hypertension, diabetes mellitus, osteoporosis, obesity, and myopathy, contribute to the five-year mortality of 50%. The low morbidity of pituitary surgery is an advantage compared with adrenalectomy. Additionally, the risk of Nelson's syndrome, reportedly 9 to 10% after adrenalectomy, is negated. The cure rate and rapidity of response after operation have made this modality superior to radiation therapy for children as well as adults.

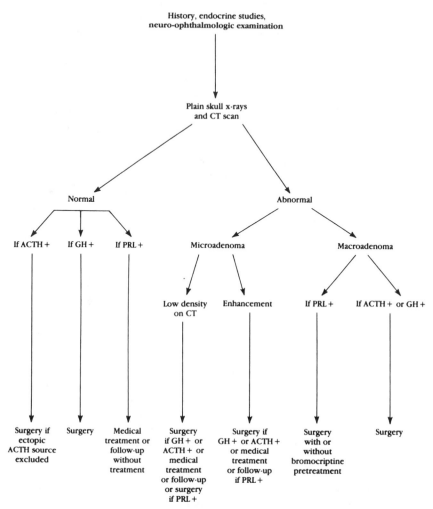

Fig. 12-2. Suggested tests for secretory tumors. ACTH = adrenocorticotropic hormone; CT = computed tomography; GH = growth hormone; PRL = prolactin.

(2) **Nelson's syndrome.** Whether developing after adrenalectomy or representing the further growth of an occult tumor initially responsible for Cushing syndrome, Nelson's syndrome has also been treated surgically. This tumor tends to have aggressive growth patterns, and early removal is suggested.

(3) **Acromegaly.** Excessive GH has many serious adverse systemic effects such as hypertension, diabetes mellitus, cardiomyopathy, cerebrovascular disease, and chronic pulmonary disease. The death rate is almost twice that expected from the

general population, making surgical removal of a GH-secreting adenoma imperative. GH-secreting adenomas are not usually as large as nonfuctional tumors when first discovered. Treatment with conventional and heavy-particle irradiation is beneficial, yet there is a significant delay before plasma GH falls and, more importantly, it may never return to normal. Similarly, medical treatment offers some benefits but does not ablate the tumor. Therefore, we consider surgery to be the therapy of choice.

(4) Prolactinomas. Prolactinomas are the most common pituitary tumor, constituting 30 to 70% of most series. If the tumor is large and causes neurologic deficit, surgery is suggested. However, recent studies with bromocriptine show significant shrinkage with relief of neural compression. Male patients who have prolactinomas generally require surgery because of visual-field defects. Women who have amenorrhea-galactorrhea syndromes often are infertile and have hyperprolactinemia and asymmetric sellae on CT scan. The efficacy of bromocriptine in normalizing prolactin and promoting pregnancy is excellent. The cure rate for microadenomas by selective adenomectomy is also high, the morbidity is extremely low, and the mortality is zero. If predictable shrinkage of tumors during treatment with bromocriptine is confirmed, then surgery may be indicated only for those patients who are medical-treatment failures or to remove the residual adenoma after shrinkage. There is no evidence to date that radiation therapy is effective enough against prolactin-secreting tumors to consider irradiation as the primary form of therapy.

3. **Pituitary apoplexy.** The sudden enlargement of a pituitary adenoma secondary to either hemorrhage or hemorrhagic infarction associated with acute neurologic deficits has been an absolute indication for surgical decompression in our clinic. Although some patients may recover spontaneously, even with the addition of high-dose glucocorticoid therapy the risks of waiting are great in relation to the risks of decompression, even in an acutely ill, elderly patient.

4. **Uncertain diagnosis.** If there is doubt as to the clinical diagnosis of a sellar lesion, specific tissue diagnosis is mandatory, especially if radiation therapy is considered. Arachnoid cysts, Rathke's cleft cysts, craniopharyngiomas, dermoid and epidermoid tumors, and chordomas may be present, which are refractory to radiation treatment.

5. **Treatment failures.** Patients who have been treated unsuccessfully with other modalities and show evidence of pituitary tumor growth or persistence of hypersecretion are operative candidates.

B. Sellar or parasellar lesions. Arachnoid cysts, Rathke's cleft cysts, small or cystic craniopharyngiomas, dermoid and epidermoid tumors, meningiomas, and chordomas may all be approached through the transsphenoidal route.

C. CSF leaks. Rhinorrhea from leakage through the sphenoid sinus may be secondary to trauma, malignant tumor, benign tumor, previous transsphenoidal operations, or increased ICP. Surgery is mandatory in such patients to seal the leak and prevent meningitis. Radiotherapy may also be required.

D. Sphenoid sinus disorders. Lesions of the sphenoid sinus such as tumor or mucocele may be approached transsphenoidally.

E. Metastatic cancer. Metastatic cancer of either the breast or the prostate may respond to hormonal ablative therapy through total hypophysectomy. Therefore, transsphenoidal surgery is often performed in these patients who are frequently debilitated and suffering from other medical problems.

III. Preoperative evaluation

A. Medical assessment. Preoperative assessment includes attention to specific problems associated with pituitary tumors including diabetes mellitus, hypertension, diabetes insipidus, hypothyroidism (rarely hyperthyroidism), and adrenal insufficiency.

B. Anatomic evaluation of sellar region. The patient's visual fields are evaluated to assess function of the optic nerves and chiasm. Neurologic evaluation is necessary to detect signs of mass effect or local invasion or compression. Otolaryngologic examination of the nasal passages and nasopharynx is important.

Radiologic studies include plain skull films, CT scans, and magnetic resonance imaging (MRI). Pneumoencephalograms are rarely performed. Carotid arteriograms are performed to exclude the presence of an aneurysm in all patients except those who have hypersecreting tumors. The CT scan is helpful in assessing the bony delineation of the sella floor. MRI is the modality of choice for tumor diagnosis and assessment of suprasellar extension. Imaging of the coronal plane can be achieved directly without reconstitution. In addition, there is neither dental nor bony artifact with MRI, and no absolute need for intravenous contrast.

C. Physiologic endocrine testing. Many tests are available for the evaluation of pituitary function. Certain investigations are indicated in the evaluation of hypopituitarism (Table 12–1), whereas others are of more relevance in presumptive states of pituitary hypersecretion (Tabel 12–2). The most useful procedures are summarized in Table 12–3. Test procedures detailed in Tables 12–1 and 12–2 can be added or interchanged, especially for pretreatment and posttreatment comparison, whereas Table 12–3 represents the basic profile. In the

Table 12-1. Diagnostic tests especially recommended for the investigation of hypopituitarism

Hormone	Test material (adult dosage)	Time of peak serum response	Comments
GH	L-Dopa (500 mg orally)	60 min	Very safe; nausea occasionally occurs; GH *falls* in acromegaly; PRL is normally suppressed (see also Table 12-2)
	Insulin (0.05–0.3 units/kg body weight IV)	60 min	To obtain a maximum response, adequate hypoglycemia must be achieved. ACTH and PRL reserve can be determined simultaneously
PRL	TRH (500 μg IV)	30 min	Very safe. TSH reserve can be determined simultaneously. A GH rise may occur in acromegaly
	Chlorpromazine (25 mg IM)	60–90 min	May produce hypotension and somnolence in hypopituitary or hypothyroid subjects. Tests for hypothalamic reserve for PRL release
ACTH	Insulin (see above)	30 min for ACTH; 60 min for cortisol	See above
	Metyrapone (30 mg/kg body weight orally at 12 midnight). The longer procedure may also be used—750 mg orally every 4 hr for 6 doses	9 A.M. for 11-deoxycortisol and cortisol and/or ACTH	Safe but may cause nausea and vomiting. Unlike the insulin challenge, metyrapone testing is vitiated by concurrent glucocorticoid administration
TSH	TSH (500 μg IV)	30–60 min	See also above under PRL. The test does not reliably separate hypothalamic from pituitary hypothyroidism
Gonadotropins	LH-RH (25–150 μg)	30–60 min	Very safe. A GH rise may occur in acromegaly
	Clomiphene (50 mg BID for 5–7 days)	LH at 5–7 days; also in females at 12–15 days for ovulatory surge	In females can cause ovarian cyst formation and "superovulation." Tests the hypothalamic reserve for gonadotropin release

Source: K. D. Post and I. M. D. Jackson, Endocrinologic Evaluation of Pituitary Tumors. In D. Long and G. Tindall (Eds.), *Contemporary Neurosurgery*, Vol. 2, No. 5. Baltimore: Williams & Wilkins, 1980.

preanesthetic evaluation, the most informative studies are those for ACTH reserve, thyroid function, and electrolyte balance.

D. Preoperative medications. Because the surgical procedure will involve either manipulation or removal of the anterior lobe of the pituitary gland, patients receive steroid replacement to provide adequate glucocorticoid concentrations during the perioperative period. We give cortisone acetate, 50 mg IM, on the night before surgery and on call to the operating room. If diabetes mellitus is present, then appropriate insulin coverage will be necessary. For the hypothyroid patient, thyroid replacement is initiated four to six weeks before elective surgery when possible to achieve a euthyroid state. Diabetes insipidus can be controlled with aqueous pitressin or with desmopressin (1-desamino-8-D-arginine vasopressin; DDAVP).

Premedication consists of diazepam, 10 to 15 mg PO, one to two hours before surgery. The use of narcotics is rarely necessary.

E. Nasal passages. A nasal culture is obtained preoperatively to identify the flora in the event of a postoperative infection. Instruction is also given for mouth breathing because the nasal passages will be occluded with packing for several days after surgery.

IV. Anesthesia

A. Preoperative considerations. In evaluating a patient who requires anesthesia for transsphenoidal surgery, the most important considerations are the nature of the patient's diagnosis and the reason for the procedure. Patients undergo transsphenoidal operations for treatment of hypersecreting pituitary tumors causing amenorrhea, galactorrhea, Cushing's disease, or acromegaly, nonfunctional pituitary adenomas, craniopharyngioma, hormone-responsive metastatic carcinoma, intractable cancer pain, sphenoid sinus lesions, and CSF rhinorrhea.

Each preoperative condition has its own constellation of systemic disorders and accompanying effects on intracranial dynamics that must be considered when selecting an anesthetic technique. Patients who have Cushing's disease may also suffer from hypertension, diabetes, osteoporosis, obesity, and friability of skin and connective tissue. Patients who have acromegaly may have hypertension, cardiomyopathy, diabetes, and osteoporosis as well as prognathism, cartilaginous and soft-tissue hypertrophy of the larynx, and an enlarged tongue, which may complicate intubation of the trachea. Patients who have panhypopituitarism require preoperative supplementation with appropriate hormones and modulation of doses of anesthetic drugs since they may be hypothyroid. Patients suffering from metastatic malignancies are frequently cachectic and debilitated and may have clotting abnormalities and pleural effusions.

B. Selection of anesthetic drugs. The size and location of pituitary and associated tumors determine their effect on intracranial dynamics. The pituitary microadenomas do not act as space-occupying lesions.

Table 12-2. Diagnostic tests especially recommended for the investigation of states of pituitary hyperfunction

Hormone	Test material (adult dosage)	Time of maximum serum response	Comments
GH	Glucose (50–100 gm PO)	60–120 min	Failure of GH suppression is diagnostic of acromegaly in the appropriate clinical setting
	L-Dopa (500 mg PO)	60–120 min	GH suppression commonly occurs in acromegaly and is suggestive of this diagnosis
	TRH (200–500 μg IV)	30 min	Positive response in acromegaly correlates with therapeutic response to bromocriptine
Prolactin	TRH (500 μg IV) (see also Table 12-1)	30 min	Failure of PRL rise may occur more frequently in prolactinomas than in other hyperprolactinemia states
	L-Dopa[a] (500 mg PO)	60–120 min	Failure of PRL to fall adequately suggests the presence of a pituitary adenoma

ACTH	Dexamethasone at a dose of 1 mg PO at 12 midnight	Cortisol[b] and/or ACTH at 9 A.M.	Failure of suppression is a useful screening test for Cushing's syndrome
	Dexamethasone at a dose of 0.5 mg every 6 hr for 2 days	Cortisol[b] and/or ACTH at 48 hr. Urine for 17-OHCS and/or "free" cortisol can also be determined	Failure of suppression suggests Cushing's syndrome[c]
	Dexamethasone at a dose of 2 mg every 6 hr for 2 days	Cortisol[b] and/or ACTH at 48 hr. Urine for 17-OHCS and/or "free" cortisol can also be determined	Suppression occurs in Cushing's disease[d] but not in other causes of Cushing's syndrome
	Metyrapone (750 mg PO every 4 hr for 6 doses). The overnight test may also be used (see Table 12-1)	ACTH and/or 11-deoxycortisol at 24 hr or urine 17-OHCS on the next day	Marked rise occurs in Cushing's disease but not in other causes of Cushing's syndrome

[a] Preceded by carbidopa, L-dopa may be helpful in the diagnosis of prolactinomas.
[b] In Cushing's syndrome due to adrenal tumor, the ACTH level is already suppressed.
[c] In some patients with Cushing's disease, "normal" suppression occurs.
[d] In some patients with Cushing's disease, higher doses of dexamethasone are required for suppression.

Source: K. D. Post and I. M. D. Jackson, Endocrinologic Evaluation of Pituitary Tumors. In D. Long and G. Tindall (Eds.), *Contemporary Neurosurgery*, Vol. 2, No. 5. Baltimore: Williams & Wilkins, 1980.

Table 12-3. Suggested tests

Tumor	Tests
Nonfunctional tumor	PRL every 15 min for 3 samples (pooled specimen). Thyroid function: T_4, T_3 resin, TSH, LH, FSH, estradiol, or testosterone. Cortisol (may be combined with Cortrosyn test). Metyrapone or ITT (if <50 years old and no cardiovascular disease)
Prolactinoma	All of the above for nonfunctional tumors, TRH stimulation test (suggestive of tumor if PRL rise is blunted)
Acromegaly	All of the above for nonfunctional tumors, GH, glucose tolerance test, L-dopa test
Cushing's disease	All of the above for nonfunctional tumors, ACTH, dexamethasone suppression test, metyrapone test

Source: K. D. Post and I. M. D. Jackson, Endocrinologic Evaluation of Pituitary Tumors. In D. Long and G. Tindall (Eds.), *Contemporary Neurosurgery,* Vol. 2, No. 5. Baltimore: Williams & Wilkins, 1980.

Craniopharyngiomas and other suprasellar tumors and pituitary tumors with suprasellar extension, however, may be large enough to exert a mass effect. Induction and maintenance of anesthesia are planned so as not to impair cerebral compliance unduly because of any untoward increase in cerebral blood flow (CBF) as a result of intubation during inadequate anesthesia, introduction of inhalation anesthetics before hyperventilation, use of drugs that increase CBF, head-down positioning, or systemic hypertension.

Because residual blood and secretions frequently remain in the posterior pharynx at the conclusion of the operation, it is important that the patient be sufficiently awake to ensure protection of the airway before extubation is accomplished. If the patient is not responsive, the trachea should remain intubated until the patient is awake. Selection of appropriate doses of anesthetic drugs and timing of their administration are particularly important in this regard because transsphenoidal explorations are relatively short procedures (two to three hours) that conclude very abruptly: Once the mucosal and abdominal incisions have been closed, the nose is packed and the operation is over.

C. **Monitoring.** The anesthesiologist monitors the patient's blood pressure, heart rate and rhythm, temperature, arterial oxygen saturation, end-tidal carbon dioxide tension, and fluid balance. Blood pressure is measured directly when indicated by preexisting medical problems. The use of a urinary catheter is not routine, but may be necessary to aid the management of patients who have diabetes insipidus.

D. **Anesthetic management**

1. **Technique.** In selecting an anesthetic technique, the major concerns are the effect of anesthetic drugs on intracranial dynamics in the presence of a space-occupying lesion, the potential difficulties

with tracheal intubation in patients who have acromegaly, the brevity of the procedure, and the patient's medical problems.

The combination of N_2O and oxygen with thiopental, a narcotic (fentanyl, sufentanil, or alfentanil by infusion), and a muscle relaxant (succinylcholine for intubation and then vecuronium or atracurium, either of which may also be used for intubation) is a satisfactory technique. Isoflurane may be added in low concentrations for blood pressure control or, alternatively, used as the primary anesthetic drug (after establishment of hyperventilation). Halothane is contraindicated because of its potential for inducing ventricular arrhythmias during infiltration of the oral and nasal mucosa with 0.5% lidocaine and epinephrine 1:200,000 or the application of 5% cocaine-soaked pledgets to the mucosa.

The patient is again reminded on arrival in the operating room about the need for mouth breathing postoperatively because of the nasal packs.

2. **Induction.** The induction sequence includes preoxygenation, *d*-tubocurarine, 3 mg, thiopental, 4 to 5 mg/kg, succinylcholine, 1.5 mg/kg, and fentanyl, 2 to 3 μg/kg. Vecuronium, 0.1 mg/kg, or atracurium, 0.5 mg/kg, may be used for intubation instead of succinylcholine, in the absence of potential airway problems. The trachea is intubated after administration of lidocaine, 1.5 mg/kg IV. If difficulty with intubation is anticipated, an inhalation induction precedes intubation during spontaneous ventilation. An assortment of tubes and blades and the use of a fiberoptic bronchoscope may be helpful.

After intubation and auscultation of the breath sounds bilaterally, the endotracheal tube is moved to the left corner of the patient's mouth and taped securely across the chin. The esophageal stethoscope and temperature probe are inserted and secured on the lower left as well, leaving the upper lip totally free. An orogastric tube is placed, aspirated, and then put to gravity drainage during the procedure. The oropharynx is then packed with moist cotton gauze. The eyes are first taped closed and then covered with cotton-padded adhesive patches to prevent corneal abrasion and seepage of cleansing solution and blood into the eyes.

3. **Subarachnoid catheter.** Access to the superior margin of a suprasellar tumor is facilitated by placement of a lumbar subarachnoid catheter (epidural catheter or #5 Stamey ureteral catheter through a Tuohy needle) after intubation and intraoperative instillation of preservative-free saline to bring the tumor down into the sella. The subarachnoid catheter should have a stopcock to prevent the excessive loss of CSF and should be within the anesthesiologist's reach.

4. **Positioning.** The patient's head, supported by a three-point pin headholder, is turned toward his or her right side and elevated 20 degrees and centered within a C-arm fluoroscopy unit for x-ray

control during surgery. Lead aprons and thyroid shields must be used by everyone, including the patient. The hoses from the anesthesia circuit are firmly secured to prevent disconnection and extubation during the operation (Fig. 12–3). The patient's arms are placed at his or her sides and padded to avoid injury to the ulnar nerves. Prophylactic antibiotics (vancomycin, 1 gm IV, and tobramycin, 80 mg IM or ceftriaxone, 1 gm IV) and corticosteroids (hydrocortisone, 100 mg/1000 ml crystalloid solution) may be given at this point.

5. **Maintenance.** Anesthesia is maintained with N_2O and oxygen narcotic (fentanyl, sufentanil, alfentanil), muscle relaxant (vecuronium, atracurium), and isoflurane. Ventilation is controlled to keep the arterial carbon dioxide tension ($PaCO_2$) between 32 and 37 mmHg to prevent a decrease in brain volume, which may withdraw the suprasellar part of the tumor out of the surgeon's reach by the transsphenoidal approach. In the presence of a large space-occupying mass or obstructive hydrocephalus, the $PaCO_2$ should be reduced to 26 to 32 mmHg. The use of mannitol is rarely necessary.

Fig. 12-3. Diagrammatic representation of operative setup for transsphenoidal approach to the sella. Note the position of the patient's head, surgeon, anesthesiologist, fluoroscope with televised image, and operating microscope. (From K. D. Post, I. M. D. Jackson, and S. Reichlin [Eds.], *Pituitary Adenoma.* New York: Plenum, 1980. By permission.)

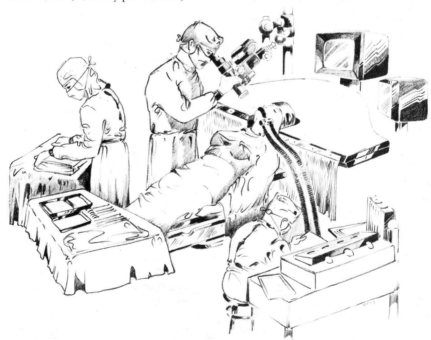

6. Emergence. At the conclusion of the operation, muscle relaxation is reversed with either neostigmine (0.04–0.05 mg/kg) and glycopyrrolate (3.5 μg/kg) or edrophonium (0.5 mg/kg) and atropine (0.01 mg/kg). N_2O is discontinued and the patient is given 100% oxygen. The use of an analgesic such as fentanyl facilitates the patient's quiet emergence from anesthesia and his or her ability to tolerate the endotracheal tube without coughing or straining. The orogastric tube is removed while suction is applied, the oropharynx is thoroughly cleared of blood and secretions, and the throat pack is taken out. The trachea is extubated when the patient is able to respond to commands. Neurologic examination including grasp, movement of the extremities, pupil size and reaction, and visual acuity is performed in the operating room and again in the recovery room.

If the patient is not responsive, the tube remains in place until the patient regains consciousness. Cardiovascular status permitting, the patient's head is elevated 30 degrees. Close monitoring including neurologic evaluation is continued in the recovery room and subsequently on the ward.

E. Fluid management. Administration of fluids during transsphenoidal procedures is calculated to include maintenance requirements and replacement of blood loss and fluid deficit. Some patients may have taken nothing by mouth for as long as 12 to 15 hours before surgery. It is therefore important that they receive additional fluid during induction of anesthesia as replacement of their deficit and in anticipation of blood loss. Operative blood loss is usually 200 to 300 ml, but can be extensive and acute. Blood should be available. If diabetes insipidus is present, the urinary losses must be replaced as well.

Ringer's lactate solution without 5% dextrose is a suitable crystalloid solution. Blood is given as necessary in the form of packed red cells reconstituted with equal volumes of normal saline. There is little indication for the administration of colloid (plasmanate, albumisol, albumin).

F. Intraoperative problems

1. Use of cocaine and epinephrine. The topical use of cocaine and the oral and nasal submucosal injection of local anesthetic solutions containing epinephrine help constrict gingival and mucosal vessels and dissect the nasal mucosa away from the cartilaginous septum. Epinephrine may produce hypertension, arrhythmias, or both; cocaine interferes with the intraneuronal uptake of catecholamines and can thus augment both the hypertensive and arrhythmogenic properties of epinephrine. The use of epinephrine is relatively safe, however, if the following conditions are met: halothane is avoided, ventilation is adequate, epinephrine is given in combination with lidocaine instead of saline, epinephrine concentrations of 1:100,000 to 1:200,000 are used, and total dose does not exceed 10 ml of 1:100,000 solution in 10 minutes for a 70-kg adult. A total dose of 250 mg of cocaine should not be exceeded. Persistent arrhythmias may require treatment with lidocaine. Hypertension may be controlled with an inhalation anesthetic or small intravenous doses of hydralazine (5-mg increments), labetalol (2.5- to 5-mg increments), or esmolol by infusion (300 μg/kg/min) [3].

2. **Bleeding.** Although an infrequent occurrence, the potential for rapid, copious blood loss from entry into either the cavernous sinus or the carotid artery is present, especially in acromegalic patients. In patients who have Cushing's disease, a steady ooze may be encountered. It is therefore important to administer adequate amounts of crystalloid solution during the early part of the procedure to prevent a significant decrease in intravascular volume should hemorrhage occur. Careful serial calculation of blood loss and immediate recognition of brisk bleeding are imperative. Replacement with crystalloid solution is usually adequate unless the patient's preoperative hematocrit is low, blood pressure is difficult to maintain, or blood loss becomes excessive.

Some anesthesiologists induce hypotension to control bleeding. In our experience, excessive blood loss is not sufficiently common to warrant the use of controlled hypotension. Raising the patient's head 20 degrees helps to reduce bleeding as well.

3. **Arterial injury.** If the carotid arteries are compressed or injured within the sella or cavernous sinus, thrombotic occlusion may occur and cause cerebral ischemia.

4. **Air embolism.** Since the site of operation is above the heart during transsphenoidal procedures, the possibility of air embolism exists [11]. The point of entry into the venous system is the vascular ring formed by the cavernous sinuses, which lie lateral to the pituitary gland, and the communicating intercavernous connections between the sinuses, which are anterior, posterior, and inferior to the gland. The opening of the veins along the path of surgical entry through the mouth and nose may also introduce intravenous air. Monitoring for air embolism with either the use of the Doppler ultrasonic precordial transducer or the measurement of end-tidal carbon dioxide tension will alert the anesthesiologist and the surgeon to entrainment of intravenous air so that the site may be identified and occluded and appropriate treatment may be instituted.

Because air embolism may occur during transsphenoidal procedures, the possibility of intravenous air should be included in the differential diagnosis of intraoperative hypotension, tachycardia, arrhythmias, hypoxia, hypercapnia, and bronchospasm.

5. **Dural manipulation.** Manipulation of the dura either anteriorly or, even more frequently, laterally along the medial aspects of the cavernous sinus often causes bradycardia. This may be due to either

a trigeminal or vagal reflex. With cessation of manipulation, the bradycardia resolves.

6. **CSF leakage.** An arachnoid pouch may extend into the sella and partially obscure the operative field. This may cause herniation of the pituitary gland or increase the risk of a dural tear and resultant leakage of CSF. The surgeon may ask the anesthesiologist to remove various amounts of CSF through the subarachnoid catheter to alleviate these problems.

7. **Visual evoked responses.** Some centers use visual evoked responses (VER) to monitor optic nerve function during surgical manipulation. Decompression of the optic nerve enhances VER, and trauma to the optic nerve distorts or abolishes them.

8. **Diabetes insipidus.** Diabetes insipidus is not an uncommon sequela of transsphenoidal procedures, particularly hypophysectomy. Although the onset is usually on the first or second postoperative day, diabetes insipidus will occasionally occur during anesthesia or in the recovery room. Measurement of urine output is important but insertion of a urinary catheter is usually unnecessary. Initial treatment includes fluid replacement with a balanced salt solution containing 5% dextrose. Five percent dextrose in water is not given because cerebral edema may be induced by the creation of an osmotic gradient between the brain and the intravascular compartment. If diabetes insipidus persists or it becomes difficult to match urinary losses, the patient may receive aqueous pitressin, pitressin tannate oil, or desmopressin. Diabetes insipidus that occurs after most transsphenoidal procedures is usually self-limited and resolves within one week to ten days.

V. Postoperative considerations
A. Immediate postoperative care

1. **Airway.** Because the nasal passages are packed, maintenance of a clear airway is of paramount importance.

2. **Nausea and vomiting.** During transsphenoidal dissection, blood and secretions run down the posterior pharynx and accumulate in the stomach. Since the presence of blood in the gastrointestinal tract is irritating, patients frequently experience nausea and vomiting in the recovery period. This can be alleviated to a certain extent once the airway has been secured by packing the pharynx with moist cotton gauze to prevent migration of blood to either the stomach or the tracheobronchial tree during surgery. The throat pack must be removed before extubation of the trachea. Aspiration of the stomach with an orogastric tube before extubation will also remove some of the accumulated air, gastric secretions, and blood, thus reducing the incidence of postoperative nausea and vomiting. The administration of metoclopramide 10 mg IV, may enhance gastric emptying as well.

3. Hypertension. Patients who have a history of hypertension (as well as some who do not) may be hypertensive in the recovery period, despite normal preoperative blood pressures. If analgesics are ineffective, blood pressure may be controlled by administering incremental doses of hydralazine, 5 mg IV, at 5-minute intervals until the desired pressure is reached. If the heart rate is greater than 70 and there is no history of either asthma or congestive heart failure, each dose of hydralazine may be given in combination with propranolol, 0.5-1 mg IV, esmolol, 300 μg/kg/min, or labetalol, 5 mg IV at 5-minute intervals, all for therapeutics and prevention of reflex tachycardia.

4. Bleeding. Bleeding from either the nose or the sublabial incision and either expectoration or vomiting of copious amounts of blood require that the neurosurgeon assess the situation and replace the nasal packing, if necessary. The application of pressure and replacement of nasal packing are usually sufficient to stop the bleeding. The nasal packing may also require adjustment if it has worked its way into the posterior pharynx, causing the patient to gag and cough.

5. Fluids. Urinary output and specific gravity are measured frequently to diagnose and treat diabetes insipidus. Serum and urine osmolalities are also measured. The treatment of diabetes insipidus is discussed in Chapter 7.

6. Medications

    a. Corticosteroid coverage is mandatory until postoperative testing shows an intact pituitary-adrenal axis. Dexamethasone is often given in the immediate postoperative period and then changed to prednisone.

    b. Thyroid replacement is given if the patient had been hypothyroid before surgery. If euthyroid preoperatively, patients need not receive replacement medication in the immediate postoperative period.

    c. Antibiotics are given in our clinic for 48 hours after surgery.

B. Long-term postoperative care

    1. Anterior and posterior pituitary function must be evaluated completely.

    2. Sinus complaints may occur and are treated symptomatically.

    3. Other modes of therapy may be necessary such as radiation therapy or medication, depending on the nature of the process.

References

1. Bergland, R. M., Ray, B. S., and Torack, M. Anatomical variations in the pituitary gland and adjacent structures in 225 human autopsy cases. *J. Neurosurg.* 23:93, 1968.
2. Costello, R. T. Subclinical adenoma of the pituitary gland. *Am. J. Pathol.* 12:205, 1936.

3. Cucchiara, R. F., Benefiel, D. J., Matteo, R. S., et al. Evaluation of esmolol in controlling increases in heart rate and blood pressure during endotracheal intubation in patients undergoing carotid erdarterectomy. *Anesthesiology* 65:528, 1986.
4. Guiot, G., and Thibaut, B. L'extirpation des adenomes hypophysaires par voir transsphenoidale. *Neurochirurgia (Stuttgart)* 1:133, 1969.
5. Hardy, J. Transsphenoidal microsurgery of the normal and pathological pituitary. *Clin. Neurosurg.* 16:185, 1969.
6. Henderson, W. R. The pituitary adenomata: Follow-up study of surgical results in 338 cases (Dr Harvey Cushing's series). *Br. J. Surg.* 26:811, 1939.
7. Kernohan, J. W., and Sayre, G. P. Tumors of the pituitary gland and infandibulum. In *Atlas of Tumor Pathology,* 1st series, Fascicle 36. Washington, D. C.: U.S. Armed Forces Institute of Pathology, 1956.
8. Kjellberg, R. N., Shintani, A., Frantz, A. G., et al. Proton-beam therapy in acromegaly. *N. Engl. J. Med.* 278:690, 1968.
9. Laws, E. R., Jr., and Kern, E. B. Complications of transsphenoidal surgery. *Clin. Neurosurg.* 23:401, 1975.
10. Messick, J. M., Jr., Laws, E. R., Jr., and Abboud, C. F. Anesthesia for transsphenoidal surgery of the hypophyseal region. *J. Anesth. Analg.* 57:206, 1978.
11. Newfield, P., Albin, M. S., Chestnut, J. S., et al. Air embolism during transsphenoidal pituitary operations. *Neurosurgery* 2:39, 1978.
12. Post, K. D., Jackson, I. M. D., and Reichlin, S. (Eds.). *Pituitary Adenoma.* New York: Plenum, 1980.
13. Post, K. D., and Jackson, I. M. D. Endocrinologic Evaluation of Pituitary Tumors. In D. Long and G. Tindall (Eds.), *Contemporary Neurosurgery,* Vol. 2, No. 5. Baltimore: Williams & Wilkins, 1980.
14. Post, K. D., and Stein, B. M. Technique for spinal drainage: A technical note. *Neurosurgery* 43:255, 1979.
15. Post, K. D., and Wolpert, S. M. Radiologic Evaluation of Pituitary Adenomas. In D. Long and G. Tindall (Eds.), *Contemporary Neurosurgery,* Vol. 2, No. 6. Baltimore: Williams & Wilkins, 1980.
16. Renn, W. H., and Rhoton, A. L., Jr. Microsurgical anatomy of the sellar region. *J. Neurosurg.* 43:288, 1975.
17. Roth, J., Gorden, P., and Brace, K. Efficacy of conventional pituitary irradiation in acromegaly. *N. Engl. J. Med.* 282:1385, 1970.
18. Tyrell, M. B., Brooks, R. M., Fitzgerald, P. A., et al. Cushing's disease: Selective transsphenoidal resection of pituitary microadenomas. *N. Engl. J. Med.* 298:753, 1978.
19. Wilson, C. B., and Dempsey, L. C. Transsphenoidal microsurgical removal of 250 pituitary adenomas. *J. Neurosurg.* 48:13, 1978.
20. Wright, A. D., Hill, D. M., Lowy, C., et al. Mortality in acromegaly. *Q. J. Med.* 39:1, 1970.

13

Head Trauma

Management

D E R E K A. B R U C E

Accidents and homicides remain the major causes of death in children and adolescents in the United States. Trauma takes more lives in those less than 45 years of age than any other single cause. Severe head injuries occur in approximately 600,000 people each year; 50,000 or more die and some significant residual disability remains in more than 20% of the survivors. Head trauma, either with or without coexisting injury to other organs, is the most commonly reported fatal injury among motor vehicle accident victims. Other causes of trauma include falls, firearm accidents, criminal assaults, birth trauma, and sporting accidents. Clearly, the ideal way to treat this problem is to eliminate the injuries. This has proven impossible in our automobile-oriented society, and thus the burden is on the medical profession to improve the outcome of the patient who has sustained head trauma. The efforts to educate the public about the causes of trauma, drunk drivers, and social programs to minimize child abuse are all likely to be much more effective ways to decrease mortality and morbidity from head trauma than treatment after the fact.

I. **Pathophysiology.** Improvement in the understanding of the pathophysiology of head injuries has resulted in significant changes in the treatment of patients who sustain severe craniocerebral trauma. In the past, transient concussion has been separated conceptually from prolonged unconsciousness. We now believe that a continuum of injury exists ranging from amnesia through transient concussion, prolonged traumatic unconsciousness, to sudden death from destruction of the brainstem. Even transient concussion is associated with some damage to the neurons and white matter. Severe acceleration-deceleration injury will produce damage in a radial fashion from the cortex to the brainstem, usually involving both areas pathologically.

A. **Brainstem contusion.** Primary brainstem injury that causes disruption of the pontomedullary junction, severe hemorrhage into the brainstem, or acute vascular damage to the basilar and vertebral arteries usually proves rapidly fatal before the patient even reaches the hospital. Prolonged unconsciousness (associated with bilateral, fixed, dilated pupils, and/or decerebrate posturing) is rarely the result of the primary brainstem injury but rather caused by diffuse damage to the white matter of the hemispheres and brainstem. These unconscious patients have often received inadequate care in the past because the diagnosis of a brainstem contusion implied that no therapy was available. However, such patients can develop brain swelling and brain edema leading to increased intracranial pressure (ICP) and secondary brain injury, all of which are amenable to treatment. There is no clinical value in considering an injury to be a primary brainstem contusion.

B. Intracranial hemorrhage

   1. Epidural. Epidural hematomas are most frequently due to laceration of branches of the middle meningeal artery. They are usually caused by an impact injury, most frequently to the temporal region. Venous epidural hematomas from laceration of the dural sinuses present with signs and symptoms of increased ICP and can occur from several days to weeks after injury. In adults, skull fractures are seen in association with epidural hematomas in approximately 80% of cases, whereas in children, the incidence is approximately 50%.

   2. Subdural. It is useful to separate subdural hematomas into acute, subacute, and chronic.

   a. Acute subdural hematomas are usually the result of acceleration-deceleration injury to the mobile head and are associated with injury and swelling of the underlying cerebral hemispheres. Although bleeding may be venous from torn bridging or cortical veins, it is more frequently arterial from an area of lacerated cerebral cortex. The presence of subdural hematoma is associated with increased mortality and poor outcome. Survival may be improved, however, by rapid intervention to decompress the brain [13]. Acute subdural hematomas are similar to other expanding mass lesions in presentation. They often occur after a lucid interval and can be small and spread over much of the hemisphere, or large and focal. The latter are more likely to benefit from surgical removal. In the former, usually severe underlying brain damage exists, and brain swelling is often more of a problem than the hematoma.

   b. Subacute subdural hematomas are similar to acute hematomas but are usually the result of venous bleeding. The hematoma is suspected clinically more than 24 hours after injury. In these patients, the degree of hemispheric injury is frequently less and the outcome is better than in acute hematomas since the most significant factor producing clinical deterioration is the expanding mass effect of the clot rather than any severe diffuse brain injury.

   c. Chronic subdural hematomas are liquified hematomas that frequently present with little or no definite history of specific trauma. They are generally associated with some brain atrophy and therefore tend to occur in either the elderly or the chronically alcoholic patient. The mechanism is believed to be slow accumulation of blood in the subdural space as a result of tearing of bridging cortical veins. Once the subdural blood has begun to accumulate, episodes of minor head trauma, coughing, sneezing, or straining (all of which produce venous engorgement and raise the intracranial venous pressure) can exacerbate the bleeding from either the initially damaged vein or the thin-walled vessels within the external membrane of the subdural hematoma. These lesions become important in acute trauma because fresh bleeding into the chronic hematoma results in acute expansion and exacerbation of the lesion. It is common to see acute hemorrhage in a chronic subdural hematoma on computed tomography (CT) scan. These chronic lesions present in a multiplicity of ways from transient ischemic attacks to progressive dementia.

3. Subarachnoid. Subarachnoid hemorrhage is extremely common after head trauma, especially in children. Eighty percent of children who have Glasgow coma scores (Table 13–1) of less than 5 during the first 48 hours after injury have evidence of subarachnoid hemorrhage on CT scan. Subarachnoid hemorrhage is an indication of the severity of the injury and, when extensive, increases the risk of delayed hydrocephalus.

4. Intracerebral. Intracerebral hematoma is an uncommon finding after head trauma (5% in children) and usually occurs only with severe injuries. With the use of the CT scan, however, small or even large hematomas may be seen in the absence of neurologic deficit. The typical cause of intracranial hemorrhage is a shearing injury that tears the cerebral substance and causes hemorrhage into the white

Table 13-1. Glasgow coma scale

Observation	Points
Eye opening	
Spontaneous	4
To speech	3
To pain	2
None	1
Best verbal response	
Oriented	5
Confused	4
Inappropriate	3
Incomprehensible	2
None	1
Best motor response	
Obeys commands	6
Localizes pain	5
Withdraws from pain	4
Flexes to pain	3
Extends to pain	2
None	1

matter. Frequently, more than one small hematoma is present. These lesions are generally not amenable to surgical intervention, but in patients who have high levels of alcohol, delayed hemorrhage is probably much more common than had been previously suspected. If further deterioration or a delayed increase in ICP occurs, intracerebral hemorrhage must be considered. Delayed hemorrhage will also occur occasionally with the onset of signs of increased ICP from 5 to 14 days after trauma. Local hematomas occur below the area of skull fracture, after impact to the skull, particularly with depressed fractures. Although intracerebral hematomas frequently do not require operation, large localized lesions producing pressure symptoms may.

C. Acute brain swelling. Acute brain swelling occurs more frequently, but not exclusively, in children from birth to 16 years of age. Noted even after relatively trivial injury, acute brain swelling may or may not be associated with a lucid period after trauma. Although formerly thought to be due to severe acute brain edema and often referred to as *malignant edema*, the entity has been well defined pathologically. A severely swollen brain and vascular engorgement of the white matter are evident, but rarely are any signs of primary impact injury present. Recent studies with CT scan and measurement of cerebral blood flow (CBF) suggest that acute brain swelling is due to sudden intracerebral vascular congestion and hyperemia, which can be controlled if treated early [2]. The recognition of the presence of acute brain swelling has important implications for the initial treatment of the brain-injured child and young adolescent. Unilateral brain swelling accompanied by hyperemia appears to occur in about 50% of adult injuries as well.

D. Cerebral edema. Cerebral edema is an increase in the water content of the brain, usually in the extracellular spaces of the white matter. On the initial CT scan after trauma, cerebral edema is rarely seen. Edema occurs most frequently more than 24 hours after trauma either in the areas around cerebral contusions or intracerebral hematomas or in multiple sites after diffuse impact injury. Cerebral edema is usually progressive over several days, and it is common to see a small contusion on day 1 become a large area of edema by day 3 or 4 (Fig. 13–1).

E. Cerebral ischemia. Cerebral ischemia can occur after head injury as a result of occlusion or a major vessel, vascular spasm, hypotension, shock, or severe intracranial hypertention with compression of vessels. The most common site of ischemia in the distribution of the large vessels is in the area fed by the posterior cerebral arteries. Ischemia occurs here as a result of herniation of the brain and compression of the posterior cerebral arteries. The second most common area is the antero-inferior frontal area, which is compromised by compression of the anterior cerebral arteries. It is common, particularly in children, to see areas of apparent infarction scattered throughout the thalami.

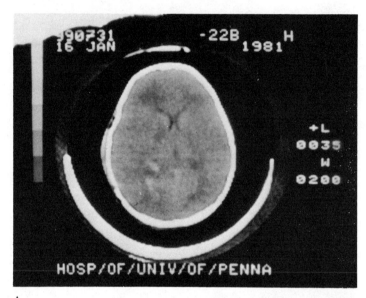

A

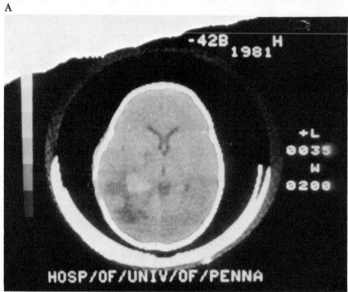

B

Fig. 13-1. *A.* CT scan in 2-year-old 24 hours posttrauma shows small deep hemorrhage in the left parieto-occipital region. The hemorrhage was seen after evacuation of an epidural hematoma. *B.* Marked increase in edema in deep parietal white matter 4 days later.

In children less than 1 year of age, focal areas of decreased density are frequently seen on the first CT scan after trauma. These usually represent areas of ischemia rather than of edema. It is important to realize that the decreased density seen soon after head trauma is of ischemic origin. A careful search should be made for vascular compression, intracranial hypertension, or systemic hypotension. The therapy and prognosis of these ischemic areas are clearly different from those for edema since edema can be expected to resolve with little problem whereas ischemia and infarction are likely to leave significant cerebral injury. Diffuse ischemia may be identified as generally low density for the supratentorial compartment with loss of the gray-white interface. This pattern is quite different from that of the swelling due to hyperemia where the normal density of the brain is preserved.

F. Craniospinal injury. When an acceleration force is applied to the freely mobile head, damage may be sustained to the cervical spine as well as to the cerebrum and cerebellum. Thus, before there is any available history as to the nature of injury, it is wise to assume that craniospinal trauma has occurred, especially in the adult, and to take all reasonable precautions to prevent excessive extension, flexion, or lateral rotation of the patient's neck during retrieval from the site of accident, transport, and resuscitation. A good history, and, if necessary, cervical spine films to include the C-7 vertebra should be obtained as soon as possible and before further movement (e.g., to the operating room or CT scanner). Evidence of spinal trauma may be identified on neurologic examination but may be difficult to diagnose in the comatose patient. Spinal trauma may only become clinically apparent as the patient begins to recover from the cerebral injury. Resuscitation should not be delayed because of the concern about spinal injury. If the patient is in a serious state because of hypercarbia or hypoxia, an adequate airway must be obtained.

G. Multiple trauma. Multiple trauma will not be specifically addressed in this chapter except to emphasize that isolated cranial trauma does not produce hypotension and tachycardia. When hypotension occurs, a careful search for another source of blood loss is necessary, which will most frequently be in the abdomen or fractured long bones. In children less than 1 year old, a large epidural hematoma can cause hypovolemia and anemia in the presence of an associated skull fracture, which permits decompression of the hematoma into the subperiosteal or subgaleal space (Fig. 13-2). Abdominal lavage may be necessary to identify a source of bleeding. Fluid not recovered from the abdomen during the lavage has to be taken into account when calculating the desired fluid balance for that 24-hour period. Increasingly, CT of the abdomen is being used to diagnose intra-abdominal bleeding, thus the problems of lavage are less frequently seen.

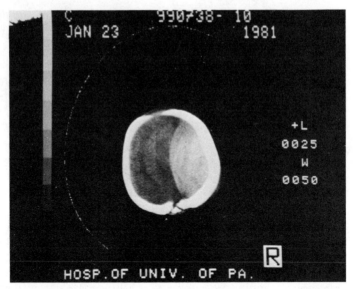

Fig. 13-2. CT scan in 9-month-old child with evidence if massive right parietal epidural hematoma and active bleeding. This child was awake and alert and had only a mild left hemiparesis.

H. Primary versus secondary injury
1. **Primary injury.** Head trauma causes primary and secondary injury to the brain. The primary injury occurs within a few milliseconds after the traumatic force is applied to the head. This injury involves the relative movement of structures inside the head, which causes immediate damage to the white matter, tearing of the arteries and veins, and contusion of the brain. What happens to neurons, dendrites, and synapses is not known. The pathology of this impact injury as it relates to the white matter includes shearing injury, tearing of axons and myelin, transient conduction abnormalities, and petechial hemorrhages. Exactly what happens to the gray matter neurons and dendrites is, at present, not understood at all. There is no treatment for this primary injury, although an artery that is torn at the moment of impact (and is therefore part of the primary injury) may cause an expanding hematoma minutes to hours later. There is overlap between the primary injury and secondary injury.
2. **Secondary injury.** The secondary injuries are a series of progressive pathophysiologic changes that can produce more damage to the brain. They are due to events set in motion by the primary insult but do not produce their deleterious effects until minutes to hours after impact. The factors contributing to the secondary injury

are hypoxia, hypercapnia, systemic hypotension, and intracranial hypertension. The apparent common denominator of the secondary injury is cerebral ischemia, both focal and global. Included within this secondary injury are the various syndromes of transcallosal, transtentorial, and cerebellar tonsillar herniation.

II. Emergency management. Current emergency management of head-injured patients is based on maximal effort from the earliest possible time to prevent the secondary injury. All of the events that lead to secondary injury of the brain can, theoretically, be prevented, setting the stage for maximal recovery.

A. Airway. From the first moments of resuscitation, a patent airway must be ensured. In severely head-injured patients, opening the airway will usually result in moderate hyperventilation, although hypoxia may persist. First, the mouth must be cleaned out manually to remove debris, vomitus, or teeth, and the tongue must be kept forward. In adults, preservation of an open airway without an artificial airway is frequently difficult, whereas in children an airway can usually be easily maintained. Hyperextension of the neck should be avoided in both groups, if possible, until the integrity of the cervical spine has been ascertained. There is no need to hyperextend the child's neck to ventilate, whereas it may be difficult to establish an adequate airway in an adult (especially someone who has a short, fat neck) without moderate hyperextension or an artificial airway.

Although endotracheal intubation may be the ideal method of airway control in the severely head-injured patient, the trachea must be intubated only when suction and oxygen are available, and when the dangers of a cervical fracture, a full stomach, and intracranial hypertension are taken into account. Until preparations can be made for endotracheal intubation, ventilation with bag and mask and supplemental oxygen (40–60%) is usually adequate, the object being to maintain the arterial carbon dioxide tension ($PaCO_2$) between 30 and 35 mmHg and the arterial oxygen tension (PaO_2) above 80 mmHg. In the presence of severe facial injuries, an emergency tracheotomy may be necessary. Apart from this situation, few other indications exist for tracheotomy, and attempts at nasal or oral endotracheal intubation should be made.

Much of the secondary injury results from poor ventilation. Decrease in the PaO_2 below 50 mmHg increases CBF, cerebral blood volume (CBV), and ICP. Increased $PaCO_2$ also increases CBF, CBV, and ICP. Brain swelling, brain edema, and mass lesions all raise ICP, which is further aggravated by hypercapnia and hypoxia. Most adults and children who have Glasgow coma scores of less than 8 (Table 13-1) will require endotracheal intubation at least in the early postinjury period. Endotracheal intubation not only permits control of arterial gas tensions but also enables the patient to be transported safely from the emergency room to the CT scanner, intensive care unit (ICU), or operating room and allows the use of muscle paralysis to obtain good CT scans. Whether to continue intubation beyond this time is based on each patient's needs. Both the level of consciousness and the results of the CT scan will help in making this decision.

In unconscious patients (Glasgow coma scores of 8 or less), endotracheal intubation is performed after administration of 100% oxygen, pancuronium or vecuronium, thiopental, and the use of cricoid pressure to prevent gastric regurgitation and aspiration. Uncuffed endotracheal tubes that permit a small leak are used for children. Once the endotracheal tube is secured, the stomach is emptied with a large-bore nasogastric tube. The nasogastric tube is then left in place and connected to straight drainage.

It is our practice to obtain a lateral x-ray film of the cervical spine if time permits before endotracheal intubation, particularly in patients who have sustained acceleration-deceleration injuries. The C-7 vertebra must be seen, and although the x-ray film does not definitively rule out spinal injury, it will identify dislocations or fractures and may suggest that nasotracheal intubation may be preferable, particularly in adults, to avoid hyperextension of the neck. The adult who has a short neck and cervical spine injury may require tracheotomy to establish an airway safely.

Once the endotracheal tube is in place, we continue moderate hyperventilation to a $PaCO_2$ of 30 mmHg in adults and 25 mmHg in children. Since it is likely that areas of disruption of the blood-brain barrier are present, the higher the end-capillary pressure and the blood flow, the greater the amount of edema that will form. Decreasing the $PaCO_2$ will reduce CBF by producing arteriolar constriction and decreasing end-capillary pressure and will prevent edema formation. Hyperventilation will also decrease CBV and lower ICP. Children who have had acceleration-deceleration injuries develop a true hyperemia in about 50% of cases. This acute brain swelling is due in large part to vasodilatation; because of this, we prefer to keep $PaCO_2$ between 25 and 30 mmHg.

B. Cardiovascular status. The head injury itself is rarely the cause of hypotension, and the source of bleeding must be sought. Resuscitation from shock should be accomplished with isotonic fluid, normal saline or Ringer's lactate solution, or colloid if blood is not readily available. Glucose and water should not be used as this decreases serum osmolality and can aggravate the cerebral swelling. The ideal replacement, of course, is blood. Since the cerebral vessels are already dilated because of the hypotension, rapid restitution of the normal arterial pressure will precipitate brain swelling. It is extremely valuable to insert an ICP monitor during resuscitation in the emergency room so that both systemis arterial pressure and ICP can be measured and controlled, thus avoiding potentially lethal elevations of ICP.

It is frequently necessary to take children directly to the operating room because of intra-abdominal hemorrhage. Here again, the ability to measure and control ICP during resuscitation, transport, and surgery is only possible when ICP is monitored directly. In patients who have circulatory collapse, the insertion of an intra-arterial cannula and an ICP monitor is vital early in the course of resuscitation: Only then can the correct balance between arterial pressure and ICP be maintained.

C. **History and examination.** Frequently, little or no history is available when the patient arrives in the emergency room and when resuscitation must begin. It is always valuable to assign one person to talk to whatever witnesses are available or to the ambulance personnel. The history should be brief but should include, if possible, the type of injury (e.g., fall, pedestrian or automobile injury); the course of events since the time the patient was first observed (i.e., improving, worsening, or the same); and the presence of any period of apnea or evidence of seizure activity. Usually any past history is unobtainable at this point.

1. **The neurologic examination** of the comatose patient is, of necessity, limited and can be performed in a few minutes and need not interfere with the resuscitative efforts. The Glasgow coma score (Table 13–1) is a good initial measurement of the degree of insult sustained. Once the patient is stabilized, the scale is helpful in making some predictions of likely outcome. The simplicity of the scale makes interobserver agreement on examination possible. The results of the assessment of pupillary responses, cold caloric responses, spontaneous ventilation, and gag reflexes will define the state of the brainstem, pons, and medulla, as well as the hemispheres. The symmetry of the motor examination, both side-to-side and proximal-to-distal, also gives information on the localization of the lesion within the brain, spinal cord, and peripheral nervous system. After head trauma, a single examination is less helpful than repeated examinations over a period of time. Changes in the patient's score can be used to define neurologic deterioration or improvement.

2. **Pupillary responses** are tested by using a bright light, and both **direct** and **consensual** responses must be assessed in each upper brainstem, mesencephalon, and second and third cranial nerves are all intact. Unilateral loss of direct response with preservation of consensual response suggests optic nerve injury. Loss of bilateral response is usually caused by injury either to the area of the superior colliculus or to the optic chiasm. When the third

nerve is involved, the pupils are usually large. With lesions in the tegmentum, the pupils are frequently in the midposition and unreactive. Small unresponsive pupils signify pontine lesions, whereas small reactive pupils are most commonly seen with hemorrhage into and around the third ventricle.

3. **Oculovestibular responses.** Because of the risk of cervical spine injury, we prefer to use the cold caloric test to assess the oculovestibular response instead of the doll's eyes or oculocephalic maneuver, in which the head is rotated from side to side and the movements of the eyes are noted. Cold caloric testing is performed with cold water irrigation of the ears. Before the test, the ear canals must be examined. If there is no leakage of cerebrospinal fluid (CSF), if the eardrum is intact, and if the canal is not filled with blood or wax, the test can be performed safely. Ideally, the head should be elevated 30 degrees from the horizontal, but this may be contraindicated if there is any question of cervical spine injury. Ice water, 100 to 200 ml, is used to irrigate each ear over several minutes to obtain maximal stimulation. A response is expected within 2 to 3 minutes. If no response is obtained, several minutes must elapse before the other side is tested.

   The normal conscious response is mild deviation of the eyes to the cooled side with rapid nystagmus back to the midline. In comatose patients, the nystagmus component is lost, and intact response involves bilateral tonic deviation to the cooled side. Lesions of the medial longitudinal fasciculus will prevent the adducting eye from crossing the midline; this may be observed either unilaterally or bilaterally. More destructive lesions will result in bilateral loss of eye movement in response to either unilateral or bilateral cooling. These findings signify severe involvement of the pons and midbrain but may be associated with recovery from head injury, especially in children.

4. **Ventilatory and gag responses.** The lowest pathways in the medulla involve the gag response and spontaneous ventilation. These responses should always be evaluated. When checking the gag response, care must be taken not to induce vomiting before endotracheal intubation. Gag response is tested by gently stimulating either side of the posterior soft palate or by placing a cotton-tipped applicator against the posterior pharyngeal wall. Spontaneous ventilation is tested by ensuring an open airway and observing the patient's spontaneous ventilatory efforts. If resuscitation has been performed and hyperventilation has been part of that resuscitation, CO_2 will have to rise to the normal range before the absence of spontaneous ventilation can be satisfactorily diagnosed. Patients who do not have spontaneous ventilatory effort will rarely, if ever, make a significant recovery, and the absence of spon-

taneous ventilation coupled with the absence of the other brainstem responses signifies brain death.

III. Special studies. Once the patient's condition is stabilized, the next step is to determine the need for further diagnostic studies. The patient's level of consciousness, the clinical examination, and the history of the trauma are all considered in selecting necessary studies.

  A. Plain x-ray films of skull and spine. In those patients who have Glasgow coma scores of 8 or more, skull x-ray films can diagnose linear or depressed fractures, the presence of which will heighten concern about possible epidural hemorrhage. X-ray studies may demonstrate pneumocephalus, which indicates a basal fracture, and in children (particularly those less than 1 year), plain skull x-ray films after trauma may show evidence of splitting the sutures. The combination of split sutures and a linear skull fracture is frequently associated with an intracranial mass lesion, most commonly an epidural hematoma, and should be an indication for obtaining a CT scan. Skull x-ray films are rarely helpful in patients who have coma scores of less than 8. These patients require CT scan (or arteriogram if CT scan is unavailable). All patients who are unconscious after head trauma who do not show signs of rapid recovery require neuroradiologic investigation to rule out the presence of a mass lesion. The most frequent cause of avoidable death after head trauma continues to be a missed mass lesion.

  To establish normal alignment of the cervical spine, lateral x-ray films of the spine, including C-7, are obtained as soon as possible in any patient who has had acceleration-deceleration trauma. Although a single lateral x-ray film will not rule out all cases of cervical fracture or dislocation, it is a good screening test before the head is moved to facilitate intubation of the trachea.

  B. CT scan. The CT scan is the single most useful study for the examination of patients who have severe head injury or a deteriorating level of consciousness. In demonstrating the state of the soft tissues, sinuses, bones, brain, and CSF spaces, the CT scan clearly defines hematomas and contusions. In restless patients, a good scan cannot be obtained because of movement artifact. The danger of missing a significant mass lesion on the CT scan is small, but the presence of motion artifact can obscure small subdural and epidural hematomas and cortical contusions. If the scan is necessary, then either sedation or endotracheal intubation and general anesthesia will be required. It is dangerous to accept a poor scan; a false sense of security may be imparted to those caring for the patient. With the new fast scanners, movement is a much less serious problem, and good scans can often be obtained without anesthesia.

  With the new rapid scanners, the problem of movement artifact has been minimized. The CT scan is now capable of demonstrating all of the pathologic lesions associated with head injury from diffuse impact injury to intracerebral hematomas. We do not generally use contrast during the first CT study.

C. **Arteriography.** When the CT scan is available, arteriography is rarely used in the study of acute head trauma patients. If a CT scan is unavailable, however, then cerebral arteriography remains the investigation of choice in the unconscious, severely head-injured patient. The arteriogram does not define the traumatic pathology as well as the CT scan, but it demonstrates the vascular pathology much more effectively. Thus, in patients in whom either cerebral arterial spasm or arterial occlusion is suspected, arteriography may still be the procedure of choice. When arteriography is considered necessary, the integrity of the cervical spine must be established. The patient must be stable enough to undergo the procedure. The safest way to accomplish the study is with the use of an endotracheal tube, muscle paralysis, controlled ventilation, and sedation with narcotics. Under these conditions, good arteriograms without movement artifact are obtained, and the patient's airway, blood pressure, and ventilation are carefully controlled during the procedure.

D. **Magnetic resonance imaging (MRI)** is now widely available in the United States. The scans obtained are particularly sensitive for small subdural hematomas and cortical contusions. They are also an excellent way for looking for residual cerebral injury post trauma. Evidence exists that the MRI scan has a better correlation with cognitive outcome then does the CT scan. Nonetheless, because of the slowness of the MRI scan, the difficulties of anesthesia within it, and the possibility of missing blood in the very early phase, the CT scan remains the procedure of choice in the acute stages of trauma. After a few days when scans are being repeated, the MRI scan may be a more sensitive way of looking for small hematomas and cerebral injury.

IV. **Further management.** After emergency resuscitation with the establishment of an airway and the correction of any cardiovascular instability, the further management of the patient is determined by the results of the neurologic examination and the CT scan, as well as any associated injuries.

A. **Scalp lacerations.** All scalp lacerations should be liberally irrigated and gently examined, using a gloved finger to seek evidence of a depressed skull fracture. If a depression is present, the wound is covered with sterile saline-soaked sponges and x-ray films are obtained. If indeed there is a compound depressed skull fracture, surgical correction is required. If either no fracture or a linear fracture is present, surgery is rarely necessary, and the wound is then closed primarily.

B. **Skull fractures.** The majority of skull fractures need no therapy. Fractures involving the base of the skull with CSF otorrhea or rhinorrhea rarely necessitate any kind of emergency surgery. Usually these CSF leaks will stop over several days, and rarely do they require surgical repair. The major disagreement in management of these basal fractures involves the administration of antibiotics. We do not administer prophylactic antibiotics to patients who have CSF leaks.

Depressed skull fractures and compound depressed fractures are likely to require surgical correction. Usually these fractures occur in patients whose neurologic state is quite good since the fractures result from localized injuries to the head. Closed depressed skull fractures rarely require emergency operation. It is often better to allow 24 to 48 hours to pass to enable the patient's level of consciousness to recover before subjecting the patient to a surgical procedure.

The reasons for operating on closed depressed skull fractures are (1) cosmetic correction, particularly in the frontal areas; (2) if the fracture is depressed more than the thickness of the table of the skull since there is a high likelihood of dural laceration; and (3) if the patient has evidence of focal neurologic deficit or of injury of the brain underlying the fracture site. In these circumstances, the CT scan can be extremely valuable in demonstrating the degree of depression of the inner table of the skull, the condition of the underlying brain, and more important the presence of other lesions.

Compound depressed skull fractures require emergency surgical correction. The decision to undertake surgery depends on the patient's neurologic state, the degree of skin laceration, and the position and location of the fractures. The CT scan is helpful before surgery for compound depressed skull fractures to determine the degree of internal displacement of the bone fragment, the condition of the underlying brain, and equally important, evidence of any other associated cerebral injury. Our technique of repairing compound depressed skull fractures is as follows: (1) try to save all fragments of bone; (2) perform a circular craniotomy that includes the area of fracture; (3) remove the bone pieces; (4) debride the brain; (5) repair the dura (an important step); and (6) replace the various pieces of bone after they have been steeped in antibiotic solution. If the dura is left open, significant cerebral herniation can occur through the defect with secondary ischemia, infarction, and increase in cerebral damage.

C. **Physiologic monitoring.** In adults who have Glasgow coma scores of 8 or less and in children who have Glasgow coma scores of 5 or less (Table 13–1), it is advisable to insert an intra-arterial cannula and an ICP monitor when the patient is in the emergency room. The blood pressure and ICP can then be monitored on portable equipment during transfer to CT scan, operating room, or ICU. For children in whom we recommend a low $PaCO_2$ as part of the early management, it is useful to have a portable capnograph to monitor end-tidal CO_2. This group of patients will also require a urinary catheter provided there is no evidence of perineal trauma. If perineal trauma is present, a urethrogram may be necessary before catheterization to rule out urethral fracture. All unconscious patients require at least one large-bore intravenous catheter. A nasogastric tube is usually inserted after the endotracheal tube is in place; the only real contraindication is the presence of severe facial, frontal, or basal skull fractures.

Once the patient's condition is stabilized in the ICU, further monitoring may include the use of a Swan-Ganz catheter if there is any cardiovascular instability or evidence of pulmonary edema. The insertion of a jugular bulb catheter permits measurement of CBF and cerebral metabolic rate ($CMRO_2$), which may be helpful if extreme hyperventilation ($PaCO_2$ of 20–25 mmHg) is necessary to control brain swelling.

Continuous monitoring of the electroencephalogram is not useful in patients who have head injury. The monitoring of visual, somatosensory, and brainstem-evoked responses is relatively new, but useful information may be obtained [8]. Blood should be drawn for type and cross match, clotting studies, baseline serum electrolytes, amylase, and osmolality. Studies in adults suggest that a good correlation exists between the disturbance of clotting studies early in the course of the head injury and final outcome. In comatose children, inappropriate antidiuretic hormone secretion is a common problem, and a sudden drop in serum sodium can occur within the first 24 to 48 hours despite fluid restriction. Thus, frequent measurement of serum electrolytes and osmolality and careful control of fluid balance are necessary in this particular group of patients.

D. **Management of increased ICP.** In unconscious patients it is extremely difficult to judge whether ICP is elevated. Therefore, all early therapy during resuscitation is designed to lower raised ICP or, at least, to prevent further increases in ICP. Simple maneuvers such as a 15- to 20-degree **head-up tilt,** keeping the head in the midline position and not rotated to either side to maintain open jugular veins; relative restriction of fluid intake; and maintenance of normal, rather than increased, arterial pressure will all help control ICP. **Endotracheal intubation** is performed using adequate supplemental oxygen and medication to ensure good oxygenation and low $PaCO_2$ and to prevent coughing and straining during laryngoscopy and intubation.

In the noncomatose patient, there is rarely need for any specific medication or therapy to reduce ICP. If the patient requires a CT scan, the findings will determine whether therapy is required (e.g., corticosteroids because of an intracerebral hematoma). In patients who have a deteriorating level of consciousness after admission, it is imperative to ascertain the cause of the altered neurologic state. Is the patient having seizures? Is the deterioration from intracranial hypertension, systemic hypotension, or hypoxia? Is there evidence that an increasing mass lesion is producing herniation with either pupillary dilatation or contralateral hemiparesis or hemiplegia? Therapy should be directed toward the cause of the problem (e.g., adequate ventilation and anticonvulsant drugs of a patient who is having seizures) rather than specifically concerned with lowering ICP (e.g., mannitol).

In patients in whom intracranial hypertension is suspected, either from an epidural or subdural hematoma or diffuse brain swelling, emergency treatment to reduce ICP is the rational course. Ideally a definitive study to identify the cause of clinical deterioration is obtained prior to therapy. This is not always possible. The first and most rapidly effective therapy is **hyperventilation.** In a patient who has multiple trauma and reduced blood volume, care must be taken during controlled ventilation to avoid increasing the intrathoracic pressure, thus decreasing cardiac return and producing secondary hypotension. Corticosteroids (dexamethasone or methylprednisolone) are of little benefit in trauma, and, certainly, these drugs should not be relied on to lower the ICP rapidly.

Although **mannitol** will effectively lower the ICP within minutes after administration, its use remains controversial. The drug is indicated, however, when either elevated ICP or a mass and herniation are responsible for the patient's deteriorating state. The risk of increasing the size of hematoma is negligible compared to the disastrous effects of untreated progressive uncal herniation. If decompression of transtentorial herniation is delayed, secondary hemorrhage into the brainstem can occur and cause irreversible neurologic deficit. Once mannitol is given and the ICP is reduced, the specific intracranial disorder must be identified as soon as possible to prevent a recurrence of the patient's deterioration.

Occasionally, the diagnosis of an epidural hematoma will be obvious, and immediate operation will be required because of rapid deterioration of the patient's level of consciousness. More frequently, the use of hyperventilation and mannitol gives the surgeon time to obtain a CT scan to define the intracranial disorder. The use of exploratory burr holes is not advocated, because if no definitive lesion is found, the patient still requires further neurodiagnostic studies. Two recent studies suggest that in the situation of unilateral fixed dilated pupil, either a twist drill hole or emergency burr hole is likely to be both diagnostic and therapeutic. Thus, depending on the rapidity with which the CT scan can be obtained, the ability of medical management of intracranial hypertension, and the availability to get to the operating room rapidly, twist drill evacuation or immediate burr hole evacuation may have a role to play. This is rarely, if ever, true in the child. If a surgical lesion is found after additional diagnostic procedures, the patient must again be returned to the operating room.

The extra time may also be determined since good recovery depends on the rapidity with which a hematoma is evacuated. The CT scan is clearly invaluable in the efficient diagnosis and treatment of severely head-injured patients. In children, acute deterioration is much less frequently due to surgically correctable lesions. Such deterioration is most often caused either by generalized brain swelling and increased ICP or by seizure activity. Thus, the use of radiologic study before any surgical intervention in children is even more important than in adults. Since acute deterioration seems to be associated with a swollen congested brain rather than with cerebral edema, we do not recommend mannitol for children unless the presence of an epidural hematoma is strongly suspected. The initial therapy for deterioration in children, then, is hyperventilation and head-up tilt of 15 to 30 degrees. If an epidural hematoma is suspected, mannitol may be given after the CO_2 has been lowered.

In both adults and children, the initial dose of mannitol is 0.5 to 1.0 gm/kg given over 3 to 5 minutes by intravenous infusion rather than by direct intravenous bolus injection. When mannitol is given rapidly to unanesthetized patients, a rise in blood pressure usually occurs and is frequently accompanied by a rise in ICP. This elevation of blood pressure and ICP can be prevented if the drug is given slowly. The reason for avoiding mannitol or other osmotic diuretics in children during the early resuscitative period is that mannitol increases CBF independent of its effect on ICP. If the diffuse swelling in children is due to hyperemia, it is possible that mannitol could exacerbate this condition and produce a further increase in ICP and clinical deterioration. The best way to treat the initial deterioration is to monitor the ICP of comatose patients from the earliest phase of resuscitation. In this way, the ICP, its response to therapy, and the need for further intervention can be measured accurately, and appropriate treatment can be initiated.

E. Corticosteroids. Corticosteroids have not been demonstrated to be of value in improving the outcome after head injury. Although the complications of corticosteroid therapy are minor over the first few days (hyperglycemia is the most frequent problem in adults), most centers have abandoned the administration of large doses of dexamethasone or methylprednisolone to comatose patients as part of the early treatment.

F. Barbiturates. The use of barbiturates in large doses to reduce ICP in head-injured patients is not part of the initial resuscitation. Their administration is usually reserved for situations in which other measures to control the ICP have failed. Large doses of barbiturates are dangerous because they lower peripheral resistance and may have deleterious effects on cardiovascular function resulting in hypotension. This reaction occurs most often in hypovolemic patients. Therefore, we do not suggest the routine use of these drugs.

If the patient shows signs of rapid deterioration in the emergency room because of intracranial hypertension, the insertion of an ICP monitor and intra-arterial cannula allows sensible management. Under these circumstances, if hyperventilation and osmotic agents fail to lower the ICP, barbiturates, initially thiopental and then pentobarbital, may be administered. In children who have severe diffuse injury, marked swelling, and high ICP, the use of barbiturates will frequently reduce the ICP when other methods have proven ineffective. If the damage to the brain is too extensive, the ICP will rise again rapidly (Fig. 13–3). In patients whose injuries are less severe, the ICP will be controlled. Barbiturates in large doses should not be used to treat intracranial hypertension unless systemic arterial pressure, central venous pressure, and ICP are monitored continuously.

G. Hypothermia. Hypothermia to 32°C is associated with a 40 to 50% decrease in the cerebral metabolic rate and a concomitant reduction in CBF, CBV, and ICP. When barbiturates are given in large doses, the patient's temperature frequently falls to the 32 to 34°C range; we make no effort to restore the temperature to normal. The benefit of hypothermia is reduction in ICP by decreasing metabolic rate and CBF and CBV. Although hypothermia has been shown to be protective against ischemia, this is not true at the levels that are obtained clinically. The

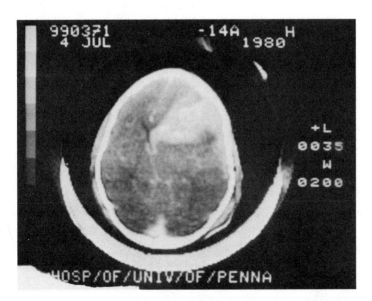

Fig. 13-3. CT scan in 8-year-old who was ejected 100 feet in the air from the cockpit of an airplane. CT scan reveals large right frontal intracerebral hemorrhage, subarachnoid hemorrhage, and brain swelling. Despite surgical evacuation, hyperventilation, barbiturates, and hypothermia, intracranial pressure rose to equal systemic arterial pressure and the child died of intracranial hypertension.

dangers of hypothermia, however, are multiple: peripheral vasocon-striction, impaired white cell phagocytosis, increased incidence of pneumonia, decreased ciliary function of the bronchi, and, if the tem-perature goes below 30°C, an increased risk of cardiac arrhythmia. Nonetheless, we believe that mild hypothermia to 32°C, whether in-duced or as a concomitant to barbiturate therapy, is a useful adjunct to patients in whose ICP is difficult to control by other means.

V. **The anesthesiologist's role in severe head injury.** The anesthesiolo-gist's involvement in the care of the head-injured patient begins immedi-ately on arrival of the patient in the trauma unit, or, if there is an outgoing ambulance retrieval system, at the site of the collection of the patient. The need to stabilize the patient before transfer from hospital to hospital is axiomatic; yet frequently, patients are transferred without provision of an adequate airway, in shock with no large-bore intravenous catheter, or with clear evidence of abdominal bleeding. Under these circumstances, the transfer is frequently detrimental to the patient's welfare. In children, not only is there a problem with inexperienced examiners overlooking sig-nificant blood loss, but frequently smaller hospitals do not have the equipment required for endotracheal intubation of small tracheas.

The Children's Hospital of Philadelphia sends their own transport team directed by an anesthesiologist who works with a pediatric resident and a nurse to collect the child at the outlying hospital. Equipment for ventila-tion and suction is carried in the ambulance. The child is not transported before an adequate airway, intravenous infusion, and intra-arterial pres-sure monitoring are established. It is likely that such transport support will become increasingly prominent in the critical care of brain-injured pa-tients. In some areas of the country, well-trained paramedics can perform a similar sort of stabilization before transfer from the site of the accident. Good on-the-spot care has been shown to decrease the incidence of hypoxia on arrival in the emergency room significantly and should be the goal in all communities.

Systemic Effects

JANE MATJASKO

The systemic effects of head injury are diverse and affect nearly all organs. In addition, they may be responsible for morbidity and even mortality in the severely head-injured patient. They thus require active prevention and prompt, thorough treatment [5]. Table 13-2 lists the organs and disease processes that are related to head injury.

I. **Cardiopulmonary effects of head injury**
   A. **Initial management and resuscitation.** Severe head injury may cause apnea and hypoxia at the time of concussion or after the develop-ment of massive brain swelling, which can lead to intracranial hyper-tension and tentorial herniation. Airway obstruction may occur from

Table 13-2. Peripheral sequelae of acute head injury

Cardiopulmonary
  Abnormal breathing patterns
  Airway obstruction
  Hypoxia
  Shock
  Adult respiratory distress syndrome (ARDS)
  Neurogenic pulmonary edema
  Fat embolism
  Venous thromboembolism
  Electrocardiographic changes
Hematologic
  Inhibition of neutrophil phagocytosis
  Trauma and coagulation
  Disseminated intravascular coagulation (DIC)
Endocrinologic
  Anterior pituitary insufficiency
  Posterior pituitary dysfunction
    Diabetes insipidus
    Syndrome of inappropriate ADH (SIADH)
Metabolic
  Cerebrospinal fluid (CSF) metabolic changes
  Nonketotic hyperosmolar hyperglycemic coma (NHHC)
Gastrointestinal
Skeletal
  Cervical spine injuries
  Maxillofacial injuries

neck flexion, loss of muscle tone, or the presence of debris in the mouth. Aspiration of gastric contents predisposes the patient to chemical pneumonitis, atelectasis, and bronchopneumonia. There seems to be no relation between abnormal breathing patterns and the site or extent of neurologic injury; persistent spontaneous hyperventilation from either cerebrospinal fluid (CSF) lactic acidosis or brainstem dysfunction carries a poor prognosis.

When admitted to the hospital, 30 to 50% of head-injured patients will have a PaO_2 of less than 60 mmHg in the absence of airway obstruction or prior pulmonary disease. Minute ventilation may be twice normal, particularly if CO_2 production is above normal, as it is in the decerebrate patient. Severe refractory hypoxia is associated with a poor prognosis. A large intrapulmonary shunt ($\dot{Q}s/\dot{Q}t$) indicates an ill-defined effect of acute intracranial hypertension on ventilation-perfusion relationships.

The primary concern is to establish ventilatory support and a patent, protected airway using a cuffed endotracheal tube and controlled ventilation. Neurologic and cardiopulmonary resuscitation includes:

1. Intubation: cuffed endotracheal tube (low-pressure cuff)

2. Mechanical ventilation

    a. PaO_2, 100 mmHg; $PaCO_2$, 25 to 30 mmHg; optimal positive end-expiratory pressure (PEEP) if neurologic condition permits

    b. Consider sedation or muscle relaxation in restless or decerebrate patients

3. Cardiovascular support

    a. Maintain cerebral perfusion pressure (CPP) at normal levels with crystalloid or colloid

    b. Blood transfusion to maximize O_2 carrying capacity

    c. Inotropic and vasopressor drugs as indicated

4. Monitoring. Mean arterial pressure (MAP), intracranial pressure (ICP), CPP, PaO_2, $PaCO_2$, hemoglobin, neurologic status, fluid and electrolyte balance, and chest x-ray

5. Drugs

    a. Intubation. Rapid sequence induction with thiopental, 1 to 3 mg/kg IV, and/or lidocaine, 1 mg/kg IV, to prevent an acute rise in ICP during laryngoscopy, and succinylcholine, 1.5 mg/kg IV, or pancuronium, 0.2 mg/kg IV

    b. Mannitol. 0.25 to 1.0 gm/kg rapidly

    c. Pancuronium. 0.1 mg/kg initially; then 0.02 to 0.03 mg/kg/hour if muscle paralysis is to be maintained

    d. Sedation. Diazepam, 5 to 10 mg every 2 to 3 hours, and fentanyl, 0.7 to 1.4 µg/kg/hour

B. Shock and adult respiratory distress syndrome (ARDS). As many as 50% of head-injured patients will have multisystem trauma and hemorrhagic shock; as many as 10% may have concomitant cervical spinal cord injury and spinal shock. Cardiogenic shock may be caused by either direct or secondary myocardial injury or by a protracted low-flow state from hemorrhagic shock. Neurogenic shock related to collapse of the vasomotor center rarely occurs and is almost always fatal. ICP and pupil size should be monitored in head-injured patients who are anesthetized for emergency operations of the abdomen, face, chest, or extremities since progressive neurologic deterioration may otherwise be undetectable.

    1. Approximately 20% of head-injured patients may develop **ARDS** characterized by

        a. Progressive hypoxia

        b. Reduced functional residual capacity

        c. Reduced compliance

        d. Pulmonary hypertension

        e. Diffuse patchy consolidation of chest x-ray film

    f. Hyaline membrane formation

    g. Pulmonary fibrosis

2. The **combination of hypoxia and shock** may exacerbate the initial neurologic injury because the resultant reduction in CPP causes cerebral ischemia. Treatment includes

    a. Optimal inspired oxygen tension (FiO_2).

    b. Careful fluid balance based on measurement of pulmonary capillary wedge pressure, central venous pressure (CVP), cardiac output, and urine output.

    c. Chest physiotherapy and prompt treatment of pulmonary infection.

    d. Optimal PEEP, the lowest PEEP that will produce maximum oxygen availability (arterial oxygen content × cardiac output). The increased airway pressure produced by PEEP may increase intrathoracic pressure, increase CVP, and hence increase ICP while simultaneously reducing CPP because of reduced cardiac output and MAP. When PEEP is discontinued, the sudden increase in central blood volume and MAP may increase cerebral blood volume and cerebral edema, particularly when cerebral autoregulation is impaired [1]. The effect of PEEP is most critical in patients who have reduced intracranial compliance. Optimal PEEP implies achieving the greatest increase in PaO_2 without reducing cardiac output or raising ICP.

3. Criteria for **weaning from mechanical ventilation** [2]

    a. Vital capacity of greater than 10 ml/kg

    b. Maximum inspiratory force of greater than -20 cm H_2O

    c. $V_D/V_T < 0.6$

    d. $P(A-a)\,O_2 < 300$ mmHg

    e. Cardiovascular stability

    f. Normal metabolic state

C. Neurogenic pulmonary edema. Various forms of noncardiogenic pulmonary edema have been explained by the presence of hypoxic pulmonary vasoconstriction that causes pulmonary arterial hypertension, pulmonary arteriolar wall rupture, and leakage of protein-rich edema fluid into the interstitium and alveoli [8]. There are similarities between the pathologic and clinical pictures of ARDS and neurogenic pulmonary edema. Perfusion of the brain with hypoxic blood leads to a lung lesion that is pathologically similar to shock lung and is associated with increased pulmonary venular resistance, vascular congestion, and interstitial and intraalveolar edema and hemorrhage. Neurogenic pulmonary edema is associated with a high mortality, and it is not clear whether reversal of the pulmonary hypertension in its early stages by the use of vasodilators such as sodium nitroprusside or nitroglycerin could be beneficial.

1. Characteristics
   a. Association with a variety of insults to the central nervous system (CNS) including head injury
   b. Presence of intracranial hypertension
   c. Marked pulmonary vascular congestion of rapid onset
   d. Massive neural discharge from injured brain or hypothalamus leading to pulmonary hypertension
   e. Increased pulmonary blood volume and pulmonary edema and hemorrhage

2. Therapy
   a. Immediate reduction in ICP through pharmacologic or surgical intervention, or both
   b. Hyperventilation: $PaCO_2$ of 25 to 30 mmHg with continuous positive pressure ventilation and high inspired oxygen tension

D. Fat embolism. Fat embolism may occur hours or days after the fracture of any bone containing marrow. Failure to recover consciousness after general anesthesia may suggest this diagnosis; secondary deterioration in a head-injured patient may be a consequence of fat embolism. No laboratory test is pathognomonic.

1. Characteristics
   a. Hypoxia
   b. Fluffy infiltrates on chest x-ray film
   c. Anemia, thrombocytopenia, hypocalcemia

2. Symptoms and signs appear 24 to 48 hours after trauma
   a. Changes in mental status ranging from restlessness to coma
   b. Seizures, paralysis
   c. Evanescent petechial rash (anterior axillary folds, neck, abdominal wall, conjunctiva)

3. Treatment.
Therapy is directed primarily to correct hypoxia with PEEP and increased FiO_2. Massive fat embolism is associated with high mortality.

E. Venous thromboembolism. The incidence of fatal pulmonary embolism in head-injured patients is unknown. There is a higher incidence of thromboembolic complications among patients who have suprasellar masses than among those who do not have suprasellar masses; a relationship between suprasellar masses and hypothalamic-associated hypercoagulability has been implied. Dehydration, obesity, and/or immobilization, all of which may be associated with hypothalamic malfunction, also predispose the patient to thromboembolism.

Minidose heparin therapy (5000 units SC every 12 hours as long as the patient is bedridden) can be used safely after a variety of surgical procedures. Whether this approach can prevent deep-vein thrombosis and pulmonary embolism in the neurosurgical population, including head-injured patients, without increasing the incidence of hematoma, is unknown.

F. Electrocardiographic changes. Arrhythmias and cardiac arrest may occur after head injury. Bradycardia, shortened Q–T interval, elevated S–T segment, nodal rhythm, increased T wave amplitude, and atrial fibrillation have occurred after head injury, in the presence and absence of intracranial hypertension. The pathogenesis is obscure. Atropine (for bradycardia), digoxin (for atrial fibrillation), and correction of metabolic and electrolyte abnormalities may be required.

II. Hematologic abnormalities

A. Inhibition of phagocytosis. Many disease states, including anoxic brain damage and head injury, are associated with the inhibition of the phagocytic function of neutrophilic granulocytes. Severe disturbances in phagocyte function have been observed in some head-injured patients who have clear consciousness and posttraumatic diabetes insipidus, implying a hypothalamic mechanism. There is a correlation between elevated serotonin levels in the CSF of head-injured patients and the inhibition of phagocytosis. Corticosteroids also stimulate serotoninergic metabolism in the brain.

B. Trauma and coagulation. The patient may be in a hypercoagulable and fibrinolytic state during the first few hours after trauma, probably from the release of tissue thromboplastin for hemostatic purposes. An abrupt rebound antifibrinolysis may also occur to facilitate hemostasis. Multiple transfusions, shock, sepsis, and unknown factors can also influence coagulation. Aspirin, phenylbutazone, chlorpromazine, penicillin, general anesthetics, furosemide, and many other drugs, as well as head trauma, impair platelet aggregation.

C. Disseminated intravascular coagulation (DIC). DIC is a physiologic response to a variety of stimuli that provoke a generalized activation of the hemostatic mechanism, leading to the intravascular consumption of clotting factors with subsequent thrombosis, bleeding diathesis, or both. DIC can be the result of three processes: endothelial cell injury, tissue injury, or red cell or platelet injury. The pathogenesis of DIC in cases of head injury is uncertain. The severity of the coagulopathy correlates with the severity of the head injury and systemic trauma. Shock, sepsis, extensive surgery, and fat embolism have all been associated with DIC. In addition, the brain is rich in tissue thromboplastin, and high levels of fibrinolytic activity are present in the highly vascular connective tissue of the choroid plexus and meninges. The mortality from DIC associated with head injury is high; death may be a consequence of intractable cerebral edema, intracerebral or intraventricular hemorrhage, multiple organ failure from microthrombosis, uncontrollable systemic hemorrhage, or a combination of these factors.

1. Diagnostic criteria for DIC include abnormal results of at least three screening tests: prothrombin time, fibrinogen, and platelets. If only two of these three factors are abnormal, one of the following should be abnormal to establish the diagnosis: thrombin time, euglobulin clot lysis, or fibrin split products.

2. Management

 a. Coagulation profile routinely on admission of head-injured patients

 b. Treatment of the underlying disease process

 c. Administration of cryoprecipitate (fibrinogin, factor VIII), fresh frozen plasma (factor V), platelet concentrates, and fresh red blood cells to correct the hemostatic defects

 d. Heparin therapy

  (1) May produce dramatic effects within a few hours, raising fibrinogen and plasminogen levels to normal, shortening thrombin time, and allowing resynthesis of consumed clotting factors

  (2) May predispose the head-injured patient to intracranial hemorrhage

III. Endocrinologic abnormalities

 A. Anterior pituitary insufficiency. Signs of anterior pituitary insufficiency after head trauma are rare; recognizable pituitary or hypothalamic damage is commonly found postmortem, however. Anterior pituitary insufficiency may be caused by traumatic rupture of the pituitary stalk, interruption of the vascular supply to the stalk at the time of head injury, traumatic hemorrhage into the pituitary gland, or systemic vascular collapse from hemorrhagic shock. More likely to occur in a patient who has a fracture of the middle cranial fossa, anterior pituitary insufficiency is frequently accompanied by transient or permanent diabetes insipidus. The diagnosis of anterior pituitary insufficiency should also be considered when there is a basal skull fracture, secondary amenorrhea, galactorrhea, or regression of secondary sexual characteristics or the persistence of poor recovery, posttraumatic psychosis, or general malaise. Appropriate replacement therapy is indicated when specific deficiencies are proved through endocrinologic testing: prednisone, 5 mg PO each morning and 2 to 5 mg each afternoon; levothyroxine (Synthroid) 0.1 to 0.15 mg PO each day.

 B. Posterior pituitary dysfunction

 1. Diabetes insipidus. Diabetes insipidus commonly occurs after craniofacial trauma and skull fracture [6]. It can be permanent or transient and may be related to hypoxic brain damage, drug overdose, hemorrhagic shock, or fat embolism. **Signs** of antidiuretic hormone (ADH) deficiency are as follows:

  a. Polyuria (2–15 L/day)

  b. Polydipsia (unless hypothalamus is destroyed)

  c. Hypernatremia

  d. Serum hyperosmolality (320–330 mOsm/L)

e. Dilute urine (specific gravity 1.001–1.005, 50–150 mOsm/L)

f. Urine/serum osmolality of < 1

The **diagnosis** is usually obvious but it can be confirmed by determining the plasma level of ADH or neurophysin (ADH carrier protein) in relation to changes in plasma and urine osmolality induced by water restriction or administration of synthetic ADH.

Essentials of **management** include determination of daily weight, careful fluid balance, and serial measurement of serum BUN, electrolytes, and osmolality, and urine specific gravity and osmolality. The hourly urine output and the usual estimate for insensible fluid loss are replaced with solutions containing water and little or no electrolytes. Administering sodium-containing solutions may lead to severe hypernatremia. Water intoxication (lethargy, confusion, seizures, and coma) can occur if excess vasopressin is administered [7]. When the patient is awake and able to take fluids orally, fluid balance can often be maintained satisfactorily. If urinary output exceeds either 250 ml/hour for two consecutive hours or 6 to 7 L/day, or if the patient is unable to maintain fluid balance, then aqueous vasopressin (5–10 IU IM or IV every 4–6 hours) or vasopressin tannate in oil (5 IU IM every 24–72 hours) may be used. A long-acting synthetic vasopressin nasal spray (desmopressin; DDAVP) is convenient for patients who develop permanent diabetes insipidus. It is supplied in 2.5-ml bottles of 100 μg/ml; the usual dose is 10 to 20 μg intranasally every 12 to 24 hours.

2. **Syndrome of inappropriate ADH (SIADH).** Many disorders of the CNS have been associated with SIADH. Anesthesia and surgery can cause elevation of plasma ADH secondary to pain, stress, and various drugs. In neurosurgical patients, all the features of SIADH may be produced by the administration of aqueous vasopressin during overvigorous therapy of diabetes insipidus. SIADH after head trauma probably results from either the overproduction or excessive release of ADH in response to irritation of the hypothalamic-pituitary axis [3]. Secretion of ADH may also be increased by stimulation of the intrathoracic volume receptors when patients are nursed in the head-up position; this position may exacerbate SIADH as well. Fluid restriction may prevent the syndrome from becoming full-blown.

The typical **signs** of SIADH include:

a. Hyponatremia

b. Serum hypoosmolality

c. Urine/serum osmolality of > 1

d. Normal renal and adrenal function

e. Absence of signs of volume depletion (normal skin turgor and blood pressure)

f. Signs of water intoxication (anorexia, nausea, vomiting, irritability, neurologic abnormalities, i.e., muscle weakness or convulsions)

Treatment involves water restriction, with or without the administration of hypertonic saline. In patients whose serum sodium is < 110 mEq/L, hypertonic saline may be necessary (3% saline, 513 mEq/L). Hyponatremia can also occur after prolonged diuresis from mannitol if sodium losses are not replaced, but total osmolality is increased and circulatory volume is reduced.

IV. Metabolic abnormalities

A. Water and electrolyte balance. Sodium retention is a normal response to bodily injury; it generally lasts from 2 to 4 days and appears to be related to hypothalamic stimulation, aldosterone secretion, and subsequent release of ACTH. There is no relationship between the severity of the sodium retention and the location of the brain damage. Major trauma may also cause a mild degree of ADH-mediated water retention, which lasts for 2 or 3 days. Despite the sodium retention, head-injured patients may be mildly hyponatremic because of the concomitant water retention.

B. Glucose metabolism. Glucose intolerance commonly develops after trauma. High catecholamine levels inhibit the release of insulin. ACTH, serum cortisol, and growth hormone levels may be elevated post trauma, as well. Exogenously administered corticosteroids are diabetogenic since they promote gluconeogenesis and increase hepatic production of glucose. Severe diabetes mellitus develops in only a few patients receiving corticosteroids; and only in those patients who have a reduced insulin reserve (e.g., the adult-onset diabetic) is the diabetogenic action of corticosteroids extreme. Latent diabetes mellitus may be unmasked by trauma and may be detrimental to the patient's recovery if it goes unrecognized.

C. CSF metabolic changes. Brain injury results in CSF lactic acidosis. The severity of CSF acidosis relates directly to the severity of the head injury and seems to depend on the amount of lactic acid produced by the injured and hypoxic brain tissue. Marked intracranial hypertension causes a reduction in cerebral blood flow (CBF) and is accompanied by long-lasting but reversible lactic acidosis of cerebral tissue. Low CSF pH promotes spontaneous hyperventilation. Serotonin levels in the CSF rise after head trauma in proportion to the severity of the trauma. CSF cAMP levels are lowest in patients in the deepest grades of coma after either head injury or spontaneous intracranial hemorrhage.

D. Nonketotic hyperosmolar hyperglycemic coma. Nonketotic hyperosmolar hyperglycemic coma (NHHC) complicates many primary illnesses, including neurologic disorders, in diabetic and nondiabetic patients. The average age of patients who have NHHC is 57 years; two-thirds have no previous history of diabetes mellitus. Many predisposing factors to NHHC are present in neurosurgical patients: they are receiving corticosteroids, prolonged mannitol therapy, hyperosmolar tube feedings, and limited water replacement. The mortality is 40 to 70%. Causes of death include renal failure, arrhythmias, cerebrovascular accidents, and systemic thromboembolic complications.

1. **Diagnostic criteria for NHHC**
   a. Hyperglycemia (400–2700 mg/100 ml)
   b. Glucosuria
   c. Absence of ketosis
   d. Hyperosmolality ($>$ 330 mOsm/L)
   e. Dehydration
   f. CNS dysfunction

2. **Characteristics.** Severe potassium depletion may result from the osmotic diuresis. Patients may also exhibit leukocytosis, hemoconcentration, and azotemia with a BUN-to-creatinine ratio of greater than 30:1. Many patients are febrile, in shock, and in coma; they may or may not have focal neurologic signs. Coma and subsequent death are attributed to either total-body sodium depletion or cellular dehydration, particularly in the brain.

3. **Pathogenesis.** The pathogenesis of NHHC is not clear. The absence of ketosis may reflect either the antiketogenic effects of severe hyperglycemia or the effect of insulin on fat and carbohydrate metabolism. At low concentrations of insulin in the plasma, insulin has no effect on the uptake of glucose by cells but can still inhibit the release of free fatty acids from adipose tissue. Before initiating therapy, appropriate laboratory data must be obtained (serum Na^+, osmolality, pH, blood urea nitrogen, glucose, K^+, lactate). Plasma osmolality can be estimated and followed during therapy ($Posm = 2\,Na^+ + glucose/18$).

4. **Treatment.** Hypovolemia and hypertonicity are the immediate threats to life. Hypotonic saline administration may not improve sodium and water deficits rapidly enough; therefore, normal saline may be used until blood pressure and urine output are stabilized. If a patient is in hypovolemic shock, administration of isotonic sodium chloride or plasma may be necessary, regardless of the osmolality. The volume of hypotonic fluid necessary varies, depending on the individual patient, but it is usually $>$ 5 liters during the first 12 hours of treatment and averages 500 to 1300 ml/hour until the plasma osmolality reaches 325 mOsm/L.

   Hyperglycemia usually responds dramatically to the administration of relatively small doses of insulin. Large doses of insulin reduce the serum glucose rapidly and may increase mortality by decreasing the plasma volume before there has been adequate fluid and salt repletion. The recommended dose is 25 units of regular insulin each hour until sodium deficits have been replaced.

V. Gastrointestinal abnormalities. Seventeen percent of head-injured patients may have esophageal, gastric, or duodenal ulceration and hemorrhage. The frequency of gastrointestinal bleeding is positively correlated with the severity of injury: severely injured patients receiving glucocorticoids have a higher incidence of bleeding than have less severely injured patients receiving corticosteroids. Hypothalamic stimulation, gastric mucosal disruption, ingestion of aspirin or ethanol, hyperacidity, and hemorrhagic shock are among the etiologic factors. Signs and symptoms include epigastric pain, abdominal distention, ileus, hypotension, hematemesis, and melena. In the unconscious patient, perforation of a viscus may be asymptomatic.

Treatment includes nasogastric suction, cold saline lavage, fluid and blood replacement, and cimetidine (to block histamine H_2 receptor and reduce parietal cell hydrogen ion secretion). Cimetidine may offer preventive therapy in patients who have preexisting ulcer disease or predisposing conditions, since it reduces acid secretion and elevates gastric pH. In one study, however, prophylactic antacid therapy was found to be more efficacious in the general category of stress ulceration, although cimetidine seemed to offer advantages to neurosurgical patients [4].

VI. Skeletal abnormalities

    A. Cervical spine injuries. Ten percent of head-injured patients have associated cervical spine injury. Fifty percent of patients who have cervical spine fracture also have concurrent evidence of head trauma. Head-injured patients should therefore be considered to have cervical spine injury until it is proven otherwise. Hyperextension of the neck during laryngoscopy and endotracheal intubation may displace an unstable fracture and cause or exacerbate spinal cord compression. All diagnostic and therapeutic maneuvers must therefore be performed with extreme caution until the stability of the cervical spine is established.

        High transection of the spinal cord (above the C-3 level) is most often fatal owing to the cessation of diaphragmatic and intercostal muscle function and to subsequent hypoventilation and secondary infection. The absence of sympathetic tone leads to hypotension, bradycardia (cardiac output may be high, low, or normal), and an increase in alveolar dead space from a reduction in pulmonary perfusion.

        Mechanical ventilation may be indicated for the management of ventilation-perfusion abnormalities (atelectasis secondary to hypoventilation, infection, "shock lung") and hypercapnia (increased alveolar dead space without compensation). Continuous application of positive pressure breathing may decrease cardiac output by reducing venous return in a patient who cannot compensate by increasing venous tone. Treatment includes replacement of intravascular volume and maintenance of adequate hemoglobin levels. Minute volume, PEEP, and chest physiotherapy are adjusted to achieve maximum acceptable oxygen availability with minimal interference with venous return. Weaning of such patients must be accomplished on an individual basis, although the usual criteria apply (see section **I.B.3**).

B. Maxillofacial injuries. Blunt trauma in the cervical region can cause carotid artery injury. Compression or stretching of the vessel may lead to thrombosis, transient ischemic attacks, Horner's syndrome, or hematoma of the lateral neck and airway obstruction. Horner's syndrome may develop after neck trauma as a result of pressure or direct injury to the sympathetic neural supply to the face. The unilateral pupillary constriction that results or the pupillary dilatation that accompanies direct trauma to the eye may lead to confusion and overtreatment of a suspected intracranial mass. Subcutaneous emphysema resulting from frontal or ethmoid sinus fractures must be distinguished from emphysema resulting from thoracic injury. Fractures of the cribriform plate may allow a nasogastric tube to enter the intracranial space; these tubes must be placed through the mouth under direct vision; gastrostomy may be indicated.

Anesthesia

PHILIPPA NEWFIELD

ROBERT D. McKAY

The anesthesiologist has an important role in the care of head-injured patients in the emergency room, operating room, and neurosurgical intensive care unit (ICU). The anesthesiologist's skills in airway management, fluid resuscitation, monitoring, and support of the cardiac and respiratory systems are invaluable. Many patients who have head injury will require anesthesia; the procedures may be neurosurgical or nonneurosurgical, such as repair of long bone fractures, facial fractures, or laparotomy for hemorrhage. A successful outcome in these situations depends on both the anesthesiologist's knowledge and application of relevant physiologic, pathophysiologic, and neuropharmacologic principles and meticulous attention to detail.

I. Pathophysiology

   A. Primary head injury is damage sustained as a direct, immediate result of the trauma [3]. Acceleration-deceleration head injuries without impact tend to produce subdural hematomas from tearing of bridging veins, as well as diffuse cortical injury with contusions or lacerations from impact of the brain with bony prominences or sharp edges of the falx cerebri or tentorium. Injury from skull impact is more likely to consist of skull fracture with associated contusion of the brain. Hematoma formation occurs in a number of cases, particularly if the fracture line crosses either an artery or a venous sinus. Acute subdural hematoma is the most common intracranial hematoma of traumatic origin requiring surgical evacuation. Mortality may be 50%, mainly secondary to malignant brain swelling [12]. Categories of primary head injury are listed in Table 13-3.

   B. Secondary head injury is a brain injury that occurs after the initial traumatic event. It is potentially preventable. Theoretically the patient should survive, but the quality of survival is determined by the severity of the primary injury. The factors involved in secondary head injury may be initiated either by intracranial, systemic, or iatrogenic events. Factors that produce secondary head injury include the following:

   1. Disturbances in the regulation of cerebral blood flow (CBF). CBF, normally coupled closely with cerebral metabolism, is regulated by several mechanisms including neurogenic (the autonomic nervous system), myogenic (auto-regulation), metabolic (changes in the concentrations of acid metabolities such as lactic acid), and chemical (arterial oxygen and carbon dioxide tensions). Head trauma may disrupt some or all of these regulatory

Table 13-3. Categories of primary head injury

Scalp
    Contusion
    Abrasion
    Laceration
    Subgaleal hematoma
Skull fractures (open or closed)
    Linear
    Comminuted
    Depressed
    Stellate
Meninges
    Epidural hematoma
    Subdural hematoma (acute, subacute, chronic)
    Basal dural tear
    Rhinorrhea
    Otorrhea
    Pneumocephalus
Brain
    Concussion
    Contusion
    Laceration
    Hematoma

mechanisms, leading to imbalances in the delivery of O_2 to brain tissues relative to the O_2 demanded by those tissues.

CBF in excess of metabolic demands (hyperemia or luxury perfusion) may lead to increases in cerebral blood volume, intracranial pressure (ICP), and edema formation. If autoregulation is impaired, CBF becomes a passive function of cerebral perfusion pressure (CPP), the difference between mean arterial pressure and ICP (MAP-ICP). Inadequate CBF, produced by hypotension, compression of the arterial supply, or vasospasm, causes a shift from aerobic to anaerobic metabolism, increased lactate production, and vasomotor paralysis. Failure of chemical regulation of CBF after head trauma is associated with loss of CO_2 reactivity by the cerebral vessels. In addition, sympathetic stimulation as a homeostatic response to hemorrhage may constrict cerebral vessels and reduce CBF.

2. **Hypoventilation.** Hypoventilation from brainstem injury, airway obstruction, aspiration, thoracoabdominal injury, or shock may contribute to secondary brain injury. Resultant hypoxia and hypercapnia, demonstrated in 70% of otherwise healthy people who had major head trauma [6], increase CBF and cerebral blood volume and compromise O_2 delivery to the injured brain. Indeed, the degree of hypercarbia closely correlates with the severity of head trauma [22].

3. **Cardiovascular dysfunction.** Cardiovascular dysfunction may produce secondary brain injury, particularly when autoregulation is impaired. Hypertension will increase CBF and cerebral blood volume, causing brain swelling and edema, whereas hypotension will lower CPP and exacerbate cerebral ischemia and acidosis.

4. **Cerebral swelling.** Cerebral swelling is an increase in CBF. This occurs most commonly in children 24 to 48 hours after head injury. Cerebral edema, an increase in brain tissue water, and intracranial mass lesions, such as epidural, subdural, and intracerebral hematomas, all reduce intracranial compliance and increase ICP. The relationship among the intracranial fluid volumes—brain tissue, brain tissue water, cerebrospinal fluid (CSF), and cerebral blood volume—and ICP is defined by the Munro-Kellie doctrine: An increase in the volume of one of the fluid compartments must be matched by a decrease in one or all of the remaining volumes or the ICP will rise.

5. **Increased ICP.** An increase in ICP causes further compression of tissue, decreases CPP, and increases ischemia. If this reduction of CPP is not reversed, a vicious cycle may develop, culminating in either inadequate cerebral perfusion (ICP > MAP) or herniation and compression of vital structures (Fig. 13-4).

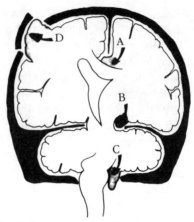

Fig. 13-4. Four sites of brain herniation. *A.* Cingulate. *B.* Uncal. *C.* Cerebellar or tonsillar. *D.* Transcalvarial.

II. CNS effects of anesthesia. Anesthetic drugs have substantial effects on CBF and cerebral metabolism. Other interventions such as intubation, positioning, and airway pressure may also affect the central nervous system (CNS).

A. Intravenous anesthetics. With the exception of ketamine, the intravenous anesthetics tend to decrease ICP, as long as CO_2 retention is prevented. CBF remains coupled with cerebral metabolism. The systemic and CNS effects of these drugs are summarized in Table 13-4 and Fig. 13-5.

1. The **barbiturates** produce the greatest reduction in CBF and $CMRO_2$. Autoregulation remains intact and the formation of cerebral edema after experimental head injury is limited. The metabolic depression with barbiturates affects the cells' energy requirements for neuronal function, rather than the requirements to maintain cellular integrity. The primary cardiovascular effects of thiopental are hypotension from venodilatation, decreased CNS sympathetic outflow, and decreased cardiac output. Reflex attempts to correct hypotension include increases in heart rate and total peripheral resistance. The hypotension may be attenuated by slow administration. The decrease in ICP from the fall in CBF is usually greater than the decrease in MAP, resulting in an increased CPP. This may not be true in the hypovolemic patient; in this situation the decrease in MAP may exceed the decrease in ICP and cause a reduction in CPP.

2. **Narcotics** including fentanyl, morphine, and meperidine in anesthetic doses cause a modest decrease in CBF and $CMRO_2$ when

Table 13-4. Effects of anesthetic drugs on CBF, ICP, MAP, and CPP

Drug	CBF	ICP	MAP	CPP
Thiopental	↓ ↓	↓ ↓	↓	↑
Fentanyl	↓	↓	SL ↓	↑
Diazepam	↓	↓ ?	SL ↓	↑ ?
Droperidol	↓	↓	↓	SL ↓
Ketamine	↑ ↑ ↑	↑ ↑ ↑	↑	↓
Halothane	↑ ↑	↑	↓	↓
Enflurane	↑	↑	↓	↓
Isoflurane	↑	↑	↓	↓
N_2O	↑	↑	NC	↓

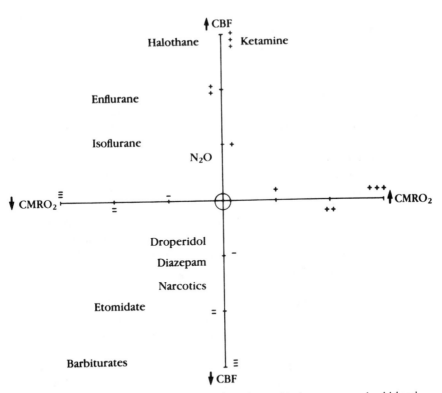

Fig. 13-5. Effect of anesthetic agents on the relationship between cerebral blood flow (CBF) and metabolism ($CMRO_2$). Increases and decreases in CBF are indicated along the vertical axis while increases and decreases in $CMRO_2$ are indicated along the horizontal axis. A drug that has no effect on CBF or $CMRO_2$, such as sodium chloride, would occupy the intersection point.

CO_2 retention is prevented; this decrease tends to reduce ICP. As with the barbiturates, autoregulation remains intact, and formation of edema in response to injury is reduced. Cardiovascular changes associated with narcotics include mild hypotension, primarily from venodilatation and bradycardia. Morphine produces more hypotension than does fentanyl. ICP is decreased to a greater extent than MAP, however, so the end result is an increase in CPP.

The administration of sufentanil and alfentanil to patients who had supratentorial tumors anesthetized with $N2_0$, 60% in O_2, caused lumbar CSF pressure to increase $89 \pm 31\%$ SE $(p < 0.05)$ and $22 \pm 5\%$ SE $(p < 0.05)$, respectively [18]. In primates, however, sufentanil preserved cerebral autoregulation and caused a dose-dependent fall in CBF and $CMKO_2$ $(p < 0.05)$ in both normal and noncompliant brains; anesthesia included 50% N_2 and 50% O_2 and muscle relaxation [4]. Hypertension is a fairly common development during anesthesia with a narcotic. The administration of naloxone to reverse the narcotic may result in hypertension and tachycardia as well as an increase in CBF, $CMRO_2$, and ICP.

3. **Diazepam, midazolam, and lorazepam** cause a modest decrease in CBF and $CMRO_2$, theoretically decreasing the ICP. The reduction of CBF and $CMRO_2$ with diazepam may be potentiated by $N2_O$. The cardiovascular effects of these drugs are mild; the slight decrease in MAP is more than offset by the reduction in ICP, resulting in an increase in CPP; however, there was no change in ICP reported when diazepam was used as the induction drug; CBF was not measured [30].

4. **Droperidol** causes a moderate reduction in CBF and ICP. The metabolic effects of this drug are not as well documented. $CMRO_2$ is either unchanged or slightly decreased. Droperidol produces hypotension primarily through alpha-adrenergic blockade and also by decreasing CNS sympathetic outflow. The degree of hypotension is variable. In some cases, particularly in hypovolemic patients, the reduction in MAP may exceed the reduction in ICP and cause a decrease in CPP.

5. **Etomidate,** in induction doses of 0.2 to 0.3 mg/kg, decreases CBF and ICP. The minimal cardiovascular effects of this drug cause CPP either to remain unchanged or to increase slightly [20].

6. **Ketamine** is the only intravenous anesthetic that increases CBF; this increase is of a most impressive magnitude. The effect of ketamine on cerebral metabolism is not as dramatic; there is either a slight increase or no change in $CMRO_2$. The increase in MAP by ketamine does not compensate for the increased ICP so that the CPP is reduced. The effects on CBF may be blocked by diazepam and thiopental. Ketamine also abolishes autoregulation.

B. **Inhalation anesthetics.** The inhalation anesthetics increase CBF while reducing $CMRO_2$. This uncoupling of flow and metabolism does not occur with the intravenous anesthetics. The CNS and cardiovascular effects of the inhalation anesthetics are shown in Tabel 13-4 and Fig. 13-5.

1. **Halothane** causes a significant dose-related increase in CBF and a significant decrease in $CMRO_2$. The increased CBF increases cerebral blood volume and ICP. This rise in ICP is dose-related and may be attenuated by introducing the drug only after hyperventilation to a $PaCO_2$ of 25 to 30 mmHg for 10 minutes. The increase in ICP with halothane can be reduced by thiopental. Halothane also impairs autoregulation in a dose-dependent fashion. Formation of edema in response to experimental cerebral cold injury is increased. The effects of halothane on the cardiovascular system include myocardial depression and vasodilatation, leading to hypotension. This, combined with the increase in ICP, causes a fall in CPP. Halothane also sensitizes the heart to catecholamines, which is important if infiltration of the scalp with a solution containing epinephrine is planned.

2. **Enflurane** is a weaker cerebrovasodilator than halothane but a more potent depressant of cerebral metabolism. ICP may be increased and, because its effect on MAP is similar to halothane, CPP is reduced. Enflurane may also produce seizures, particularly in the presence of hypocapnia. These seizures can cause increases in both CBF and $CMRO_2$.

3. **Isoflurane** increases CBF and ICP while decreasing $CMRO_2$. The increase in CBF is not as great as with halothane. Hyperventilation instituted simultaneously with isoflurane may not be adequate to block the increase in ICP in the presence of a mass lesion large enough to cause a midline shift in intracranial contents [7]. Isoflurane also causes hypotension and decreases CPP. The effect on MAP appears to be primarily from vasodilation rather than from reduced cardiac output.

4. **Nitrous oxide (N_2O)** increases cerebral metabolic oxygen demand and thus increases CBF and ICP when intracranial compliance is compromised [2]. Aside from its effect on CBF, N_2O can increase ICP in the presence of pneumocephalus by diffusing into the trapped air faster than nitrogen can diffuse out [17]. N_2O may also interfere with the protective effect of barbiturates [10].

C. **Muscle relaxants** differ in their CNS effects. Succinylcholine can increase ICP because of the vasodilatory effect of the preservatives methylparaben and propylparaben [9]. The rise in ICP can be blocked by prior administration of a nondepolarizing muscle relaxant [19]. The use of curare may be associated with a rise in electrical impedance and ICP, most likely because of histamine release. The release of histamine also plays a role in producing systemic hypotension. Pancuronium does not seem to affect ICP; it may produce hypertension and tachycardia. Dimethyl curare also does not increase ICP, at least in doses where histamine release is not seen. Vecuronium and atracurium do not increase ICP, even in situations in which intracranial compliance is reduced. Laudanosine, a metabolite of atracurium, does produce an arousal pattern on electrocardiogram (EEG) and increases the minimum alveolar concentration in animals [26].

Succinylcholine causes potassium release. Elevations of serum potassium sufficient to cause lethal arrhythmias have been reported when succinylcholine was administered to head-injured patients in the absence of paresis.   The time between injury and the onset of susceptibility to hyperkalemia has not been established. Patients who have flaccid paralysis, spasticity, or clonus after head injury may be susceptible, as may those who move extremities in response to pain but not to command. In the absence of massive muscle trauma, the use of succinylcholine in the head-injured patient within three days of injury should not cause significant hyperkalemia.

D. Nonpharmacologic interventions

1. **Laryngoscopy and intubation,** in addition to significantly raising the blood pressure, may cause a substantial increase in ICP. This response can be demonstrated in the absence of coughing and straining, which of themselves will aggravate the increase in ICP.

2. Placing the patient in the **Trendelenburg position** with the head down will decrease cerebral venous return, increase ICP, and promote the formation of cerebral edema. Cervical rotation or flexion may compress a jugular vein, which will have the same effect. Care must be taken when inserting internal jugular intravenous catheters. Puncture of the carotid or vertebral artery and laceration of the jugular vein may create a hematoma that compresses the jugular vein, again decreasing venous return and increasing ICP.

3. **Positive airway pressure** may be transmitted to the pleura and vena cava, which may decrease jugular venous return. The effect of positive end-expiratory pressure (PEEP) on ICP is unpredictable so that the need for PEEP in a head-injured patient is an indication for ICP monitoring. Although PEEP *may* increase ICP, it should be remembered that hypoxia *will* increase ICP. The positive airway pressure may also reduce venous return enough to decrease stroke volume, cardiac output, MAP, and CPP; these reductions will be of greater magnitude in the hypovolemic patient.

III. The anesthesiologist's evaluation.

The anesthesiologist should evaluate the patient on arrival in the emergency room, without waiting to see whether the patient will come to the operating room. The anesthesiologist can make a significant contribution to the patient's care through airway management, fluid resuscitation, cardiorespiratory support, and monitoring, even if surgery is not necessary.

A. Evaluate the airway. This is of paramount importance and is discussed in section **IV.**

B. Evaluate the CNS status. The Glasgow coma scale (see Table 13-1) has been an important advance in the neurologic evaluation and monitoring of the head-injured patient. The value of this system is its reproducibility from observer to observer, the ease with which changes can be documented, and the demonstration of trends in recovery or exacerbation. Other pertinent neurologic findings include focal deficits, signs of herniation, or signs of brainstem dysfunction. Spinal cord injury fairly often accompanies head injury.

C. Obtain patient history. If the patient is awake, a history should be obtained. Many patients unfortunately will be unable to provide any information because of the severity of their injury or the influence of alcohol, prescription drugs, or street drugs, or a combination of these factors.

   1. Ascertain time and nature of **last oral intake.**

   2. Obtain **description of the injury** if the patient can recall. The description may provide clues as to potential associated injuries. Approximately 1 out of 3 patients who have head injury will also have at least one other associated injury.

   3. Obtain **drug and alcohol** history from family members, friends, or witnesses. Ethanol intoxication worsens the prognosis of severe head injury.

D. Perform physical examination. A thorough physical examination is essential because positive nonneurologic findings will suggest sites of associated injury. For example, fractured ribs may indicate lung contusion, or ecchymosis over the right upper quadrant may suggest liver laceration. An estimate of the patient's intravascular volume should be made, using the "Tilt test" (determination of pulse and blood pressure while the patient is supine and then with the head elevated).

E. Monitor the patient. After initial evaluation and stabilization, many patients undergo computed tomography (CT) or cerebral angiography during which time the anesthesiologist should establish monitoring, ensure adequate intravenous accesss, and check on laboratory results and blood bank support. These patients will be closely monitored in the operating room and neurologic ICU; they should receive the same close attention while in transport or in the radiology suite. Precordial or esophageal stethoscope and blood pressure cuff should be routine. If an arterial cannula is in place, a portable transducer and oscilloscope or an aneroid manometer (Fig. 13-6) can be used to monitor MAP.

IV. Airway management

A. Basic principles. Securing the airway of the head-injured patient may present many potential problems. Since 5 to 10% of patients will also have cervical spine injuries, hyperextension of the neck should

Arterial line

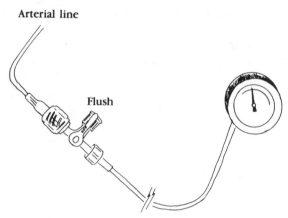

Flush

Fig. 13-6. A gas sterilized aneroid manometer connected to an arterial line. This system may be useful for monitoring blood pressure during transport. The needle fluctuations correspond to mean arterial pressure.

be avoided when opening the airway. The possibility of an unsuspected fracture of the basal skull or the cribriform plate makes the insertion of nasopharyngeal airways, nasogastric tubes, or nasotracheal tubes hazardous, since the object may pass intracranially rather than into the pharynx. Fractures into nasal sinuses that are accompanied by dural tears and CSF rhinorrhea present another problem: Positive pressure ventilation transmitted to the nasal sinuses may push contaminated material into the CNS, creating a serious infection.

Mask fit may be difficult in the patient who has serious craniofacial trauma; the mouth may not open well and laryngoscopic exposure may be poor because of bleeding into the airway. A hematoma in the neck can compress and shift the larynx and trachea, making visualization and intubation difficult. Preexisting conditions such as receding mandible, protruding teeth, or a short, thick neck may also make intubation difficult.

Awake intubation has hazards also. Attempts at awake intubation, with or without a fiberoptic laryngoscope, may cause coughing and straining, leading to increases in ICP or spinal cord injury from unstable fractures or dislocations of the cervical spine. A rapid sequence induction may be associated with wide swings in blood pressure or inability to insert the endotracheal tube or ventilate the patient once anesthesia and muscle relaxation have been induced.

B. Criteria for airway support. In the absence of pulmonary complications, airway injury, thoracoabdominal injury, or shock, patients who are awake and following commands will not need endotracheal intubation. Unresponsive patients who have an impaired gag reflex will require intubation. Patients who fall in between these points on the spectrum need close evaluation. The Glasgow coma scale (see Table 13-1) may be helpful in making the decision: endotracheal intubation of all patients who have a Glasgow coma score of 7 or less is a safe approach.

C. **Establishing the airway.** Airway management must begin at the scene of the accident, since hypoxia and hypercapnia are important factors in secondary head injury. Clearing the airway of mucus, blood, vomitus, and broken teeth, pulling the jaw foward, and administering supplemental oxygen will usually correct hypercapnia and hypoxia.

1. **Assisted ventilation.** If air exchange is inadequate, then respirations must be assisted. An oropharyngeal airway and oxygen delivery with positive pressure may be used. If an oral airway is used, then cricoid pressure will minimize gastric distention and regurgitation. All patients who have head injury have a full stomach. Once the airway is secure, radiologic evaluation of the cervical spine including C-7 can then be performed. Care is indicated to avoid spinal cord injury if the radiographs showing no evidence of a fracture or dislocation are incomplete.

2. **Monitoring.** Basic monitoring should be established, using precordial stethoscope, blood pressure cuff, and electrocardiogram (ECG).

3. **Intubation**

   a. **Stable vital signs.** If vital signs are stable, if hypovolemia is not present, and if intubation does not appear difficult, anesthesia can be induced with thiopental, 3 to 6 mg/kg. Muscle relaxation can be achieved using either succinylcholine (after pretreatment with a nondepolarizing muscle relaxant to prevent fasciculations) or pancuronium. A nerve stimulator should be used to ensure the presence of good muscle relaxation before laryngoscopy. Lidocaine, 1.5 mg/kg IV, 90 seconds before intubation may prevent an increase in ICP with laryngoscopy and intubation.

   b. **Unstable vital signs.** If the vital signs are unstable or if significant hypovolemia is suspected, a smaller dose of thiopental (1–2 mg/kg) should be used. Diazepam, 0.1 to 0.2mg/kg, midazolam, 0.1 to 0.2 mg/kg, or etomidate, 0.2 to 0.3 mg/kg, are suitable alternatives. These drugs can be given with lidocaine and a muscle relaxant. A flow chart for the airway management of a head-injured patient is illustrated in Fig. 13-7. Adequate preparation for intubation includes suction, monitoring, oxygen, and a selection of laryngoscopes, blades, and endotracheal tubes.

   c. **Difficult intubation.** If a difficult intubation is suspected, muscle relaxants should not be used until either the larynx has been visualized or the endotracheal tube has been placed. Sedation with droperidol, fentanyl, and/or diazepam may be used. Superior laryngeal nerve blocks or transtracheal instillation of lidocaine should not be used with a full stomach. Lidocaine, 1.5 mg–kg IV, may be used to minimize coughing and rise in ICP. Nasotracheal intubation while the patient is awake may be used in the absence of a direct communication between the nasal passages and the brain. A "blind" approach may be used or the tube may be placed under direct vision. Alternatively, a suction catheter, ureteral catheter, or other guide can be inserted through the larynx and the tube passed over it. Flexible fiberoptic instruments, optical stylets, prisms, and the retrograde technique have all been used successfully. Tracheotomy or cricothyroidotomy is necessary when there is no access to the larynx perorally or pernasally or when the trachea communicates with the outside. Once the endotracheal tube is in place, intravenous sedatives, narcotics, and muscle relaxants should be administered to prevent coughing and straining, and to facilitate controlled ventilation.

V. Anesthetic management for neurosurgical procedures. Operative procedures include craniotomy for evacuation of epidural, subdural, or intracerebral hematoma, placement of ICP monitors, elevation of

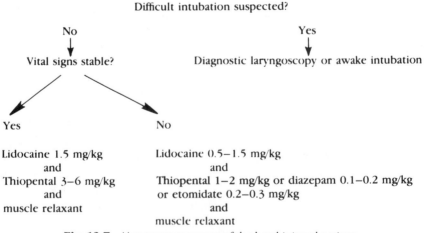

Fig. 13-7. Airway management of the head-injured patient.

depressed skull fractures, and decompression operations such as craniectomies or excision of portions of the frontal or temporal lobe.

A. Monitoring. Monitors can be divided into two classes: noninvasive and invasive. Invasive monitors are indicated when the benefit of the information to be gained outweighs the risk to the patient that the monitor entails, or more simply, when the risk of not having the information outweighs the risk of getting the information. Noninvasive monitors pose minimal risk to the patient; the decision to use them is based in part on the cost-effectiveness of the monitor. Ideally, the considerations for monitoring the patient during emergency neurosurgical procedures should be the same as those for the patients undergoing more elective procedures. However, the patient who has an epidural hematoma and impending herniation has compromise of viable brain tissue. Delay in evacuating the hematoma may produce irreversible damage. The best way to avoid delay in the operating room is to use the time in the emergency and neuroradiology areas to establish intravenous access and monitors. The patient can then be brought to the operating room, anesthetized (if not already under anesthesia), and prepared as quickly as possible for the surgical procedure.

1. **A precordial or esophageal stethoscope** is useful during transport as well as in the operating room to monitor heart and breath sounds. The esophageal stethoscope is particularly important in neurosurgery because the connections between the anesthesia machine and endotracheal tube may be hidden by drapes.

2. **The ECG** is essential since patients who have head injury may manifest electrocardiographic changes. The ECG may also show abnormalities from basic medical problems and cardiovascular complications of trauma.

3. **Blood pressure** may be measured by an indwelling arterial catheter or a blood pressure cuff; placement of a Doppler device may facilitate the cuff measurements. Direct arterial measurement offers several advantages, including beat-to-beat pressure monitoring capability, monitoring in transit, and accessibility of blood for arterial blood gases, hematocrit, blood chemistries, and coagulation profiles.

4. **A urinary catheter** provides measurement of urine output and urine samples for determination of specific gravity, osmolality, and chemistries.

5. **CVP and pulmonary artery catheters.** An indication of preload can be helpful. In the absence of left ventricular dysfunction, measurement of central venous or right atrial pressure is adequate. A Swan-Ganz pulmonary artery catheter should be used when there is left ventricular dysfunction or high cervical spinal

cord injury. This catheter can also provide cardiac output measurements and information necessary to calculate peripheral and pulmonary vascular resistance, which can be useful information, particularly in patients receiving high doses of barbiturates. A central venous catheter can be easily exchanged for a pulmonary artery catheter using the Seldinger technique. Acceptable veins for placing the catheters include antecubital, subclavian, internal and external jugular, and femoral.

6. Esophageal thermistor.

7. Ventilator monitors include FIO_2 analysis, a disconnect alarm, end-tidal CO_2, and O_2 saturation via pulse oximetry.

8. Monitors for the **detection of venous air-embolism** (Doppler, end-tidal CO_2, Swan-Ganz catheter) are indicated for procedures in which veins in the operative site are above the level of the heart. Surgical positioning (particularly the seated position), hypovolemia with low venous pressure, potential venous sinus injury, or other factors may predispose to venous air embolism.

B. Induction of anesthesia in neurosurgical emergencies is inseparable from securing the airway (see section **IV**). If succinylcholine is used for intubation, pancuronium, vecuronium, or atracurium should be administered before the patient has recovered enough neuromuscular function to cough or strain.

C. Maintenance of anesthesia. Close attention to the airway is required during positioning and preparation to avoid dislodging, kinking, or advancing the tube into a main-stem bronchus.

   1. Ventilation should be controlled. A $PaCO_2$ of 25 to 30 mmHg will promote brain relaxation for surgical exposure without producing ischemia from hypocapnic vasoconstriction. A higher $PaCO_2$ (30–35 mmHg) is recommended for patients who require burr holes for evacuation of chronic subdural hematomas, particularly after decompression, since a slack brain may encourage recurrence. Despite evidence that a prolonged decrease in $PaCO_2$ loses its CBF-lowering effect in normal animals [24], evidence in head-injured humans demonstrates that the sensitivity to changes in CO_2 may increase the longer the hyperventilation is continued [21, 25].

   2. Anesthetic drugs for head-injured patients are determined by the patient's condition. If the patient is unconscious in the absence of a drug overdose, the ICP is probably elevated. Then a barbiturate and a narcotic (possibly excluding sufentanil and alfentanil) in combination with O_2 or air O_2 and a muscle relaxant are appropriate. A similar technique is indicated for the patient whose CT scan demonstrates obliterated basal cisterns, dilated fourth or lateral ventricles, or a midline shift of 10 mm.

   Although hyperventilation will attenuate the increase in ICP with

volatile anesthetics, in the head-injured patient, cerebrovasoconstriction in response to hypocapnia is not a dependable response.
The introduction of volatile agents in these patients may increase
ICP and exacerbate the formation of edema. The volatile anesthetics in low concentrations may have a role in the treatment of
intraoperative hypertension, however.

Muscle relaxation should be maintained with pancuronium,
vecuronium, or atracurium and monitored by a peripheral nerve
stimulator. Administration of only 100% oxygen to unresponsive
patients who have unstable cardiovascular systems should be
avoided. Surgical decompression may improve these patients'
level of consciousness enough for them to cough, with disastrous
consequences.

Patients who have chronic subdural hematoma and are alert and
responsive may have burr holes for evacuation under local
anesthesia and moderate sedation. Some depressed skull fractures
may also be elevated under local anesthesia with sedation. This
technique must be used cautiously in the patient placed in the pin
headholder who has a full stomach.

3. **Administration of fluid** is guided by the amount required to
   maintain satisfactory organ perfusion, as indicated by heart rate,
   blood pressure, urine output, and cardiac filling pressures.

Although fluid restriction had been recommended in the past as a
means of controlling brain edema and ICP, such cerebral volume
control does not preclude ensuring the adequacy of the circulating
intravascular volume. Trauma patients often arrive in the operating
room in a volume-depleted state, and, as such, are at increased risk
for intraoperative cardiovascular instability, including hypotension
(with compromise of cerebral perfusion), hypertension (with increased brain swelling and edema formation), and inadequate depth
of anesthesia and hypoxemia. Intraoperative brain swelling will also
limit the surgeon's ability to expose the surgical site with minimal
retraction.

The blood-brain barrier is the major determinant of water movement into the normal brain. It is permeable to water but has a
relatively small pore size, which restricts the passage of ionized
molecules. There is thus minimal hydrostatically mediated movement of fluid in the normal brain from the intravascular compartment
to the brain's interstitium. Most of the water movement is occasioned
by changes in the blood-to-brain osmotic pressure gradient. The
brain also has a relatively low hydraulic conductivity, which further
limits entry of water. Consequently, a decrease in plasma osmotic
pressure produces an increase in the brain water content. The administration of fluids that are isosmotic to plasma causes no change in
brain water content and little change in ICP.

When the brain is normal, isovolemic hemodilution with solutions that are isosmotic to plasma cause minimal change in brain water and ICP, compared with hypoosmotic solutions, provided that the hemoglobic concentration is kept constant. As such, normal saline, 5% albumin, and 6% hetastarch have minimal effects on the brain's water content or ICP. The administration of large volumes of lactated Ringer's solution, on the other hand, has been associated with an increase in brain water and ICP [33].

When the blood-brain barrier is interrupted, as with neurotrauma or experimentally through a cryogenic lesion to the brain surface, the response to intravenous fluids is altered. Because the pore size is increased, the permeability to sodium, chloride, and colloids, such as albumin, is increased, as well. Consequently, an increase in the hydrostatic pressure gradient will increase the movement of water into the brain. Saline, 5% albumin, and 6% hetastarch produce equivalent increases in brain water and ICP when the blood-brain barrier is disrupted. In contrast, prolonged reduction of colloid osmotic pressure in the presence of cryogenic injury was not associated with further increase in brain water on the injured side [13]. The water content on the normal side was unchanged, but tissue water in peripheral muscle and jejunum was markedly increased.

Hemodilution with hypertonic lactated Ringer's solution caused an increase in CBF and a decrease in brain water and ICP [32], whereas the administration of normal saline in the same experimental model increased CBF, increased ICP slightly, and did not change brain water content. The increase in ICP was most likely secondary to the increase in CBF attendant on hemodilution. In animals who had cryogenic lesions, the administration of lactated Ringer's solution and hypertonic lactated Ringer's solution both increased the ICP, the former to a greater extent than the latter, but brain water content on the injured side was equal in both groups. The difference in ICP presumably reflected the decreased water content on the normal side in the group receiving the hypertonic solution [35]. In another experimental model, the increase in ICP caused by resuscitation from hypovolemic shock with lactated Ringer's solution was prevented by the use of 3% hypertonic saline [8, 23].

For fluid resuscitation of the head-injured patient, the infusion of fluid that maintains the plasma osmolality will have minimal effect on CBF and ICP [34] and will decrease the involvement of water into the normal areas of brain. Although fluid restriction in and of itself will reduce the water content of normal brain (but not reduce peritumoral edema) and the total intracranial volume, inadequate circulating volume must be corrected before the induction of anesthesia to avoid hypotension and hypoxemia. Lactated Ringer's solution is appropriate if small volumes are required, since lactated Ringer's solution, with an osmolality of 254 mO5m/kg, is hypoosmotic relative to blood. Normal saline has a measured osmolality of 300 to 305 MOgm/kg, is more closely isotonic to plasma, and is preferable if the patient is hypertonic, either because of prolonged fluid restriction or administration of mannitol. Small volumes of hypertonic, hypernatremic solutions, such as 7.5% saline, may be indicated initially to restore circulating blood volume after the extensive blood loss. (See chapter 7.)

Once the patient's deficit is restored, lactated Ringer's solution may be administered for maintenance at 2 to 4 ml/kg/hour. Colloid and hetastarch can be used to replace small amounts of blood, but larger blood loss requires transfusion. Besides the expense, the amount of hetastarch administered is limited to 1.0 to 1.5 liters by the development of a coagulopathy. The optimal hematocrit to maintain CBF remains in question. Isovolemic hemodilution increases cerebral perfusion in humans, whereas nondilutional hypervolemia does not increase CBF [11]. Although there is an inverse relationship between the hematocrit and CBF in humans, this does not necessarily produce an increase in brain O_2 transport (O_2 content XCBF) [16]. The balance of evidence leans in favor of maintaining the hematocrit at a lower than normal level (32–35%). Blood is administered if the amount of intraoperative blood loss will reduce the hematocrit below 30%.

The use of glucose-containing solutions is avoided because of the evidence for a worsened outcome from global cerebral ischemia in the presence of an elevated serum glucose. This exacerbation is attributed to the development of intracellular lactic acidosis, which causes the formation of free radicals and the interference with intracellular metabolism and ionic homeostasis. Hyperglycemia is also not necessary to elicit the adverse effect: Small doses of glucose produced a significantly worsened neurologic outcome in primates subjected to a reversible global ischemic insult. Furthermore, neurosurgical patients who did not receive glucose intraoperatively maintained adequate serum glucose levels and did not become hypoglycemic [27]. Diabetics and neonates require frequent monitoring of sugar-containing solutions.

VI. Anesthetic management for nonneurosurgical procedures. The same considerations for anesthesia for neurosurgical procedures apply to nonneurosurgical procedures. These patients may be at even greater risk than patients undergoing neurosurgical procedures. The brain of a patient undergoing a neurosurgical procedure may be decompressed by the operation, whereas the patient who has severe head injury and is undergoing a nonneurosurgical procedure gains no improvement in intracranial dynamics. This is not the situation in which to administer an inhalation anesthetic with spontaneous ventilation.

The use of **regional anesthesia** in these patients is controversial. Peripheral nerve blocks (such as digital or ankle blocks) or blocks of a major plexus (such as brachial, sciatic, or femoral) may be acceptable as long as sedation is not so heavy that respiratory depression occurs, unless of course the patient has an endotracheal tube and the ventilation is controlled. Care must also be taken to avoid a local-anesthetic–induced seizure. In the absence of patient cooperation, a nerve stimulator can be used to identify nerves. Spinal anesthesia would appear to be unsuitable, since there is potential for sudden changes in CSF volume and pressure. Epidural anesthesia shares this potential problem because of possible entry into the subarachnoid space. In addition, epidural injection may reduce intracranial compliance by compressing the spinal subarachnoid space, diminishing the ability of this space to accept CSF translocated from above.

The need to administer anesthesia for a nonneurosurgical procedure to a patient after craniocerebral trauma is a strong indication to monitor ICP. Only then can elevations of ICP be diagnosed and treated appropriately. Monitoring of EEG and evoked potentials may prove useful in these situations.

VII. Pediatric considerations. The brains of children and teenagers have significantly better recuperative powers than adults; the mortality after severe head injury in patients under 19 years of age is only a fourth of that for adults. The reason for this difference is not completely clear, although some differences in pathophysiology are apparent. Within 24 hours after head injury, children manifest cerebral swelling from hyperemia more frequently than adults. Whereas this makes mannitol less useful, hyperventilation to a $PaCO_2$ of 20 to 25 mmHg may be effective in reducing ICP without causing cerebral ischemia. Children who are unresponsive in the emergency room and who have dilated pupils and gasping respiration may respond after intubation and ventilation alone. The time to peak formation and resolution of cerebral edema is also much shorter in children than in adults.

The choice of anesthetic technique for the pediatric patient who has severe head injury is the same as for adults. Close attention to the position of the endotracheal tube, fluid and blood replacement, and temperature control is essential. Moderate hypothermia is acceptable and perhaps even beneficial.

Small children can lose a significant percentage of their blood volume into an intracranial hematoma. Initially, hypotension may not be apparent because of the hypertension induced by an increase in ICP. The surgical evacuation of the hematoma and subsequent decompression of the brain under anesthesia may unmask the hypovolemia and cause severe hypotension.

VIII. Treatment of intraoperative complications

A. Hypotension in the presence of increased ICP will reduce cerebral perfusion. The most likely causes of intraoperative hypotension in patients who have severe head injury are hypovolemia, anesthetic overdose, and neurogenic changes. Cardiogenic, anaphylactic, endocrinologic, and septic causes are rare. Hypovolemia may be compensated by increased sympathetic nervous system activity as a response to increased ICP. Surgical decompression can then reduce the hypertension, producing serious hypotension. Sudden hypovolemic hypotension may also be caused by rupture of a subcapsular splenic hematoma or an aortic dissection.

Treatment of hypovolemia consists of restoring the circulating blood volume with balanced salt solutions and blood products, guided by heart rate, blood pressure, urine output, and cardiac filling pressures. Treatment of hypotension secondary to anesthetic overdose and neurogenic causes combines fluid therapy with pharmacologic intervention such as ephedrine, 0.1 to 0.5 mg/kg, or calcium chloride, 5 to 10 mg/kg.

B. Arterial hypertension is caused by hypercapnia, surgical stimulation, light anesthesia, Cushing's response to increased ICP, excessive fluid resuscitation, preexisting hypertension, or surgical stimulation of the cerebellum or the sensory branches of the trigeminal nerve. The heart rate may be helpful in determining the cause because bradycardia is usually associated with the Cushing response and trigeminal stimulation, whereas tachycardia can accompany hypercapnia, light anesthesia, and fluid resuscitation. With preexisting hypertension, the heart rate is variable.

Hypertension secondary to hypercapnia can best be treated by lowering $PaCO_2$. The ideal drug to treat other forms of hypertension during anesthesia for head-injured patients—potent, fast-acting, and of short duration—should not increase ICP or alter the neurologic status. Unfortunately such an agent is not yet available. The drugs in

Table 13-5. Pharmacologic agents useful in the treatment of hypertension during surgery in head-injured patients

↑ ICP	No ↑ ICP
Hydralazine	Alpha-adrenergic blockers
Sodium nitroprusside	Beta-adrenergic blockers
Nitroglycerin	
Trimethaphan	
Volatile anesthetic agents	

current use have cerebrovascular effects: those that increase CBF may increase ICP in the head-injured patient (Table 13-5). The vasodilating drugs may also induce intracerebral steal and impair autoregulation.

Figure 13-8 illustrates a flow chart for the treatment of hypertension during anesthesia for the head-injured patient. The initial treatment consists of the intravenous anesthetics that are cerebrovasoconstrictors; some of them are alpha-adrenergic blocking drugs as well; next would be propranolol, esmolol, labetalol, and/or phentolamine. If these are ineffective, trimethaphan is the next agent. Disadvantages of this drug include the tendency to increase ICP when intracranial hypertension is present [14], tachyphylaxis, and cycloplegia, which may prevent the use of the pupils as neurologic monitors postoperatively. If trimethaphan is ineffective or undesired, the volatile anesthetics can be used in concentrations of less than 0.5 MAC in the hyperventilated patient ($PaCO_2$ 25–30 mmHg). The volatile anesthetics are preferable to the direct-acting vasodilators since the depression in $CMRO_2$ accompanying the use of the volatile anesthetics may be advantageous. If the blood pressure remains elevated, the direct-acting vasodilators such as sodium nitroprusside, nitroglycerin, or hydralazine may be used. The increase in ICP caused by nitroprusside and the other vasodilators may be attenuated by hypo-

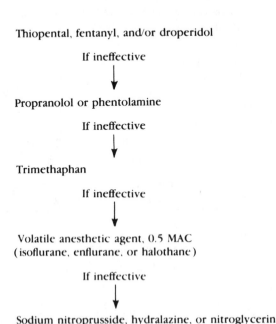

Thiopental, fentanyl, and/or droperidol

If ineffective

Propranolol or phentolamine

If ineffective

Trimethaphan

If ineffective

Volatile anesthetic agent, 0.5 MAC
(isoflurane, enflurane, or halothane)

If ineffective

Sodium nitroprusside, hydralazine, or nitroglycerin

Fig. 13-8. Treatment of intraoperative hypertension in head-injured patients. Treatment assumes hypocapnia (25–30 mmHg) has already been achieved.

capnic and hyperoxic conditions and a slow rate of administration. If at all possible, cerebrovasodilating drugs should be used either in conjunction with the monitoring of ICP or after the dura has been opened. Then at least the ICP will not increase, although brain swelling may produce poor operating conditions. A more detailed discussion of the pharmacologic treatment of hypertension is presented in Chapter 6.

C. **Intracranial hypertension** is a possible complication in every head-injured patient. The diagnosis is suspected when headache, papilledema, unilateral pupillary dilatation, oculomotor or abducens palsy, respiratory irregularities, hypertension, or bradycardia is present. Many of these signs are masked by general anesthesia. The diagnosis is confirmed either by the measurement of an elevated ICP or the finding of a tense, swollen brain at craniotomy, which can make the neurosurgical procedure extremely difficult. Failure to control intracranial hypertension will result in cerebral hypoperfusion and possible herniation. The anesthetic techniques that have been presented are designed to reduce ICP and preserve CPP after the institution of adequate hyperventilation ($PaCO_2$ of 25–30 mmHg in adults, 20–30 mmHg in children).

If, in spite of these techniques, intracranial hypertension persists, avenues of therapy remain that can produce a rapid effect. Two or more of these therapies may be used simultaneously.

1. **Augmentation of anesthesia.** Thiopental or pentobarbital, 1.5 to 5.0 mg/kg, as a bolus injection has been shown to be effective in the reduction of increased ICP (Fig. 13-9). Although the CPP in most patients will increase because the magnitude of the decrease in ICP exceeds the magnitude of the decrease in MAP, close monitoring of both pressures is indicated. In situations in which there is either hypotension or hypovolemia, lidocaine, 1.5 mg/kg, may be useful in reducing ICP while maintaining MAP. Failure of intracranial hypertension to respond to barbiturates usually indicates a poor prognosis.

2. **Diuretics.** Loop diuretics such as furosemide and ethacrynic acid have been used to reduce ICP. Mechanisms of action include general diuresis, decreased rate of CSF production, and resolution of cerebral edema. The osmotic diuretics work primarily by re-

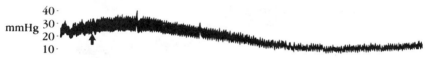

Fig. 13-9. Reduction of elevated intracranial pressure by barbiturates. Pentobarbital, 200 mg, was administered intravenously at the arrow. The reduction occurred approximately 5 min after the pentobarbital was given.

moving water from normal brain tissue. Of the osmotic diuretics, mannitol is the most widely used for acute control of intracranial hypertension (Fig. 13-10). Rapid administration may lead to vasodilatation, increased CBF, and a transient rise in ICP. The initial increase in ICP may be diminished by prior administration of furosemide. The reduction of ICP begins shortly after administration and lasts 4 to 6 hours, depending on the dose. The usual dose of mannitol is 0.25 to 1.0 gm/kg. Continued use of mannitol may lead to hyperosmolality and electrolyte imbalance. This problem may be reduced when the loop diuretics are combined with mannitol (Fig. 13-11).

D. **Hypoxia.** The causes of hypoxia during anesthesia for head-injured patients include aspiration, atelectasis, decreased cardiac output, pneumothorax, neurogenic pulmonary edema, lung contusion, fluid overload, embolism of fat or thrombi, and mechanical problems such as a kinked endotracheal tube or endobronchial intubation. As an initial step in treatment, the FIO_2 should be increased to provide adequate oxygenation. If this cannot be achieved by an FIO_2 of less than 0.55, the use of PEEP may be indicated. Optimal management includes monitoring the effect of PEEP on ICP, MAP, and CPP since PEEP may increase ICP and decrease MAP and CPP. This effect may be attenuated by elevation of the head.

E. **Diabetes insipidus** is suspected when polyuria with dilute urine occurs. The differential diagnosis includes diabetes mellitus, complications of diuretic therapy, ethanol intoxication, mineralocorticoid deficiency, and mobilization of fluids given during volume resuscitation for multiple trauma. Diagnostic studies include urine and serum chemistries and osmolalities and a monitor of right-sided or left-sided cardiac filling pressures. Failure to treat diabetes insipidus will result in serum hypernatremia and hyperosmolality. Urinary output is replaced with 0.45 normal saline since 5% dextrose in water may lead to superimposed diabetes mellitus or increased cerebral edema.

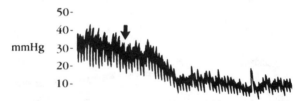

Fig. 13-10. Reduction in elevated intracranial pressure by mannitol, 0.8 gm/kg, administered intravenously at arrow.

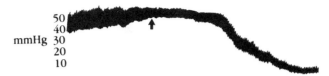

Fig. 13-11. Reduction in elevated intracranial pressure by mannitol, 0.4 gm/kg, and furosemide, 0.6 mg/kg, administered intravenously at arrow.

Aqueous vasopressin, 5 IU subcutaneously, will usually relieve the symptoms of diabetes insipidus for 3 to 4 hours. Overzealous treatment with vasopressin may cause water intoxication, which will promote the formation of edema.

IX. Postanesthetic care. An important question regarding the transition between the operating room and recovery area is whether the patient should go to the recovery room first or directly to the neurologic ICU. This decision depends on the level of care offered, availability of monitoring, and distances involved.

   A. Airway management. Whether to maintain controlled ventilation, endotracheal intubation, or both in the postoperative period is influenced by many factors including age, preexisting pulmonary disease, thoracoabdominal trauma, severity of the head injury, anticipated level of consciousness, and anticipated edema formation. There is a spectrum ranging from, for example, the young patient undergoing elevation of a depressed skull fracture, who was alert and responsive before anesthetic induction and has minimal underlying brain contusion, to the older patient who had evacuation of a large subdural hematoma and who has severe underlying brain injury.

   If extubation is planned, the muscle relaxant should be reversed and the trachea extubated when spontaneous ventilation is adequate. Administration of narcotic anesthetics may facilitate tolerance of the endotracheal tube. Lidocaine, 1.5 mg/kg, may attenuate the coughing response to the tube but may also potentiate the action of the nondepolarizing muscle relaxants, possibly interfering with reversal. Controversy exists as to whether recovery from anesthesia and extubation should be in the operating room or special care unit. If it is to be in the ICU, precautions should be taken to prevent the patient from coughing and straining during transport. Appropriate monitoring is required during transit. If hypothermia has developed, shivering should be prevented. As the patient recovers from anesthetic effects, painful stimulation should be minimized to prevent elevation of ICP (Fig. 13-12).

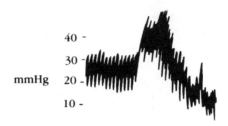

Fig. 13-12. Increased intracranial pressure in response to painful stimulus.

B. Communication in this transition phase is important. Discussion of the postoperative plans and equipment needs with the special care unit will ensure that a monitor and ventilator will be ready when the patient arrives in the unit. Communication between the anesthesiologist and the neurosurgeon is also essential to delineate and facilitate understanding of the effects of fluid balance, ventilator settings, vasoactive drugs, residual anesthetics, and muscle relaxants. Meticulous attention to detail is necessary for successful outcome in patients who have severe head trauma.

References

MANAGEMENT
1. Adams, H., Mitchell, D. E., Graham, D. I., et al. Diffuse brain damage of immediate impact type. Its relationship to "primary brain-stem damage" in head injury. *Brain* 100:489, 1977.
2. Bruce, D. A., Alavi, A., Bilaniuk, L. T., et al. Diffuse cerebral swelling following head injuries in children: The syndrome of "malignant brain edema." *J. Neurosurg.* 54:170, 1981.
3. Bruce, D. A., and Schut, L. The value of CT scanning following pediatric head injury. *Clin. Pediatr.* 19:719, 1980.
4. Bruce, D. A., Gennarelli, T. A., and Langfitt, T. W. Resuscitation from comas due to head injury. *Crit. Care Med.* 6:254, 1978.
5. Davis, K. R., Taveras, J. M., Robeson, G. H., et al. Computed tomography in head trauma. *Semin. Roentgenol.* 12:53, 1977.
6. Dolinskas, C. A., Bilaniuk, L. T., Zimmerman, R. A., et al. Computed tomography of intracerebral hematomas. 1. Transmission CT observations of hematoma resolution. *Am. J. Roentgenol.* 129:681, 1977.
7. Galbraith, S. C. Age distribution of extradural hemorrhage without skull fracture. *Lancet* 1:1217, 1973.
8. Greenberg, R. P., Becker, D. P., Miller, J. D., et al. Evaluation of brain function in severe human head trauma with multimodality evoked potentials. Part 2: Localization of brain dysfunction and correlation with posttraumatic neurological conditions. *J. Neurosurg.* 47:163, 1977.
9. Greenberg, R. P., Mayer, D. J., Becker, D. P., et al. Evaluation of brain function in severe human head trauma with multimodality evoked potentials. Part I: Evoked brain-injury potentials, methods, and analysis. *J. Neurosurg.* 47:150, 1977.
10. Lewis, A. J *Mechanisms of Neurological Disease.* Boston: Little, Brown, 1976.
11. Lindenberg, R., Fischer, R. S., Durlacher, S., et al. The Pathology of the Brain in Blunt Head Injuries of Infants and Children. In *Proceedings of the Second International Congress of Neuropathology.* Amsterdam: Excerpta Medica, 1955. Vol. 1. Pp. 477–479.

12. Ommaya, A. K., and Gennarelli, T. A. Cerebral concussion and traumatic uncon-sciousness: Correlation of experimental and clinical observations on blunt head injuries. *Brain* 97:633, 1974.
13. Seelig, J. M., Becker, D. P., Miller, J. D., et al. Traumatic acute subdural hematoma: Major mortality reduction in comatose patients treated within four hours. *N. Engl. J. Med.* 304:1511, 1981.
14. Windle, W. F., Groat, R. A., and Fox, C. A. Experimental structural alterations in brain during and after concussion. *Surg. Gynecol. Obstet.* 79:561, 1944.
15. Zimmerman, R. A., Bilaniuk, L. T., and Gennarelli, T. A. Computed tomography of shearing injuries of the cerebral white matter. *Radiology* 127:393, 1978.

SYSTEMIC EFFECTS
1. Aidinis, S. J., Lafferty, J., and Shapiro, H. M. Intracranial responses to PEEP. *Anesthe-siology* 45:275, 1976.
2. Feeley, T. W., and Hedley-Whyte, J. Weaning from controlled ventilation and sup-plemental oxygen. *N. Engl. J. Med.* 292:903, 1975.
3. Fox, J. L., Falik, J. L., and Shalhoub, R. J. Neurosurgical hyponatremia: The role of inappropriate antidiuresis. *J. Neurosurg.* 34:506, 1971.
4. MacDougall, B. R. D., Bailey, R. J., and Williams, R. H_2-receptor antagonists and antacids in the prevention of acute gastrointestinal hemorrhage in fulminant hepatic failure. *Lancet* 1:617, 1977.
5. Matjasko, M. J. Peripheral Sequelae of Acute Head Injury. In J. E. Cottrell and H. Turndorf (Eds.), *Anesthesia and Neurosurgery.* St. Louis: Mosby, 1980. Pp. 211–247.
6. McLaurin, R. L., and King, L. R. Recognition and treatment of metabolic disorders after head injuries. *Clin. Neurosurg.* 19:281, 1972.
7. Shucart, W. A., and Jackson, I. Management of diabetes insipidus in neurosurgical patients. *J. Neurosurg.* 44:65, 1976.
8. Theodore, J., and Robin, E. D. Pathogenesis of neurogenic pulmonary edema. *Lancet* 2:749, 1975.

ANESTHESIA
1. Albin, M. S. Anesthetic management of the patient with head injury. *Int. Anesthesiol. Clin.* 15:297, 1977.
2. Archer, D. P., Labrecque, P., Tyler, J. L., et al. Cerebral blood volume is increased in dogs during administration of nitrous oxide or isoflurane. *Anesthesiology* 67:642, 1987.
3. Bruce, D. A. Management of Severe Head Injury. In J. E. Cottrell and H. Turndorf (Eds.), *Anesthesia and Neurosurgery.* St. Louis: Mosby, 1980. Pp. 183–210.
4. Bunegin, L., Albin, M. S., Ernst, P. S., and Garcia, C. Cerebrovascular responses to sufentanil citrate (SC) in primates with and without intracranial hypertension. *J. Neurosurg. Anesthesiology* 1(2):138, 1989.
5. Butler, S. H., and Freund, P. R. Regional anesthesia as a safe alternative to general anesthesia in the multiple-trauma patient. *Reg. Anaesth.* 6:26, 1981.
6. Frost, E. A. M., Arancibia, C. U., and Schulman, K. Pulmonary shunt as a prognostic indicator in head injury. *J. Neurosurg.* 50:768, 1979.
7. Grosslight, K., Colahan, A., and Bedford, R. F. Isoflurane anesthesia—risk factors for increase in ICP. *Anesthesiology* 63:533, 1985.
8. Gunnar, W., Jonasson, O., Merlotti, G., et al. Head injury and hemorrhagic shock: Studies of the blood brain barrier and intracranial pressure after resuscitation with normal saline solution, 3% saline solution, and dextran-40. *Surgery* 103:398, 1988.
9. Hamilton, J. T., Zhou, Y., and Gelb, A. W. Paraben preservatives but not succinyl choline are vasodilators. *Can. Anaesth. Soc. J.* 585, 1989.
10. Hartung, J., and Cottrell, J. E. Nitrous oxide reduces thiopental-induced prolon-gation of survival in hypoxic and anoxic mice. *Anesth. Analg.* 66:47, 1987.

11. Henrikson, L., Paulson, O. B., and Smith, R. J. Cerebral blood flow following normovolemic hemodilution in patients with high hematocrit. *Ann Neurol.* 9:454, 1981.
12. Jones, N. R., Blumberg, P. C., and North, J. B. Acute subdural hematomas. Aetiology, pathology and outcome. *Aust. N.Z. J. Surg.* 56:907, 1986.
13. Kaieda, R., Todd, M. M., and Warner, D. S. Prolonged reduction of colloid oncotic pressure does not increase brain edema following cryogenic injury. *Anesthesiology* 69:A622, 1988.
14. Karlin, A., Hartuna, J., and Cottrell, J. E. Rate of induction of hypotension with trimetaphan modifies the intracranial pressure in cats. *Br. J. Anaesth.* 60:161, 1988.
15. Keylen, H. J., Graham, R., Fenske, A., et al. The Role of Tissue Pressure and Bulk Flow in the Formation and Resolution of Cold-induced Edema. In H. M. Pappium and W. Feindel (Eds.), *Dynamics of Brain Edema.* Berlin: Springer-Verlag, 1976. Pp. 103–112.
16. Kusunoki, M., Kimura, K., Nakamura, M., et al. Effects of hematocrit variations on cerebral blood flow and oxygen transport in ischemic cerebrovascular disease. *J. Cereb. Blood Flow Metab.* 1:413, 1981.
17. Latinen, L. V., Johansson, G. G., and Tarkkanen, L. The effect of nitrous oxide on pulsatile impedance and cerebral blood flow. *Br. J. Anaesth.* 39:781, 1967.
18. Marx, W., Shah, N., Long, C., et al. Sufentanil, alfentanil, and fentanyl: Impact on cerebrospinal fluid pressure in patients with brain tumors. *J. Neurosurg. Anesth.* 1:3, 1989.
19. Minton, M. D., Stirt, J. A., and Bedford, R. F. Increased intracranial pressure from succinylcholine: Prevention by prior nondepolarizing blockade. *Anesthesiology* 63:165, 1986.
20. Moss, E., and McDowall, D. G. ICP increases with 50% nitrous oxide in oxygen in severe head injuries during controlled ventilation. *Br. J. Anaesth.* 51:757, 1979.
21. Obrist, W. D., Gennarelli, T. A., Segawa, H., et al. Relation of cerebral blood flow to neurological status and outcome in head injured patients. *J. Neurosurg.* 51:292, 1979.
22. Pfenninger, E., Ahnefeld, F. W., Kilian, J., et al. Blood gases at the scene of the accident and on admission to hospital following cranio-cerebral trauma. *Anaesthetist* 36:570, 1987.
23. Prough, D. S., Johnson, J. C., Poole, G. V., Jr., et al. Effect on intracranial pressure of resuscitation from hemorrhagic shock with hypertonic saline versus lactated Ringer's solution. *Crit. Care Med.* 13:407, 1985.
24. Raichle, H. E., Posner, J. B., and Plum, F. Cerebral blood flow during and after hyperventilation. *Arch. Neurol.* 23:394, 1970.
25. Raley, R. A., Schlobom, R. M., Pitts, L. M., et al. Mechanical hyperventilation in patients with head trauma potentiates the ICP response to $PaCO_2$. *Anesthesiology* 57:3, 1982.
26. Shi, W. Z., Fahey, M. R., Fisher, D. M., et al. Lautanosine (a metabolite of atracurium) increases the minimum alveolar concentration of halothane in rabbits. *Anesthesiology* 63:584, 1985.
27. Sieber, F. E., Smith, D. S., Crosby, L., et al. The effects of intraoperative glucose on brain metabolism and serum glucose levels in patients with supratentorial tumors. *Anesthesiology* 64:453, 1986.
28. Sieber, F. E., Smith, D. S., Traystman, R. J., et al. Glucose: A reevaluation of its intraoperative use. *Anesthesiology* 67:72, 1987.
29. Stevenson, P. H., and Birch, A. A. Succinylcholine-induced hyperkalemia in a patient with a closed head injury. *Anesthesiology* 51:89, 1979.
30. Tateishi, A., Maekawa, T., Takeshita, H., et al. Diazepam and intracranial pressure. *Anesthesiology* 54:335, 1981.
31. Teasdale, G., and Jennett, B. Assessment of coma and impaired consciousness. *Lancet* 2:81, 1974.

32. Todd, M. M., Tommasino, C., and Moore, S. S. Cerebral effects of isovolemic hemodilution with a hypertonic solution. *J. Neurosurg.* 63:944, 1985.
33. Tommasino, C., Moore, S. S., and Todd, M. M. Cerebral effects of isovolemic hemodilution with crystalloid or colloid solutions. *Crit. Care Med.* 16:862, 1988.
34. Wood, J. H., Snyder, L. L., Simeone, F. A. Failure of intravascular volume expansion without hemodilution to elevate cortical blood flow in region of experimental focal ischemia. *J. Neurosurg.* 56:80, 1982.
35. Zornow, M. H., Scheller, M. S., Shackford, S. K., et al. Effect of a hypertonic lactated Ringers solution on cerebral edema and intracranial pressure following cryogenic brain injury. *Anesthesiology* 67:A654, 1987.

14

Spinal Cord Injury

JOSEPH P. GIFFIN
KENNETH GRUSH
ANDREW KARLIN
JAMES E. COTTRELL
PHILIPPA NEWFIELD

Each year approximately 10,000 survivors of spinal cord injury (SCI) enter our national health care system. About two-thirds are males, and 70 to 80% are between 11 and 30 years old [12,62]. Although mortality before reaching the hospital remains about 30% [61,62], mortality during the first year of treatment has decreased to 10% or less because of advances in resuscitation, supportive care, and rehabilitation [113]. After the first year, the life expectancy and cause of death of many SCI patients, — paraplegics, for example, — are relatively normal. The overall result has been an expanded population of long-term survivors [26,113]. As one might expect, the economic impact is huge: Costs of care plus lost wages amount to more than $1,000,000 per patient [113].

I. **Pathophysiology.** Spinal cord trauma results in both primary and secondary injuries. The primary injury, if severe enough, will result in functional or anatomic disruption of the cord at the scene of the accident with a correspondingly dismal prognosis. The uniformly encountered anatomic and histologic findings associated with such primary injury include direct neurilemmal and neuronal disruption and/or destruction, petechial hemorrhages, gross hematomyelia, or even total cord transection, a rare event. The areas rendered nonviable by this primary insult will go on to develop a cavitating necrosis and ultimately glial scar formation.

The observation that areas of the spinal cord not immediately destroyed by traumatic force subsequently undergo progressive hemorrhagic necrosis, edema, and inflammation at a rate proportional to the severity of the lesion has produced the concept of a secondary injury, perhaps mediated and propagated by mechanisms initiated by but distinct from the initial mechanical deformation.

The extension of tissue necrosis from the initial gray matter involvement to include the white matter, producing the clinical picture of quadriplegia or paraplegia, is preceded by endothelial damage with platelet adhesion, platelet aggregation, microvascular occlusion, and embolization of microthrombi. On a macroscopic scale, corresponding vascular stasis, decreased spinal cord blood flow (SCBF), and ischemia are noted. Axonal degeneration (hydropic and then granular), myelinolysis, cell necrosis, inflammatory infiltrate, and neuronophagia ensue. A striking feature is the occurrence of intra-axonal calcium hydroxyapatite crystals and mitochondrial calcification. Similar degenerative changes have been observed following exposure of rat spinal cords to calcium or calcium in the presence of an ionophore [5].

Biochemical events coinciding with this process of progressive autodestruction include (1) a massive translocation of calcium from the extracellular to the intracellular space; (2) the loss of intracellular potassium; (3) decreased Na^+-K^+-ATPase activity; (4) activation of phospholipase A_2 leading to arachidonic acid release and its metabolism to lipid peroxides (via free radical attack), prostaglandins (via cyclo-oxygenase), or leukotrienes (via lipoxygenase); (5) increase in total thromboxane as well as its ratio to prostacyclin; (6) the degradation of axonal and myelin proteins by neutral proteinases; (7) the failure of energy metabolism and protein synthesis; and (8) hypoxia and lactic acidosis [4,5].

It is possible to organize these events into a positive feedback cascade mechanism activated by the release of certain catalysts from the blood and their initial intracellular flux caused by the endothelial and neuronal membrane disruption at the initial site of maximal tissue trauma. Calcium [51], bradykinin, thrombin, ferrous ion [4], and norepinephrine [67] have been cast in such a role.

The basic scheme of such a secondary injury hypothesis is the activation of membrane phospholipase A_2 by calcium, thrombin, or bradykinin to catalyze hydrolytic cleavage of arachidonic acid and other free fatty acids from the cell membrane. Metabolism of arachidonic acid to prostaglandins (mostly thromboxane) and leukotrienes can account for microcirculatory thrombosis and stasis, vasogenic edema, ischemia, and chemotaxis. Free radicals generated during hypoxia, by neutrophils, or during prostanoid biosynthesis react with polyunsaturated lipids during oxidative degradation to produce lipid peroxides. Iron catalyzes both free radical generation and lipid peroxidation. Lipid hydrolysis and peroxidation fragment membrane phospholipids, which would have a positive feedback effect on the influx of calcium or other mediators and further phospholipase activation. Increased prostaglandin F_2 alpha production and thrombin generation may also augment phospholipase activity. Lipid peroxidation in itself tends to be a geometrically progressive chain reaction [4,44,51].

Calcium overloading of the intracellular space, in particular the mitochondria, secondary to influx through damaged membranes and further membrane lipid destruction as described previously should have obvious deleterious effects on cellular energy metabolism and maintenance of integrity and function. Na^+-K^+-ATPase has been shown to be phospholipid-dependent and very susceptible to free radical attack and lipid peroxidation [67]. This enzyme is needed to maintain normal cellular volume and ion content, membrane potential, and cellular function. Cellular swelling secondary to loss of this enzyme and membrane integrity in general can further worsen ischemia and result in enlargement of the area of lipid destruction and necrosis. Finally, the neutral proteinase, which is the predominant source of increased proteolytic activity in experimental SCI, is calcium activated [51].

The feasibility of such secondary injury mechanisms is supported by a number of additional observations. The time course of change in tissue concentration of some of the proposed mediators closely matches that of the histologic, biochemical, and physiologic processes described before. In the case of calcium, neurologic deficit scores have also been shown to be proportional to the extent of calcium influx, the rise in phospholipase-generated metabolites, vascular damage, and increased tissue water content [56]. In addition, as mentioned before, exposure of the spinal cord to calcium chloride solution results in similar prostaglandin (thromboxane) generation, proteolysis, and morphologic changes in proportion to the solution molarity [51].

Recently the excitotoxin hypothesis of neuronal injury has been expanded to include trauma in addition to ischemic or degenerative disorders. Excitatory neurotransmitters such as glutamate or aspartate have experimentally documented neurotoxic properties, perhaps acting through such observed effects as acute cellular swelling produced by a depolarization-induced influx of sodium and chlorine and a more delayed influx of calcium. The calcium might conceivably participate in secondary injury models such as those examined above. Faden and Simon [32] found that MK-801, a selective, noncompetitive N-methyl-D-aspartate (NMDA) antagonist, improved neurologic recovery in SCI rats whereas exogenous NMDA worsened it.

Finally, Faden and colleagues [30] had previously demonstrated an increase in the endogenous opioid *kappa* receptor agonist, dynorphin, as well as an increase in receptor-binding capacity after experimental SCI in rats, which correlates closely with neurologic dysfunction. No change in *mu* or *delta* receptor binding was found. Since intrathecal dynorphin A, but not other opiate agonists, can produce dose-related hind limb paralysis in the rat, it has been postulated that this opioid system may contribute to the pathophysiology of secondary SCI when activated during the beta endorphin surge that occurs after SCL [30,63] and that is believed to also play a role in spinal shock.

However, caution must be exercised in equating close correlation with causation, and further investigation continues. Nevertheless, it has been clearly documented that in the period following primary SCI, a progressive decrease in SCBF occurs, resulting in marked ischemia associated with a morphologic and biochemical cascade as detailed before [91]. The fact that this sequence may not begin for over an hour, in some cases as much as four hours after the primary injury, suggests the possibility of intervention to prevent or alter the ischemic sequence [94].

The normal mean SCBF of 40 to 50 ml/100 gm/min is partitioned in a ratio of 3 : 1 between gray and white matter, respectively [89]. Autoregulation of SCBF between 60 and 150 mmHg has been demonstrated in rats [50]. SCBF has been shown to vary in direct proportion (1 : 1) with $PaCO_2$ [39]. Although conflicting results have been reported [59], the preponderance of researchers agree that total SCBF decreases significantly from one to four hours after subtotal experimental injury, with most of the decrease occurring in the central cord region [91].

SCI in cats has been shown to abolish autoregulation with the onset of ischemia [95]. This would be expected to render the spinal cord susceptible to increased hemorrhage and edema in the face of significantly increased blood pressure, as has been shown experimentally in cats [87]. Such a hypertensive phase has been documented for three to four minutes after experimental SCI [2,86,113]. Spinal shock, in which endorphin-mediated parasympathetic stimulation has been implicated, would decrease SCBF in the absence of autoregulation [95].

In addition, vasoconstriction of resistance vessels would more readily result in ischemia. Such vasoconstriction may be secondary to some of the mediators already mentioned: a preponderance of thromboxane over prostacyclin. PGF_2 alpha, and slow-reacting substance of anaphylaxis [5]. Although the originally proposed increase in spinal cord catecholamines (as a cause of ischemia and hemorrhagic necrosis [81,82] has not been verified by subsequent investigators, norepinephrine has been shown to significantly reduce SCBF when the cord-blood barrier has been disrupted [19]. More recent investigations already mentioned have enumerated a number of membrane-damaging factors, operating by way of free radical attack and lipid peroxidation, that may disrupt the cord-blood barrier and that correlate with cord edema. Norepinephrine has been shown to be capable of activating similar membrane lipid peroxidation [67]. Acute ethanol intoxication (blood level of 100 mg/dl) worsens spinal cord hemorrhage and the extent of anatomic damage and impairs recovery of function [3]. Possible reasons for this include the direct effects on neuronal conduction, vascular congestion, and increased permeability (altered blood-cord barrier), increased lactate production, increased free radical peroxidation catalyzed by iron, and toxic aldehyde metabolite effects.

On a gross physiologic scale, spinal cord impulse transmission, as assessed by evoked potentials, disappears immediately with complete transection and after a variable delay period in less severe lesions. Somatosensory evoked potentials (SSEPs) studied in humans distinguished complete anatomic lesions with little or no hope of recovery from patients with complete or incomplete functional deficits but could not predict the degree of functional deficit [16]. On the other hand, motor evoked potentials (MEPs) or corticomotor evoked potentials (CMEPs) have been shown in both rat and cat dynamic SCI models to be more sensitive indicators of the onset of injury [73] as well as good predictors of the extent and anatomic distribution of tissue damage and the prognosis for functional recovery [72,96].

II. Treatment

A. Physical and surgical. Procedures to relieve cord compression, ischemia, and edema must be accompanied by steps to realign, stabilize, and immobilize the injured elements of the vertebral column [102]. Stabilization of the cord is achieved by traction (skull tongs or halo for cervical injury, halopelvic or halotibial traction for thoracic and lumbar injuries) and by adjustments in posture using bolsters of different shapes and sizes. Surgical reduction may be indicated for dislocations that cannot be reduced by traction or manipulation because of bone fracture and impaction, extensive disruption, or incorporation of soft tissue into the dislocated elements. When instability persists, surgical fixation is necessary after an adequate period of immobilization by external fixation.

Whereas the timing of surgical decompression in the management of acute partial cord injury is controversial, neurosurgeons seem to agree that decompression and exploration of the spinal canal are indicated for a complete lesion less than 48 hours old, when a foreign body is present in the canal, and when patients who have incomplete SCIs deteriorate neurologically [15,47,85]. In the latter instance, the evacuation of a subdural or epidural hematoma may reverse the patient's deficit.

In most cases of trauma, the spinal canal is compromised anteriorly. Consequently, the anterior approach is preferable when spinal decompression is necessary, both for accomplishing decompression and for achieving spinal stability. If the laminae or facets have been fractured and driven into the canal, posterior surgical decompression is required.

In complete SCIs, early surgical stabilization allows aggressive rehabilitation, but such surgery should be delayed until the patient is medically stable.

If anatomic reduction can be achieved and maintained, the healing of the fractured bone and torn ligaments often produces a stable spine within three to six months [85].

B. Pharmacologic. Pharmacologic attempts to preserve spinal cord function parallel the approach to preservation of the brain after head injury. A number of animal studies have demonstrated that corticosteroids given before or shortly after injury appear to reduce the degree of spinal cord damage [64,114]. Despite this animal evidence, an initial multicenter study failed to show any benefit of steroids [14]. A second study by the same group using higher doses, however, revealed improved motor and sensory function at six weeks and six months.

Methylprednisolone was administered in a dose of 30 mg/kg over 15 minutes; after another 45 minutes the patients received an infusion of methylprednisolone at 5.4 mg/kg/hour over 23 hours. The benefit was statistically significant only when treatment began within eight hours of the injury. Steroid therapy did not increase the incidence of septic complications [13].

Mannitol is now a mainstay of neurologic intensive care and is used to reduce intracellular fluid by creating an osmotic gradient between the intracellular and extracellular spaces and thus reduce parenchymal volume. Mannitol also causes a vigorous osmotic diuresis. Therefore, intravascular volume must be maintained to ensure perfusion of the cord [83].

C. **Spinal cord perfusion.** After experimental SCI, autoregulation appears to be lost. Hypotension results in hypoperfusion [95], whereas hypertension leads to increased cord edema and hemorrhage [87]. Concern that the same process may occur in humans leads us to believe that blood pressure control is an important part of treatment and that mean arterial pressure (MAP) be maintained at or above the midpoint of normal autoregulatory range.

D. **Experimental.** Experimental methods of preserving cord function include the use of hypothermia, hyperbaric oxygenation, catecholamine antagonists, dimethyl sulfoxide, and endogenous opiate antagonists (naloxone). We will not elaborate the experimental evidence for and against the efficacy of these treatments, but only point out that none of them have consistently demonstrated clinical benefits in humans.

1. **Hypothermia.** Localized cooling of the spinal cord will reduce cord metabolism at the site of injury [1]. Optimal results are obtained when cooling is instituted within two hours after injury. The effects of hypothermia are temporary, however, and spinal cord damage may subsequently progress.

2. **Hyperbaric oxygenation.** In animals that sustained impact injury to the cord, hyperbaric oxygenation (3 atm) improved when compared to controls [46].

3. **Dimethyl sulfoxide.** Dimethyl sulfoxide has been shown to decrease central hemorrhage and edema of the white matter in experimental SCI [57].

4. **Opiate antagonists.** Following the demonstration that the opiate antagonist naloxone improved arterial pressure and survival in hemorrhagic and septic shock, investigators studied its effect in spinal shock and in enhancing recovery from SCI [28,45]. Intravenous naloxone has effectively prevented or reversed spinal shock in rat and cat cervical cord transection models, significantly increasing MAP, increasing respiratory rate, and decreasing hypothermia [52,53]. Also, naloxone in doses of 2 to 10 mg/kg has been shown to yield significant improvement in SSEPs [34] and neurologic function

[29]. Recently, Faden and colleagues [31] have demonstrated a dose-related improvement in neurologic recovery of rats after traumatic SCI when nalmefene, a relatively specific kappa receptor antagonist, was administered 60 minutes after injury.

Although these and many other animal studies supported the effectiveness of naloxone, a human phase I clinical trial of naloxone was less encouraging. This trial showed some clinical improvement only with the highest loading dose of 5.4 mg/kg IV followed by continuous hourly infusion of 75% of this amount for 23 hours, but the results fell short of statistical significance. The mortality rate was not greater than expected in similar injuries, but awareness of pain was significantly increased. A possible contributing factor limiting success may be the average interval of 6.6 hours from admission until the start of therapy [33]. However, a number of recent studies in animals [43,107,108] have challenged the effectiveness of naloxone, as did the second human methylprednisolone study previously mentioned [13]. Since the naloxone dose used was less than the dose used in successful animal studies, further clinical trials are needed.

Potentially significant effect of naloxone therapy in a patient undergoing general anesthesia was reported. The patient had received the 5.4 mg/kg regimen already mentioned 30 minutes before presenting for a stabilization procedure of the thoracolumbar spine. Fentanyl (25 meg/kg), isoflurane (2.0–3.5%), thiopental (700 mg), diazepam (10 mg), morphine (15 mg), and sufentanyl (0.5 meg/kg) were used during and immediately after surgery to manage hypertension and hyperventilation. This resistance to normally effective anesthetic doses was attributed to antianalgesic and analeptic effects of the naloxone treatment [8].

Experimental work on the possible sites and mechanisms of action of opiate antagonists has been reviewed [45]. Briefly summarized, evidence indicates that naloxone interacts stereospecifically at a central site to inhibit opiate receptor-mediated stimulation of the parasympathetic nervous system in achieving improvement of MAP and SCBF. A central outpouring of beta endorphin following SCI has been found at the time of cord ischemia, and naloxone may antagonize its effects. In addition, naloxone elevates peripheral dopamine levels 300 to 400%, partially contributing to naloxone's hemodynamic effects after SCI. Other catecholamine levels remain unaltered. This is thought to be an indirect effect, possibly mediated by the central parasympatholysis. Finally, because naloxone is only effective in doses of magnitude greater than that required for mu receptor agonist reversal, it is possible that it is acting at a receptor, perhaps the kappa receptor, for which it has marginal affinity. Naloxone and a specific kappa receptor antagonist have prevented experimental cord damage induced by dynorophin, a kappa receptor agonist [31]. In fact, some evidence exists that naloxone acts through nonopioid mechanisms, involving its ability to inhibit membrane damage by free radical-induced lipid peroxidation, to act as an antioxidant, to modulate calcium fluxes, and to increase cyclic-AMP activation of prostaglandins.

5. **Others.** Recent studies have demonstrated potential effectiveness of GM-1 ganglioside [11] and a combination of triethanolamine and cytosine arabinoside [42] to markedly stimulate axonal growth in spinal cord–transected rats. Continuously applied weak electrical fields achieved similar results in guinea pigs [10]. A series of investigations has shown that peripheral nerve grafts or central nervous system implants derived from the embryonal neuraxis can stimulate axonal outgrowth and may prove useful in repairing disrupted intraspinal circuits [88].

III. Associated hazards and complications

A. **Airway management.** A patient who has a fracture of the vertebral column and proven or potential SCI requires skilled, meticulous care at the accident site, during transport, and in the hospital. Adequacy of airway, oxygenation, and perfusion pressure must be maintained to avoid additional injury to the spinal cord from hypoxia or hypercarbia. It must be remembered that even patients with low-level injuries will have decreased respiratory function if the abdominal muscles are affected [74,75].

Obtunded patients who breathe spontaneously may require an airway only; during insertion, care is necessary to avoid laryngospasm, aspiration, and movement of the neck. When the patient has a normal level of consciousness, intact pharyngeal reflexes, and a patent airway, the rescue team should provide supplemental oxygen and assist ventilation as necessary with bag and mask. These patients require observation, however, to detect progressive loss of ventilatory ability as a result of either evolving diaphragmatic or intercostal muscle paralysis or medullary ischemia involving the respiratory center.

The apneic patient requires immediate ventilatory support. It may be assumed that comatose patients have unstable spine injuries until x-ray films exclude such lesions. Consequently, aspiration, respiratory muscle failure, or marked airway obstruction at the scene of the accident necessitates either intubation or passage of an esophageal obturator.

Endotracheal intubation of patients who have cervical spine injuries is a classic problem in anesthesia, and we can offer no easy solutions. During intubation the patient's head should be maintained in a neutral position. Traction used acutely in a nonincremental fashion and uncontrolled by radiology may worsen the extent of injury and does not prevent deleterious movement of the affected region [9].

Nasal fiberoptic or blind nasal intubations may be attempted in spontaneously breathing patients if basal skull injuries have been ruled out. Both these methods may induce coughing and bucking, so laryngeal anesthesia by superior laryngeal nerve block or direct application of a local anesthetic via the fiberoptic laryngoscope's suction port should be considered and weighed against the increased risk of aspiration.

In the presence of an associated head injury or complete apnea, or if a patient is so uncooperative that attempted intubation may cause further injury, rapid sequence induction and intubation are indicated.

Tracheostomy, cricothyroidotomy, transcricothyroid membrane jet ventilation [98], and retrograde intubation are alternatives if a difficult intubation is anticipated. Trauma patients are often brought to the operating room without examination to rule out SCI. We consider *all* unconscious patients and all patients with abdominal, thoracic, or neck injuries compatible with SCI to have SCI until proven otherwise.

B. Respiratory complications. Depending on the level and degree of SCI, respiration may be impaired by paralysis of abdominal, intercostal, diaphragmatic, and accessory muscles of respiration progressively as the site of trauma moves from low thoracic to high cervical or even brainstem levels. Loss of motor function originating at C-3 to C-5 giving rise to the phrenic nerves, results in diaphragmatic paralysis (major contribution from C-4) as well as the loss of intercostal and abdominal motor function. High quadriplegia (C-4 or above) results in a severe, life-threatening decrease in all standard measures of respiratory mechanics and dynamics: forced vital capacity, forced expiratory volume in one second, peak inspiratory and expiratory force and flow, and total pulmonary compliance. Only the accessory muscles of inspiration (sternocleidomastoid, scalenes, and trapezius) function during inspiration. Lower rib cage and abdominal paradox is seen as the hemidiaphragms passively respond to the changes in intrathoracic pressure caused by accessory muscle activity. As the upper rib cage expands (less than with intact intercostal muscles), upward diaphragm motion decreases intra-abdominal pressure, resulting in inward movement of it and the lower rib cage. The reverse occurs during expiration. The paradoxical diaphragm motion and its cephalad displacement decrease the efficiency of already diminished muscle activity in effecting gas exchange [75]. Tidal volume, inspiratory and expiratory reserve volumes (IRV and ERV), and functional residual capacity (FRC) are critically reduced; residual volume is increased [22].

Alveolar hypoventilation results in hypercarbia. Hypoventilation, atelectasis, and airspace collapse associated with the decrease in FRC relative to closing volume produce ventilation-perfusion ($\dot{V}/\dot{Q}$) mismatching and cause hypoxemia. Respiratory function in the case of total diaphragmatic paralysis is worst in the supine or Trendelenburg positions, as abdominal contents displace the diaphragm further cephalad, and improves if other variables (e.g., blood pressure) permit some degree of head and thorax elevation. Global hypoventilation often worsens further during sleep, occasionally progressing to sleep apnea, which has been attributed to diminished CO_2 responsiveness [20,49].

Sighing and coughing are essential to maintain alveolar patency and pulmonary toilet. A near-normal inspiratory reserve is required in the former case; the generation of pressure against a closed glottis and maintenance of flow following glottic opening are essential in the latter. Decreases in IRV, ERV, FVC, peak inspiratory and expiratory force and flow, as well as inability to "splint" the diaphragm accompanying diaphragmatic, intercostal, and abdominal paralysis cause inability to cough and clear airway secretions or to sigh and diminish atelectasis in proportion to the level of injury [74].

Low quadriplegic patients with partial or complete integrity of diaphragmatic innervation will have variable diaphragmatic strength. However, the diaphragms are prevented from achieving their optimal, steeply domed fiber length-tension position at end expiration because of intercostal and abdominal muscle paralysis; hence, their inspiratory efficiency is impaired. The Trendelenburg position, by shifting the diaphragms cephalad to a more mechanically advantageous starting fiber length, actually increased IRV and FVC an average of 300 ml [36]. Adding to this effect is the upper rib cage's paradoxical *inward* motion during inspiration (compare this to lower rib cage and abdominal paradox in high quadriplegics) [74]. The resulting decrease in respiratory capacity may produce $\dot{V}/\dot{Q}$ mismatching and hypoxemia. Spirometric assessment of lower cervical (C-5–C-7) level SCI patients from 24 hours through 3 weeks post injury revealed average initial decreases in FVC to 22% of the predicted values, further deterioration through the fourth postinjury day, then gradual improvement to 30% of what was expected [55].

The extent of diaphragmatic paralysis is an important determinant of morbidity. A study compared quadriplegics with complete cord lesions at the C-5 to C-6 level, with an average initial FVC of 1.5 L (24% of predicted), to those with complete lesions at C-4, with one of 1.3 L (21% of predicted). Four of eleven patients with C-5 to C-6 lesions required oxygen, but only two required mechanical ventilation. All five patients with C-4 lesions received oxygen and were ventilated. Although both groups approximately doubled their vital capacities over the next three months and were breathing unassisted, two C-4-level patients displayed postural hypoxemia and hypercarbia [70].

Training directed at both expiratory and inspiratory accessory muscles and diaphragms, combined with any functional intercostal recovery, can result in improved strength and endurance as well as decreased likelihood of fatigue [41,71].

Low quadriplegics and paraplegics, although less compromised than high quadriplegics, are still at risk for hypoventilation, V/Q mismatching, and retention of secretions paralleling the changes in respiratory parameters outlined previously. Aside from diaphragmatic and intercostal muscle strength, a key factor in overall respiratory function is the contribution of the abdominal muscles in increasing expiratory pressure directly, as well as improving the efficiency of the intercostals in forced expiration or coughing by preventing paradoxical movement of the diaphragm into the abdomen. The importance of abdominal muscle tone in optimizing diaphragmatic position for inspiration has already been discussed. The abdominal weakness or paralysis accounts for the persistence of respiratory complications, especially retained secretions and pulmonary infections seen in some paraplegics with intact diaphragms and intercostal muscles.

Ventilatory assistance is indicated in patients displaying an elevated $PaCO_2$ or a borderline PaO_2 in the face of maximal sustainable ventilatory efforts. No mode of ventilation is inherently superior [74], although synchronized intermittent mandatory ventilation has the theoretic advantages of greater hemodynamic stability, continuing exercise of functional muscles, and ease of weaning [24]. Positive end-expiratory pressure (PEEP) may be added for considerations already mentioned. The recent introduction of variable pressure support ventilation, in which all spontaneous breaths can be supported at any desired pressure level and synchronized with variable-frequency mandatory machine breaths, combines many of the advantages of synchronized intermittent mandatory ventilation with the security of controlled or assist-control ventilation in terms of compensating for potential muscle fatigue. In the exclusively pressure-support mode, fine tuning of muscle workload is possible for training and weaning purposes. A final subset of patients seems to benefit, in terms of relieving dyspnea during spontaneous ventilation, when their diaphragms are rendered inactive during negative pressure ventilation [90].

In cases of complete lesions above C-3, alternatives to chronic positive-pressure ventilation include radio frequency electrophrenic stimulation in patients with damaged phrenic nuclei but intact phrenic nerves [38], or intermittent negative-pressure ventilation in an iron lung when the phrenic nerves are interrupted. Chronic subtotal diaphragmatic dysfunction can be managed by a rocking bed, chest cuirass, or pneumobelt [75].

Respiratory complications are the most common cause of death in acute SCI, with pneumonia being the most frequent after anoxic death at the time of injury [101]. In chronic, stabilized patients, respiratory infections decrease and cause less than 10% of the febrile episodes. The importance of aggressive pulmonary toilet in addressing this problem was evidenced by a 33% decrease in prolonged ventilation as a result of such measures as careful monitoring of pulmonary function, vigorous chest physical therapy, and early bronchoscopy and lavage if lobar collapse developed on chest roentgenograms [78]. Any fever accompanied by leukocytosis or physical and/or radiographic evidence of pneumonitis should be aggressively treated.

During the early stages of injury, pulmonary edema (see subsequently) and venous thrombosis with pulmonary embolism also contribute significantly to morbidity. Pulmonary edema was seen in 44% of patients during resuscitation from spinal shock [79]. Pulmonary emboli were found in 15.2% of patients dying acutely but were never a cause of death after the first postinjury month [111].

C. Cardiovascular problems

1. Acute changes. At the moment of experimental SCI, a sudden and drastic increase in blood pressure occurs that lasts for several minutes [86]. This injury-induced hypertension is probably caused by a sympathetic discharge followed by adrenal catecholamine release [114]. The possible role of this abrupt pressor response in augmenting the extent of hemorrhagic necrosis and releasing possible mediators of secondary injury was discussed in **I** [87].

Experimental cord injury has also been shown to result in transient but significant increases in intracranial pressure, blood-brain barrier permeability, brain water, and extravascular lung water, with a marked decrease in cerebral blood flow [2]. This investigation verified the severe increase in blood pressure (to a mean of 225 mmHg) lasting for six minutes and also showed increases in pulmonary artery pressure, pulmonary artery occlusion pressure, central venous pressure, and cardiac output. However, the intracerebral and pulmonary changes occurred before the full development of the cardiovascular changes. This, along with the fact that phentolamine pretreatment sufficient to prevent the cardiovascular changes did not prevent the brain and lung events, seems to support the notion of independent but causally linked "neurogenic" mechanisms producing both processes. At any rate, this work is compatible with the clinically observed susceptibility to pulmonary and cerebral edema seen during resuscitation of patients with SCI and reinforces the advisability of early hemodynamic monitoring to guide fluid management in these patients. A possible role for beta endorphin–initiated changes together with neural influences acting to increase pulmonary capillary permeability has been well summarized by Fraser and Edmunds-Seal [37].

2. Hypotension. Because patients with SCI rarely reach medical attention within minutes of their injury, acute hypertension is seldom, if ever, observed. Most patients appear with varying degrees of hypotension. This phase, commonly called *spinal shock,* features hypotension, bradycardia, decreased total peripheral resistance, low or normal central venous pressure, and normal or mildly elevated cardiac output [79]. However, myocardial contractility may be suspected as well in view of abnormal decreases in left ventricular stroke work index (LVSWI) and cardiac index (CI) in response to volume loading observed in 26% and 18% of all patients, respectively, during spinal stabilization surgery. A reversible, enhanced sensitivity to halothane-induced myocardial depression was a contributing factor in some but not all patients [76]. In addition, the lack of sympathetically mediated increases in heart rate and contractility accompanying lesions above T1 leaves only the Frank-Starling mechanism to augment contractility, and impairment of myocardial perfusion during hypotension may also "stun" the myocardium — especially in the presence of preexisting coronary artery or hypertrophic disease [76,105]. Finally, the beta endorphin surge associated with acute SCI has been hypothesized to depress myocardial contractility either by a direct action on the heart or by central (brain) activation of the parasympathetic nervous system [37,52]. Orthostatic and other pressor reflexes are diminished or absent, dictating caution in any position changes. At the same time somatic and visceral motor and sensory loss below the level of the lesion are observed.

The extent of these changes is a result of the level of the cord injury. Injuries at or above T-1 may lead to mean blood pressures as low as 40 mmHg. The observed bradycardia may be due to unopposed vagal tone secondary to loss of the cardiac accelerator fibers (T-1–T-4), but many feel that the Bainbridge reflex caused by a fall in right atrial and cenetral venous pressures is a more important contributing factor, as bradycardia is seen with lesions below T-4. On the other hand, MacKenzie and colleagues [76] found no evidence of an active Bainbridge reflex during their observations on the responses of acutely quadriplegic patients to volume loading. The critical level above which significant hypotension will be manifest is T-6 to T-7.

This phase of spinal shock may last days to weeks but is often more abbreviated than the period of skeletal muscle flaccid paralysis. Unfortunately, no one has exactly delineated the point at which the sympathetic neurons regain their functional ability, now autonomous from higher control. It is clear that they do regain some tonic activity as well as the ability for reflex reaction, as evidence by less orthostatic hypotension and the unpredictable onset of potentially catastrophic sympathetic reflex spasticity, analogous to but possibly not simultaneous with the development of somatic reflex spasticity [21, 37].

Management of hypotension is dictated by the physiologic alterations that produce it. A conservative approach is usually indicated, the urgency of treatment being proportional to the degree of hypotension and the symptoms produced (e.g., central nervous system [CNS], cardiac, renal). Trending of such variables as lactate production, mixed-venous oxygen content, and oxygen consumption should help to verify the adequacy of tissue perfusion. The etiology of the hypotension is usually a decreased venous return following sympathetic denervation, which causes increased venous capacitance as well as some degree of decreased arteriolar tone. However, cautious addition of volume is indicated in view of decreased cardiovascular reserve. This deficit in ability to accommodate excess volume is a natural consequence of the inability to further increase venous capacitance as the venous reservoir becomes full. Central venous pressure increases relatively little until volume equals capacity; then it can rise abruptly. On the other hand, left ventricular and left atrial pressures increase proportionally with filling volume, and such indices as pulmonary capillary occlusion pressure (PCOP) will provide an early measure of volume status before central venous pressure finally rises equivalently. Limitation of the cardiac response to stress or volume loading in the Frank-Starling mechanism following loss of autonomic reflexes was discussed earlier [105]. Finally, the possibility of altered pulmonary capillary permeability to water during the acute phase of SCI, as already discussed, may increase the susceptibility to pulmonary edema during resuscitation of these patients [23,79].

In view of these findings, early use of pulmonary artery catheters in monitoring fluid resuscitation during spinal shock would seem prudent. Not only are filling pressures and volume status readily assessable, but cardiac output (CO) and total peripheral resistance can also be measured and manipulated if they are found to contribute to the hypotension. MacKenzie and colleagues [76] have used pulmonary arterial hemodynamic monitoring to categorize four groups of patients with SCI. Rapid fluid infusion (50 ml/min of colloid in 250-ml increments), leg raising, or MAST trousers were used to increase central volume. One group of patients displayed a 3- to 4-mmHg rise in PCOP, which settled to a level 2 mmHg above control, with concomitant increases in CO. A second group showed similar increases in PCOP, which then returned to baseline with no net change in CO. The third group showed progressive increases in PCOP and no change or a fall in CO. Finally, 1 of 22 subjects showed a fall in PCOP and an increase in CO. These findings were interpreted as indicating adequate volume loading in the first instance, the need for more volume in the second group, excessive volume and/or an indication for inotropic support in the third group, and improved pump function resulting from vasodilatation accompanying volume replacement in the last patient. These guidelines seem appropriate in optimizing filling pressures at the lowest value yielding adequate CO and perfusion pressures. Above a PCOP of 18 mmHg LVSWI and CI decreased; hence, this should serve as an infusion endpoint.

If, in spite of volume loading, CO and MAP are such that spinal cord and other organ hypoperfusion seems likely, inotropic support is indicated. One study compared the efficacy of either dopamine or transfusion in raising MAP and augmenting SCBF in rats. Both yielded improvements in these two variables, but transfusion alone was better than dopamine alone [23]. The demonstration that naloxone-mediated increased in systemic blood pressure and SCBF may be mediated by augmented endogenous plasma dopamine levels also suggests that this inotrope may be used where indicated without adversely affecting the potential for spinal cord recovery [45].

3. **Autonomic hyperreflexia.** Eventually, the phase of flaccid paralysis, or spinal shock, resolves, and in patients with an injury level above T-6 to T-7, blood pressure returns to slightly low or normal with episodes of severe hypertension in 85% of patients. These episodes may be triggered by everyday noxious stimuli — bladder or rectal distention, for example — or by labor or surgical pain [68]. This generalized uncontrolled response to a noxious stimulus occurs below the level of injury, where the sympathetic system has been freed of higher control and coordination and is called *autonomic hyperreflexia.*

Typical symptoms are nasal congestion, severe headache, dyspnea, and nausea. Signs include vasoconstrictive pallor, sweating, intense somatic and visceral muscle contraction, and piloerection below the level of injury [58]. Above the lesion is flushing and severe hypertension that induces bradycardia [21]. Subarachnoid and retinal hemorrhages have been observed, which lead to syncope, convulsions, and finally death if the hypertension continues unabated [68].

The neuroanatomic correlates of this syndrome include stimuli arising from somatic or visceral receptors causing afferent impulses that follow their normal course along the posterior columns and spinothalamic tracts. Spinal cord transection prevents these impulses from reaching the brain, but they do synapse with cells of the intermediolateral gray area, giving rise to efferent sympathetic discharges. Normally, these reflexes are localized, but after SCI they tend to involve much of the sympathetic system below the level of the lesion as a result of overgrowth of internuncial synapses on adrenergic neurons of the intermediolateral gray area [37]. The usual homeostatic inhibitory impulses from higher centers following the initial arrival of such afferent impulses are never triggered. Intense, unabated somatic and visceral muscle contractions, arteriolar spasm, sweating, and piloerection are caused by the unchecked sympathetic reflexes below the cord lesion. Above the cord lesion, the hypertension caused by the arteriolar spasm and adrenal secretion activates carotid sinus and aortic arch baroreceptors, as well as other CNS reflexes, to cause sympatholysis and parasympathetic activation; vagally induced bradycardia results as well as generalized vasodilation above the level of injury. These measures, however, are insufficient to reverse the hypertension which the lesion is above the origin of the splanchnic sympathetic outflow (T-4–T-6), reflecting the proportion of arterioles that remain undilated. The time at which spastic autonomic or somatic reflex activity supersedes spinal shock and flaccid paralysis is difficult to predict and may occur one to three weeks or more after injury [21,37].

Pharmacologic regimens investigated for preventing or treating autonomic hyperreflexia have included ganglionic blockers (trimethaphan, hexamethonium, pentolinium), catecholamine depleters (guanethidine), alpha-adrenergic blockers (phentolamine, phenoxybenzamine), and direct-acting vasodilators (nitroprusside). Unfortunately, many of the studies were small, lacked controls, or featured concomitant use of anesthetics. Consequently, comparison of the various drugs is difficult. Unpleasant side effects have limited these drugs' usefulness. Finally, the ability to control visceral and somatic muscle spasm is not achieved when only blood pressure is controlled.

Persistent attacks may require surgical or chemical ablation of the afferent pathways initiating the reflex through such measures as sacral neurotomy, dorsal rhizotomy, and subarachnoid phenol or alcohol.

The aim in SCI patients is, therefore, to avoid known stimuli to hyperreflexia through such measures as regular self-catheterization. If an attack does occur, any treatment that controls the arteriolar spasm and arrhythmias while maintaining cardiac output is acceptable.

4. Arrhythmias and electrocardiograph abnormalities. Cardiac arrhythmias and electrocardiographic abnormalities may also contribute to cardiovascular risk in these patients. Acute midthoracic spinal cord compression, in addition to producing hypertension, resulted in sinus or nodal bradycardia in monkeys. Moreover, this initial response often preceded the pressor response. The initial bradyarrhythmias were followed by premature atrial and ventricular contractions, atrioventricular dissociation, or ventricular tachycardias. Atropine prevented the bradycardia, whereas propranolol prevented the delayed ventricular tachyarrhythmia [27]. The electrocardiogram frequently shows STT wave changes variously interpreted as left ventricular strain pattern or consistent with subendocardial ischemia [37,74,84]. Similar arrhythmias have been reported in 75% of autonomic hyperreflexia episodes [58]. The potential for severe bradycardia, heart block, and even cardiac arrest after stimulation in these patients has already been noted [110].

Significant arrhythmias such as ventricular tachycardia are usually attendant to episodes of autonomic hyperreflexia and can likewise be prevented by adequate anesthetic depth or neural blockade in the surgical patient, or by the other modalities discussed previously for day-to-day prophylaxis. Any life-threatening tachyarrhythmia that does occur in spite of prophylactic measures should be treated with beta-adrenergic blockers (concurrent alpha-adrenergic blockade is mandatory if significant hypertension is present) or other indicated antiarrhythmic agents (such as calcium channel blockers). The baseline high vagal tone of these patients should be kept in mind, and atropine and pacemaking capability should be available if the combination of vagal tone and antiarrhythmic therapy results in sinus arrest, heart block, or too slow a rate to support adequate cardiac output. The potential need for atropine to treat the vagal reflexes attending tracheal stimulation should be anticipated.

D. Genitourinary complications. Acute renal failure may occur in acute SCI patients as a result of hypotension, dehydration, sepsis, nephrotoxic drugs, acute obstruction, associated kidney trauma, and other causes. During the chronic phase of SCI, renal failure becomes a progressively more important cause of death, accounting for 20 to 75% of mortality. In one series, renal failure caused only 4.5% of all deaths in patients surviving only 2 years but caused 60% or more of deaths among those surviving more than 10 years [101].

Urinary retention, more often a problem in the flaccid lower motor neuron bladder than in the spastic upper motor neuron type, predisposes the patient to autonomic hyperreflexia and to cystitis. Vesicoureteral reflux may result from this retention, and repetitive ascending pyelonephritis occurs, leading eventually to secondary renal and adrenal amyloidosis and insufficiency. Renal calculi also tend to be a recurrent problem in patients with urinary retention. They are most often of the triple phosphate variety associated with urease-producing bacteria (e.g., *Proteus* species), but some investigators [101] feel that hypercalciuria may play a limited role.

Proteinuria is usually the earliest sign of renal dysfunction, although it is qualitative rather than quantitative [21]. Serum creatinine may be misleading in view of the decrease in muscle mass seen in chronic quadriplegics. Intravenous pyelography allows excellent visualization of the upper urinary tract, but its usefulness is limited by potential allergic reactions, discomfort of the procedure and preparation, potential nephrotoxicity of the contrast material, cumulative radiation, and the fact that significant functional impairment may precede detectable anatomic alterations. Renal scintigraphic determination of effective renal plasma flow seems to be a sensitive indicator of renal dysfunction and also correlates with the presence of calculi and altered renal architecture; it may be used for serial follow-up of these patients and in determining the need for an intravenous pyelogram [65,66]. Various equations for estimating creatinine clearance have proven very inaccurate, and direct measurement of creatinine clearance is recommended to avoid renal or systemic toxicity of agents eliminated by or toxic to the kidneys [80].

A large proportion of surgery in chronic SCI patients is devoted to cystoscopy, urologic invasive diagnostic studies, stone removal, lithotripsy, and urinary drainage or diversion procedures.

E. **Altered thermoregulation.** Temperature regulation is impaired for a number of reasons. Afferent information to the hypothalamic thermoregulatory center may be interrupted. Sympathetic denervation causes cutaneous vasodilation, which increases heat loss. Also, inability to shiver limits the ability to increase body temperature. SCI patients, therefore, become relatively poikilothermic.

F. **Other systemic alterations.** Other abnormalities that have been described in association with SCI are known and summarized in several reviews, and the following are highlights from these authors [74,101].

1. **Fluids and electrolytes.** Apart from the problems associated with neurogenic shock and renal failure already discussed, chronic SCI patients, especially bed-bound patients with prolonged hospital confinements, are often hypovolemic. Additionally, they may suffer from nutritional anemia or from anemia of chronic disease if they have decubiti or frequent urinary and respiratory infections. Therefore, a normal or slightly low hematocrit may imply a combination of hypovolemia and reduced red-cell mass.

   Hypercalcemia and hypercalciuria have been observed in the early stages of SCI. These phenomena occur most often in young male patients and seem to result from calcium release from denervated muscle and possibly from bone stores; they occur in the first year with a peak around 10 weeks post injury. They are more common in higher-level injuries, and serum sodium and parathyroid hormone levels are normal [17]. In contrast, long-term SCI patients develop osteoporosis as a result of their paralysis and, especially in the case of supervening renal failure, become hypocalcemic.

   Last, as muscle mass atrophies, the serum creatinine goes down. A high-normal creatinine level, therefore, may be a sign of renal disease or hypovolemia.

2. **Skin, muscle, bone.** The skin of denervated areas becomes atrophic and susceptible to decubitus ulceration. Underlying bone is

then at risk for developing osteomyelitis. In addition, pathologic fractures often result from the disuse osteoporosis. Skeletal muscle spasticity or contractures complicate skin and general patient care and make surgical positioning difficult.

3. Blood. Hematologic studies in SCI patients with normal kidney function show anemia in 52%, which may be either normocytic hypochromic (56%) or normochromic (32%). Possible causes for these anemias include increased plasma water in response to over-aggressive hydration; malnutrition; or chronic infection.

4. Digestive system. Gastrointestinal bleeding may occur in up to 20% of SCI patients acutely. Gastric distention, ileus, and nonspecific liver dysfunction with a normal serum bilirubin are common complications usually occurring during the first postinjury week and then resolving over several weeks, although occasionally persisting longer. Pancreatitis also occurs, but it is unknown if this is related to the cord injury per se. Diagnosis of these and other intra-abdominal emergencies may be difficult as a result of altered sensation. Vomiting may occur without pain or nausea. The newly described syndrome of gastroduodenal motor dysfunction, possibly secondary to loss of adrenergic inhibitory control, features altered motility, pain, and vomiting. It is seen in certain SCI cases and responds to low doses of adrenergic agonist such as ephedrine [99]. Gastric and bowel distentions and the tendency toward vomiting in most of these disorders warrant a high index of suspicion of acute abdomen and preparation for airway protection on the part of the anesthesiologist. The distention itself may embarrass respiration.

5. Pain. Chronic pain is a problem in many SCI patients. It can cause and reinforce the depression that is often present. Proper management of pain and psychosocial support have proved essential for adaptation and rehabilitation of the patient.

G. Abnormal response to depolarizing muscle relaxants. Of great importance to the anesthesiologist is the massive translocation of intracellular potassium from skeletal muscle to the extracellular space following the administration of a depolarizing muscle relaxant such as succinylcholine. This phenomenon may occur as early as three days after injury and is thought to result from the denervation process of overgrowth and spread of cholinergic nicotinic receptors to include extrajunctional sarcolemma. This results in supersensitivity to depolarizing agents, whereby the entire affected muscle mass depolarizes synchronously and releases large amounts of potassium into the circulation [40].

Three important points should be emphasized. First, the magnitude of potassium release is a function more of the amount of muscle mass affected than of the amount of drug given: 20 mg of succinylcholine has been noted to result in a serum potassium concentration of 13.6 meq/L

[104]. Second, the causative overgrowth of receptors may well occur before spasticity replaces flaccid muscle paralysis. Third, pretreatment with a defasciculating dose of nondepolarizing relaxants does not reliably block the occurrence of significant hyperkalemia. Because the precise onset of supersensitivity is unpredictable, depolarizing agents should be avoided in all patients with SCI.

Should succinylcholine be inadvertently administered, electrocardiographic changes could progress from atrial conduction disturbances to prolonged PR interval (> 7 meq/L), tall peaked T waves (7–9 meq/Ll), progressive widening and aberration of the QRS complex (> 7 meq/L), and finally to sinusoidal ventricular complexes and ventricular fibrillation when serum potassium concentration reaches or exceeds 12 to 14 meq/L.

IV. Anesthetic management. Patients with SCI may come to surgery for treatment of their injury; for treatment of problems consequent to their injury, such as skin grafts over decubitus ulcers; or for problems unrelated to their SCI, such as cancer excisions or related traumatic injury. Their injury may be in its acute or chronic phase. Nevertheless surgical therapy for these reasons and for a variety of associated injuries or sequelae developing during the course of the illness resulted in 78% of the patients admitted to one spinal injury center undergoing some type of surgical procedure [112]. Therefore, we can suggest only some general principles, keeping the prior discussion of hazards and complications in mind.

Preanesthetic evaluation of the patient should be directed to the abnormalities associated with SCI as discussed and also to defining the extent of associated traumatic injuries. Between 25 and 65% of patients with SCI have associated problems, the most common being head, chest, abdominal, and skeletal injuries [1]. These may complicate ventilatory and circulatory problems resulting from the cord injury, and a high index of suspicion is necessary in evaluating these patients. As soon as feasible, appropriate roentgenographic studies should be completed. Initial laboratory determinations should include CBS, arterial blood gases, serum, electrolytes, serum creatinine, and any other study dictated by the individual patient's intrinsic illnesses or associated injuries.

Injury stability should be assessed and discussed with the surgeons. If the patient has been brought to surgery without proper spinal evaluation, he or she should be intubated as if SCI is present, and postoperative spine radiographs should be obtained as soon as possible, perhaps before the patient is reversed and extubated.

The earlier discussion of acute and chronic derangements in systemic function provides the basis for rational and safe anesthetic management as well as daily care of these patients.

In the acute phase, maintenance of normal acid-base and blood-gas parameters and adequate spinal cord perfusion pressure is paramount in importance. Experimental work in cats has suggested that there is no therapeutic advantage of either hypercapnia or hypocapnia over normocapnia in terms of both neurologic recovery and histologic tissue preservation. Although not statistically significant, mortality and tissue preservation results suggested that hypocapnia may be less harmful than hypercapnia immediately after the injury [35]. Consequently, it seems prudent to maintain $PaCO_2$ in the 35- to 40-mmHg range. Management of closed head injury with increased intracranial pressure would take precedence in this area ($PaCO_2$ maintained between 25 and 30 mmHg).

Hypoxemia must be prevented by careful attention to minimizing significant physiologic shunting, which is suggested by the inability to maintain a $PaCO_2 > 60$ mmHg with an FiO_2 of 50%. Possible contributing etiologies such as hemothorax or pneumothorax, pulmonary embolization of fat or thrombi, foreign body or gastric content aspiration, and noncardiogenic pulmonary edema should be suspected and either excluded or treated appropriately. PEEP may be required to decrease shunting and increase oxygenation, once pneumothorax or other reversible causes of hypoxemia have been excluded. However, the possible negative effect of PEEP on blood pressure, cardiac output, and intracranial pressure must be considered. In case the patient is not already intubated and this is necessary, it should be carried out as already discussed.

Cardiovascular management, as previously mentioned, most frequently requires judicious repletion of intravascular volume to restore normal venous return and filling pressures. However, it should be recalled that 4 of 22 patients in the study cited on volume loading during the acute postinjury period actually showed a decrease in CI accompanying infusion to increase PAOP, which necessitated decreasing halothane concentration from 0.55 to 0.25% to restore CI to baseline. However, both before and after infusion and at all halothane concentrations, the CI was at or above normal resting limits, and no evidence of organ hypoperfusion was noted [76]. Hence, caution but not exclusion is indicated with the use of potent inhalation agents during the acute stage of SCI, as compared to later when autonomic hyperreflexia is likely. During the phase of spinal shock lasting from three days to six weeks (average of three weeks), the advantages of pulmonary artery catheter monitoring are obvious in maintaining hemodynamics and avoiding pulmonary edema. Also, it allows quantitation of shunt and monitoring of the respiratory and hemodynamic effects of PEEP and continuous positive pressure ventilation. It is also necessary to keep in mind electrolyte, neuromuscular, and other potential systemic alterations, with management as has been outlined.

Recent investigations have documented deleterious effects of hyperglycemia resulting from dextrose infusion on neurologic outcome after cerebral [69] and spinal cord [25] ischemia. In the latter study, Drummond and Moore [25] showed that mild to moderate increases of plasma glucose averaging only 40 mg/dl tripled the incidence of paraplegia in rabbits subjected to transient spinal cord ischemia following aortic occlusion (9 of 10 dextrose-treated animals as compared to 3 of 10 control animals). Although not elucidated by the study design, the authors considered end products of hypoxic glucose metabolism, such as lactate, which has experimentally verified adverse effects on physiologic and histologic outcome after cerebral iscemia, the most likely mechanism by which enhanced glucose availability could worsen tolerance to ischemia. Of note was the lack of correlation between the magnitude of plasma glucose elevation and the extent of neurologic injury. This result was thought to be possibly attributable to differences in intracellular glucose availability not reflected by extracellular concentration, perhaps as a result of varying insulin effect. In light of these findings, routine use of dextrose-containing fluids, as part of initial resuscitation or perioperatively in cases where the development or worsening of spinal cord ischemia is possible, should be confined to those instances where a definite medical indication exists and dose monitoring and control of plasma glucose are possible. The data were not sufficient to allow recommending that an already elevated plasma glucose be lowered emergently when encountered intraoperatively.

Schonwald and colleagues [92] reported a series of 219 patients with SCIs. Of the patients with lesions at or above T-5, 33% underwent general anesthesia with halothane (37 cases) or enflurane (12 cases), and none of these developed autonomic hyperreflexia or arrhythmias. Of nine patients in this group receiving nitrous oxide-narcotic anesthesia, two developed intraoperative hyperreflexia. In 97 cases in which spinal anesthesia with tetracaine was used, no attacks occurred, but in 1 case a lidocaine spinal anesthetic apparently wore off before the end of urologic surgery, resulting in autonomic hyperreflexia. The level of injury was a major factor influencing the technical ease and feasibility of lumbar subarachnoid block. Low levels of injury resulted in failure in 3 of 19 patients, most likely as a result of previous spine surgery or other traumatic distortion of the anatomy. An alternative where surgical considerations would require high spinal levels (above T-5) is subarachnoid block followed by light general anesthesia with endotracheal intubation and controlled ventilation.

Of relevance for anesthesia during the acute phase of SCI, Cole and colleagues [18] investigated the effect of various anesthetic regimens on the susceptibility of rats to ischemic SCI. Of the four techniques investigated — halothane, fentanyl, nitrous oxide, and subarachnoid lidocaine — all increased the duration of ischemia required to produce SCI. No one technique was relatively more favorable or deleterious than the other in terms of final neurologic outcome. Possible mechanisms for this protective effect, although not clear at present, may include depression of spinal cord metabolism, effects on SCBF, alterations in endogenous catecholamine levels, alteration of opiate receptor activity, or interaction with other potential mediators of secondary SCI (for example, prostaglandins). Hence, although anesthetics have not been shown to play a role in treating SCI in this model, the anesthetized state using the cited agents seems to provide some degree of protection against its occurrence.

A study [60] in dogs showed consistent statistically significant increases in lumbosacral SCBF with a lesser, nonsignificant tendency toward increases in thoracic and cervical cord flow after subarachnoid tetracaine, as long as mean arterial pressure remained 100 mmHg or more. The favorable effect was blocked by the addition of epinephrine to the tetracaine; in fact, a nonsignificant tendency toward decreased thoracic and cervical cord flows actually occurred. Hence, spinal anesthesia may improve cord blood flow, but vasoconstrictors should not be added to the anesthetic. Although spinal or epidural anesthetics have been considered hemodynamically unpredictable in these patients [21], baseline hemodynamic stability as well as ablation of autonomic hyperreflexia has been verified by many other workers [92,106]. One study [6] showed such stability of cardiac output, stroke volume, and heart rate during cystoscopy that it was actually impossible to determine when bladder distention and emptying had occurred from the inspection of these data alone. Further, no ephedrine was required during the study. These authors emphasized the importance of judicious choice of the anesthetic dose and attention to intravascular volume as factors contributing to the noted stability. Low-dose intrathecal morphine (0.2–0.25 mg) has, incidentally, been shown effective in alleviating the symptoms of spastic bladder for up to 24 hours [48]. A note of caution is warranted in patients with subarachnoid block of cerebrospinal fluid circulation, because a 14% incidence of neurologic deterioration following removal of cerebrospinal fluid or delayed leakage through the puncture site has been reported [54]. Nitrous oxide–oxygen, narcotic-based techniques seem less recommendable in light of their failure to prevent hyperreflexia in two of nine patients. Regardless of the technique employed, direct-acting arteriolar dilators (such as nitroprusside), alpha-adrenergic blockers (such as phentolamine), antiarrhythmics (such as lidocaine, propranolol, and esmolol), new antihypertensives (such as labetalol and nifedipine), and atropine should be readily available [92]. The need to avoid succinylcholine is reiterated. However, the new, short-acting nondepolarizing agents make this constraint clinically feasible because they are a reasonable alternative.

Obstetric management of women with SCI during labor and delivery or cesarean section, as already mentioned, is complicated by the possibility of autonomic hyperreflexia, threatening both the mother and the fetus. Contractions are often felt as abdominal spasms or other symptoms similar to the bowel hyperactivity familiar to them [109]. Many anesthesiologists feel that epidural anesthetics in these circumstances, even if not needed for analgesia, are indicated for preventing hyperreflexive episodes [77,100,106], whereas others fear hypotension as a potential complication. In our practice, epidural anesthetics are used with careful titration of drug dosage and maintenance of normal cardiac filling pressures, if not contraindicated by the obstetric condition.

In the case of incomplete spinal cord lesions, SSEPs and MEPs can be useful in monitoring cord function (see **I**). This is true during surgery to relieve cord compression or to correct spinal deformity, as well as during the acute phase of SCI when neurologic status may progressively worsen. The usefulness of electrophysiologic monitoring is exemplified by a case report of verified iatrogenic posterior SCI that was immediately diagnosed by SSEP, but not by two false-negative "wake up" tests or during the admission evaluation in the recovery room [7]. The use of transcutaneous corticomotor stimulation with recording of spinal level CMEPs or electromyogram activity distal to the area at risk has also proven feasible. It often indicates injury when the ascending pathways are normal, and occasionally the reverse is true. SSEPs and CMEPs cover distinct regions of the cord and, used separately or together, can diagnose almost all injuries with more sensitivity and specificity than clinical observations alone [103].

Of possible utility during surgery in patients with incomplete lesions is the observation that etomidate improved the SSEP in patients receiving neuroleptanesthesia by increasing the latency and amplitude of the short-latency cortical responses [97]. A 0.3- to 0.5-mg/kg bolus of etomidate followed by a continuous infusion of 0.01 to 0.05 mg/kg/min was used. Areas of potential concern that should be resolved include the possibility that the improved amplitude may be associated with etomidate's tendency to produce myoclonic activity and its ability to produce adrenocortical suppression for 8 to 24 hours. The clinical significance of these two drug properties when used on a short-term basis remains to be documented, in contrast to the known adrenal insufficiency that required treatment and influenced mortality when the drug was employed for sedation in a critical care setting. Further study is needed before this technique is widely accepted; however, where SSEP monitoring is considered essential but is technically nonreproducible, etomidate may be the solution. Another recent report [93] suggests that the use of lower than usual stimulus presentation rates (1.1–2.1 Hz as compared to 5.1 Hz) resolved problems similar to those found in the first study and may provide an acceptable alternative solution.

Acknowledgment

The authors thank Grune & Stratton for giving permission to use information that was previously published in J. P. Giffin. Spinal cord injury. *Semin Anesth.* 614:246, 1987. Thanks also to Naomi W. Barker for preparation of the manuscript.

References

1. Albin, M. S. Resuscitation of the spinal cord. *Criti. Care Med.* 6:270, 1978.
2. Albin, M. S., Bunegin, L., and Wolf, S. Brain and lungs at risk after cervical spinal cord transaction: Intracranial pressure, brain water, blood-brain barrier perme-

ability, cerebral blood flow, and extravascular lung water changes. *Surg. Neurol.* 24:191, 1985.

3. Anderson, T. E. Effects of acute alcohol intoxication on spinal cord vascular injury. *Cent. Nerv. Syst. Trauma* 3:183, 1986.

4. Anderson, D. K., Demediuk, P., and Saunders, R. D. Spinal cord injury and protection. *Ann. Emerg. Med.* 14:816, 1985.

5. Banik, N. L., Hogan, E. L., and Hsu, C. Molecular and anatomical correlates of spinal cord injury. *Cent. Nerve. Syst. Trauma* 2:99, 1985.

6. Barker, I., Alderson, J., and Lydon, M. Cardiovascular effects of spinal subarachnoid anaesthesia. *Anesthesia* 40:533, 1985.

7. Ben-David, B., Taylor, P. D., and Haller, G. S. Posterior spinal fusion complicated by posterior column injury: A case report of a false negative wake-up test. *Spine* 12:540, 1987.

8. Benthuysen, J. L. Naloxone therapy in spinal trauma: Anesthetic effects. *Anesthesiology* 66:238, 1987.

9. Bivins, H. G., Scott, F., Bezmalinovix, Z., et al. The effect of axial traction during orotracheal intubation of the trauma victim with an unstable cervical spine. *Ann. Emerg. Med.* 17:25, 1988.

10. Borgens, R. B., Blight, A. R., and Murphy, D. J. Transected dorsal column axons within the guinea pig spinal cord regenerate in the presence of an applied electric field. *J. Comp. Neurol.* 250:168, 1986.

11. Bose, B., Osterholm, J. L., and Kalia, M. Ganglioside-induced regeneration and reestablishment of axonal continuity in spinal cord–transected rats. *Neurosci. Lett.* 63:165, 1986.

12. Bracken, M. B., Freeman, D. H., and Hellenbrand, K. Incidence of acute traumatic hospitalized spinal cord injury in the United States, 1970–77. *Am. J. Epidemiol.* 113:615, 1981.

13. Bracken, M. B., Shephard, M. J., Collins, W. F. et al. A randomized, controlled trial of methylprednisolone or naloxone in the treatment of acute spinal cord injury. *N. Engl. J. Med.* 322:1405, 1990.

14. Braken, M. B., Shepard, M. J., Hellenbrand, K. G., et al. Methylprednisolone and neurological function 1 year after spinal cord injury: Results of the National Acute Spinal Cord Injury Study. *J. Neurosurg.* 63:704, 1985.

15. Burke, D. C., and Murray, D. D. The management of thoracic and thoracolumbar injuries of the spine with neurological involvement. *J. Bone Joint Surg. Am.* 58B:72, 1976.

16. Chabot, R., York, D. H., and Watts, C. Somatosensory evoked potentials evaluated in normal subjects and spinal cord-injured patients. *J. Neurosurg.* 63:544, 1985.

17. Claus-Walker, J., Carter, R. E., and Campos, R. J. Hypercalcemia in early traumatic quadriplegia. *J. Chronic Dis.* 28:81, 1975.

18. Cole, D. J., Shaprio, H. M., Drummond, J. C., et al. Halothane, fentanyl, nitrous oxide, and spinal lidocaine protect against spinal cord injury in the rat. *Anesthesiology* 70:967, 1989.

19. Crawford, R. A., Griffiths, I. R., and McCulloch, J. The effect of norepinephrine on the spinal cord circulation and its possible implications in the pathogenesis of acute spinal trauma. *J. Neurosurg.* 47:567, 1977.

20. Davis, J. N., Goldman, M., and Loh, L. Diaphragm function and alveolar hypoventilation. *Q. J. Med.* 177:87, 1976.

21. Desmond, J. Paraplegia: Problems confronting the anaesthesiologist. *Can. Anaesth. Soc. J.* 17:435, 1970.

22. DeTroyer, A., Estenne, M., and Heilporn, A. Mechanism of active expiration in tetraplegic subjects. *N. Engl. J. Med.* 314:740, 1986.

23. Dolan, E. J., and Tator, C. H. The effect of blood transfusion, dopamine, and gamma hydroxybutyrate on posttraumatic ischemia of the spinal cord. *J. Neurosurg.* 56:350, 1982.

24. Downs, J. B., Klein, F. F., Jr., Desantels, D., et al. Intermittent mandatory ventilation: a new approach to interweaning patients from mechanical ventilators. *Chest* 64:331, 1973.
25. Drummond, J. C., and Moore, S. S. The influence of dextrose administration on neurologic outcome after temporary spinal cord ischemia in the rabbit. *Anesthesiology* 70:64, 1989.
26. Eisenberg, M. G., and Tierney, D. O. Changing demographic profile of the spinal cord injury population: Implications for health care support systems. *Paraplegia* 23:335, 1985.
27. Evans, D. E., Kobrine, A. I., and Rizzoli, H. V. Cardiac arrhythmias accompanying acute compression of the spinal cord. *J. Neurosurg.* 52:52, 1980.
28. Faden, A. I., Jacobs, T. P., and Holaday, J. W. Endorphin-parasympathetic interaction in spinal shock. *J. Auton. Nerv. Syst.* 2:295, 1980.
29. Faden, A. I., Jacobs, T. P., and Holadway, J. W. Opiate antagonist improves neurologic recovery after spinal injury. *Science* 211:493, 1981.
30. Faden, A. I., Molineaux, C. J., and Rosenberger, J. G. Increased dynorphin immunoreactivity in spinal cord after traumatic injury. *Regul. Pept.* 11:35, 1985.
31. Faden, A. I., Sackson, I., and Noble, L. J. Opiate-receptor antagonist nalmefene improves neurologic recovery after traumatic spinal cord injury in rats through a central mechanism. *J. Pharmacol. Exp. Ther.* 245:742, 1988.
32. Faden, A. I., and Simon, R. P. A potential role for excitotoxins in the pathophysiology of spinal cord injury. *Ann. Neurol.* 23:623, 1988.
33. Flamm, E. S., Young, W., and Collins, W. F. A phase I trial of naloxone treatment in acute spinal cord injury. *J. Neurosurg.* 63:390, 1985.
34. Flamm, E. S., Young, W., and Demopoulos, H. B. Experimental spinal cord injury: Treatment with naloxone. *Neurosurgery* 10:227, 1982.
35. Ford, R. W. J., and Malm, D. N. Therapeutic trial of hypercarbia and hypocarbia in acute experimental spinal cord injury. *J. Neurosurg.* 61:925, 1984.
36. Forner, J. V., Llombart, R. L., and Valledor, M. C. V. The flow-volume loop in tetraplegics. *Paraplegia* 15:245, 1977, 1978.
37. Fraser, A., and Edmunds-Seal, J. Spinal cord injuries: A review of the problems facing the anaesthetist. *Anaesthesia* 37:1084, 1982.
38. Glenn, W. W. L., Holcomb, B. E. E., and McLaughlin, A. J. Total ventilatory support in a quadriplegic patient with radiofrequency electrophrenic respiration. *N. Engl. J. Med.* 286:513, 1972.
39. Griffiths, I. R. Spinal cord blood flow in dogs II. The effect of the blood gases. *J. Neurol. Neurosurg. Psychiatry* 36:42, 1973.
40. Gronert, G. L. A., and Theye, R. A. Pathophysiology of hyperkalemia induced by succinylcholine. *Anesthesiology* 43:89, 1975.
41. Gross, D., Ladd, H. W., and Riley, E. J. The effect of training on strength and endurance of the diaphragm in quadriplegia. *J.A.M.A.* 68:27, 1980.
42. Guth, L., Barrett, C. P., and Donati, E. J. Enhancement of axonal growth into a spinal lesion by topical application of triethanolamine and cytosine arabinoside. *Exp. Neurol.* 88:44, 1985.
43. Haghighi, S. S., and Chehrazi, B. Effect of naloxone in experimental acute spinal cord injury. *Neurosurgery* 20:385, 1987.
44. Hall, E. D., and Wolf, D. L. A pharmacological analysis of the pathophysiological mechanisms of posttraumatic spinal cord ischemia. *J. Neurosurg.* 64:951, 1986.
45. Hamilton A. J., Black, P. M., and Carr, D. B. Contrasting actions of naloxone in experimental spinal cord trauma and cerebral ischemia: A review. *Neurosurgery* 17:845, 1985.
46. Hartzog, J. T., Fischer, R. G., and Snow, C. Spinal Cord Trauma: Effect of Hyperbaric Oxygen Therapy. In *Proceedings of the Veterans Administration Spinal Cord Injury Conference* 17:70, 1971.

47. Heiden, J. S., Weiss, M. H., Rosenberg, A. W., et al. Management of cervical spinal cord trauma in Southern California. *J. Neurosurg.* 43:732, 1975.

48. Herman, R. M., Wainberg, M. C., del Guidice, P. F., and Wilkscher, M. K. The effect of a low dose of intrathecal morphine on impaired micturition reflexes in human subjects with spinal cord lesions. *Anesthesiology* 69:313, 1988.

49. Heros, R. C. Spinal Cord Compression. In A. H. Ropper, S. K. Kennedy, and N. T. Zevas (Eds.), *Neurological and Neurosurgical Intensive Care.* Baltimore: University Park, 1982. Pp. 231–248.

50. Hickey, R., Albin, M. S., et al. Autoregulation of spinal cord blood flow: Is the cord a microcosm of the brain? *Stroke* 17:1183, 1986.

51. Hogan, E. L., Hsu, C., and Banik, N. L. Calcium-activated mediators of secondary injury in the spinal cord. *Cent. Nerv. Syst. Trauma* 3:175, 1986.

52. Holaday, J. W., and Faden, A. I. Spinal shock and injury: Experimental therapeutic approaches. *Adv. Shock. Res.* 10:95, 1983.

53. Holaday, J. W., and Faden, A. I. Naloxone acts at central opiate receptors to reverse hypotension, hypothermia and hypoventilation in spinal shock. *Brain Res.* 189:295, 1980.

54. Hollis, P. H., Malis, L. I., and Zappulla, R. A. Neurological deterioration after lumbar puncture below complete spinal subarachnoid block. *J. Neurosurg.* 64:253, 1986.

55. Holmstrom, F., and Babinski, M. Spirometry in acute spinal cord injury. *Crit. Care Med.* (Abstr.) 8:253, 1980.

56. Hsu, C., Hogan, E. L., and Gadsden, K. M. Sr. Vascular permeability in experimental spinal cord injury. *J. Neurosci.* 70:275, 1985.

57. Kajihara, K., Kawanga, H., de la Torre, J. C., et. al. Dimethyl sulfoxide in the treatment of experimental acute spinal cord injury. *Surg. Neurol.* 1:16, 1973.

58. Kendrick, W. W., Scott, J. W., and Jousse, A. T. Reflex sweating and hypertension in traumatic transverse myelitis. *Treatment Serv. Bull.* (Ottawa) 8:437, 1953.

59. Kobrine, A. I., Doyle, T. F., and Martins, A. N. Local spinal cord blood flow in experimental traumatic myelopathy. *J. Neurosurg.* 42:144, 1975.

60. Kozody, R., Palahiuk, R. J., and Cumming, M. O. Spinal cord blood flow following subarachnoid tetracaine. *Can. Anaesth. Soc. J.* 32:23, 1985.

61. Kraus, J. F. A comparison of recent studies on the extent of the head and spinal cord injury problem in the United States. *J. Neurosurg.* 53:35, 1980.

62. Kraus, J. F., Franti, C. E., Riggins, R. S., et al. Incidence of traumatic spinal cord lesions. *J. Chronic Dis.* 28:471, 1975.

63. Krumins, S. A., and Faden, A. I. Traumatic injury alters opiate receptor binding in rat spinal cord. *Ann. Neurol.* 19:498, 1986.

64. Kuchner, E. F., and Hansebout, R. R. Combined steroid and hypothermia treatment of experimental spinal cord injury. *Surg. Neurol.* 6:371, 1976.

65. Kuhlemeier, K. V., and Huan, C. T., et al. Effective renal plasma flow: Clinical significance after spinal cord injury. *J. Urol.* 133:758, 1985.

66. Kuhlemeier, K. V., Lloyd L. K., and Stover, S. L. Urological neurology and urodynamics: Long-term follow-up of renal function after spinal cord injury. *J. Urol.* 134:510, 1985.

67. Kurihara, M. Role of monamines in experimental spinal cord injury in rats: Relationship between Na+ −K= −ATPase and lipid peroxidation. *J. Neurosurg.* 62:743, 1985.

68. Kurnick, N. B. Autonomic hyperreflexia and its control in patients with spinal cord lesions. *Ann. Intern. Med. 44:678, 1956.*

69. Lanier, W. L., Stangland, K. J., Scheithauer, B. W., et al. The effects of dextrose infusion and head position on neurologic outcome after complete cerebral ischemia in primates: Examination of a model. *Anesthesiology* 66:39, 1987.

70. Ledsome, J. R., and Sharp, J. M. Pulmonary function in acute cervical cord injury. *Am. Rev. Respir. Dis.* 124:41, 1981.

71. Leith, D. E., and Bradley, M. Ventilatory muscle strength and endurance training. *J. Appl. Physiol.* 41:508, 1976.
72. Levy, W., McCaffrey, M., and Hagichi, S. Motor evoked potential as a predictor of recovery in chronic spinal cord injury. *Neurosurgery* 20:138, 1987.
73. Levy, W., McCaffrey, M., and York, D. Motor evoked potential in cats with acute spinal cord injury. *Neurology* 19:9, 1986.
74. Luce, J. M. Medical management of spinal cord injury. *Crit. Care Med.* 13:126, 1985.
75. Luce, J. M., and Culver, B. H. Respiratory muscle function in health and disease. *Chest* 81:82, 1982.
76. MacKenzie, C. F., Shin, B., and Krishnapradad, D., et al. Assessment of cardiac respiratory function during surgery on patients with acute quadriplegia. *J. Neurosurg.* 62:843, 1985.
77. McCunniff, D. E., and Dewan, D. Pregnancy after spinal cord injury: Letter to the Editor. *Obstet. Gynecol.* 63:757, 1984.
78. McMichan, J. C., Michel, L., and Westbrook, P. R. Pulmonary dysfunction following traumatic quadriplegia. *J.A.M.A.* 243:528, 1980.
79. Meyer, G. L., Berman, I. R., and Doty, I. B. Hemodynamic responses to acute quadriplegia with or without chest trauma. *J. Neurosurg.* 34:168, 1971.
80. Mohler, J. L., Ellison, M. F., and Flanigan, R. L. Creatinine clearance prediction in spinal cord injury patients: Comparison of 6 prediction equations. *J. Urol.* 139:706, 1988.
81. Osterholm, J. L., and Mathews, G. J. Altered norepinephrine metabolism following experimental spinal cord injury. I. Relationship to hemorrhagic necrosis and post-wounding neurological deficits. *J. Neurosurg.* 36:386, 1972.
82. Osterholm, J. L., and Mathews, G. J. Altered norepinephrine metabolism following experimental cord injury. II. Protection against traumatic spinal cord hemorrhagic necrosis by norepinephrine synthesis blockade with alpha methyltyrosine. *J. Neurosurg.* 36:395, 1972.
83. Parker, A. J., Park, R. D., and Stowater, J. L. Reduction of trauma-induced edema of spinal cord in dogs given mannitol. *Am. J. Vet. Res.* 34:1355, 1973.
84. Quimby, C. A., Williams, R. N., and Greifenstein, F. E. Anesthetic problems of the acute quadriplegic patient. *Anesth. Analg.* 52:333, 1973.
85. Ransohoff, J., Flamm, E. S., and Demopoulos, H. B. Mechanisms of Injury and Treatment of Acute Spinal Cord Trauma. In J. E. Cottrell and H. Turndorf (Eds.), *Anesthesia and Neurosurgery.* St. Louis: Mosby, 1980. Pp. 361–386.
86. Rawe, S. Lee, W., and Perot, P. L. Pressor response resulting from experimental contusion injury to the spinal cord. *J. Neurosurg.* 50:58, 1979.
87. Rawe, S. E., Lee, W. A., and Perot, P. L. The histopathology of experimental spinal cord trauma: the effect of systemic blood pressure. *J. Neurosurg.* 48:1002, 1978.
88. Reier, P. J. Neural tissue graft and repair of the injured spinal cord. *Neuropathol. Appl. Neurobiol.* 11:81, 1985.
89. Rivlin, A. S., and Tator, C. H. Regional spinal cord blood flow in rats after severe cord trauma. *J. Neurosurg.* 49:844, 1978.
90. Rochester, D. F., Braun, N. M. T., and Laine, S. Diaphragmatic energy expenditure in chronic respiratory failure: the effect of assisted ventilation with body respirators. *Am. J. Med.* 53:223, 1977.
91. Sandler, A. N., and Tator, C. H. Review of the effect of spinal cord trauma on the vessels and blood flow in the spinal cord. *J. Neurosurg.* 45:638, 1976.
92. Schonwald, G., Fis, K. J., and Perkash, I. Cardiovascular complications during anesthesia in chronic spinal cord injured patients. *Anesthesiology* 55:550, 1981.
93. Schubert, A., Drummond, J. C., and Garfin, S. R. The influence of stimulus presentation rate in the cortical amplitude and latency of intraoperative somatosensory-evoked potential recordings in patients with varying degrees of spinal cord injury. *Spine* 12:969, 1987.

94. Senter, H. J., and Venes, J. L. Altered blood flow and secondary injury in experimental spinal cord trauma. *J. Neurosurg.* 49:569, 1978.
95. Senter, H. J., and Venes, J. L. Loss of autoregulation and posttraumatic ischemia following experimental spinal cord trauma. *J. Neurosurg.* 50:198, 1979.
96. Simpson, R. K., and Baskin, D. S. Corticomotor evoked potentials in acute and chronic blunt spinal cord injury in the rat: Correlation with neurological outcome and histological damage. *Neurosurgery* 20:131, 1987.
97. Sloan, T. B., Ronai, A. K., and Toleikis, R. J. Improvement of the intraoperative somatosensory evoked potentials by etomidate. *Anesth. Analg.* 67:582, 1988.
98. Smith, R. B., Schaer, W. B., and Pfaeffle, H. Percutaneous transtracheal ventilation for anesthesia and resuscitation: a review and report of complications. *Can. Anaesth. Soc. J.* 22:607, 1975.
99. Sninsky, C. A., Martin, J. L., and Matthias, J. R. Effect of lidamidine hydrochloride, a proposed alpha-2 adrenergic agonist in patients with gastroduodenal motor dysfunction. *Gastroenterology* 84:1315, 1983.
100. Spielman, F. J. Parturient with spinal cord transection: Complications of autonomic hyperreflexia: Letter to the editor. *Obstet. Gynecol.* 64:147, 1984.
101. Surgarman, B. Medical complications of spinal cord injury. *Q. J. Med.* 54:3, 1985.
102. Sussman, B. J. Fracture dislocation of the cervical spine: A critique of current management in the United States. *Paraplegia* 16:15, 1978.
103. Thompson, P. D., Dick, J. P. R., Asselman, P. et al. Examination of motor function in lesions of the spinal cord by stimulation of the motor cortex. *Ann. Neurol.* 21:387, 1987.
104. Tobey, R. E. Paraplegia, succinylcholine and cardiac arrest. *Anesthesiology* 32:359, 1970.
105. Troll, G. F., and Dohrmann, G. J. Anaesthesia of the spinal cord injured patient: Cardiovascular problems and their management. *Paraplegia* 13:162, 1975.
106. Verduyn, W. H. Spinal cord injured women, pregnancy and delivery. *Paraplegia* 24:231, 1986.
107. Wallace, M. C., and Tator, C. H. Failure of blood transfusion or naloxone to improve clinical recovery after experimental spinal cord injury. *Neurosurgery* 19:489, 1986.
108. Wallace, M. C., and Tator, C. H. Failure of naloxone to improve spinal cord blood flow and cardiac output after spinal cord injury. *Neurosurgery* 18:428, 1986.
109. Wanner, M. B., Rageth, C. J., and Zach, G. A. Pregnancy and autonomic hyperreflexia in patients with spinal cord lesions. *Paraplegia* 25:482, 1987.
110. Welphy, N. C., Mathias, C. J., and Frankel, H. L. Circulatory reflexes in tetraplegics during artificial ventilation and general anesthesia. *Paraplegia* 12:172, 1975.
111. Wolman, L. The disturbance of circulation in traumatic paraplegia in acute and late stages: A pathological study. *Paraplegia* 1:213, 1965.
112. Woolsey, R. M. Rehabilitation outcome following spinal cord injury. *Arch. Neurol.* 42:116, 1985.
113. Young, J. S. Initial hospitalization cord rehabilitation costs of spinal cord injury. *Orthop. Clin. North Am.* 9:263, 1978.
114. Young, W., DeCrescito, V., and Tomasula, J. J. The role of the sympathetic nervous system in pressor responses induced by spinal injury. *J. Neurosurg.* 52:473, 1980.
115. Young, W., and Flamm, L. E. S. Effect of high-dose corticosteroid therapy on blood flow, evoked potentials, and extracellular calcium in experimental spinal injury. *J. Neurosurg.* 57:667, 1982.

15

Pediatric Neurosurgery

DIANE R. ROSNER

MARK A. ROCKOFF

I. Pathophysiology

A. Cerebrospinal fluid. The average adult has between 90 and 150 ml of cerebrospinal fluid (CSF) throughout the brain and spinal subarachnoid space. Children have lesser amounts and, in neonates, often only a few drops of CSF can be obtained from the spinal canal. CSF is produced predominantly in the choroid plexus, and total CSF replacement occurs about 4 to 5 times each day [16,46]. Under normal conditions, CSF exists in dynamic equilibrium with absorption equal to production. Production of CSF is affected little by alterations in **intracranial pressure** (ICP) [43] and is usually unchanged in children with hydrocephalus. CSF-producing tumors, such as choroid plexus papillomas, are rare but are more likely to occur during childhood. In the presence of an intracranial mass lesion or cerebral hyperemia, translocation of CSF from the intracranial to spinal compartment can act as an acute volume buffer to prevent elevation of ICP, provided no obstruction to CSF circulation exists [41].

1. **Absorbtion.** CSF absorption occurs via arachnoid villi and arachnoid granulations into the venous system. Absorption increases as ICP rises. Intracranial hemorrhage, infections of the **central nervous system** (CNS), and congenital abnormalities that obstruct CSF circulation or arachnoid granulations, or both, are conditions that decrease CSF absorption [5]. In the presence of open fontanelles and open cranial sutures, and increase in ICP may be attenuated, but not eliminated, by increasing head circumference; herniation is still possible if acute, severe increases in ICP develop.

B. Cerebral blood flow, cerebral blood volume, and cerebral metabolism. In addition to CSF translocation, an increase in ICP can be offset by a decrease in intracranial blood volume. Although **cerebral blood volume** (CBV) occupies only about 10% of the intracranial compartment, dynamic, blood volume–related changes are often initiated by anesthetic or intensive care maneuvers. As with other vascular beds, most blood is contained in the low-pressure, high-capacitance venous system. This venous blood volume can be translocated as compensation for an increase in ICP [9,58]. Accordingly, in hydrocephalic infants, a shift of venous blood from intracranial to extracranial vessels produces distended scalp veins [18]. Ultimately, increases in CBV due to increases in **cerebral blood flow** (CBF) will result in elevation of ICP.

As in adults, CBF in infants and children usually parallels **cerebral metabolic rate** (CMR); however, both parameters vary with age. Between 6 months and 11 years, CBF is approximately 100 ml/100 gm/min [33,45], which is about twice that in adults [34,35]. **Cerebral metabolic rate for oxygen** ($CMRO_2$) in children is, likewise, nearly twice that of adults [34,35] at approximately 5 ml of oxygen per 100 gm/min [33]. Little data exists regarding CBF and CMR in infants; however, in anesthetized infants, $CMRO_2$ has been found to be approximately 2.3 ml of oxygen per 100 gm/min [57]. CBF is also lowest in the neonate with a value close to 40 ml/100 gm/min [15,66].

CBF in infants and children appears to be affected by the same drugs and maneuvers that produce alterations in adults; however, as with baseline values, the limits of responsiveness may vary with age [53]. **Arterial carbon dioxide tension** ($PaCO_2$) is a potent cerebral vasodilator. In normal adults, CBF changes approximately 4% per mmHg change in $PaCO_2$ over the range of 20 to 80 mmHg [25,35,52]. Little data are available concerning the effects of $PaCO_2$ or **arterial oxygen tension** (PaO_2) on CBF in infants and children. In one study involving a small number of neonates, CBF increased less to hypercarbia and decreased more to hyperoxia [49] than in adults [35].

1. **Autoregulation.** Finally, although there are scant data on infants, animal data suggest that autoregulation (the ability to alter cerebrovascular tone to maintain CBF constant over a range of mean arterial pressures [MAP]), is present at birth, but clearly at different absolute values from adults. In the normal adult, autoregulation occurs with MAP over the range of 50 to 150 mmHg. Outside these limits, CBF is passively dependent on MAP. Decreases in MAP may then result in ischemia, while elevations increase CBF, CBV, and, therefore, ICP. Normal MAP may not reach 50 mmHg until several months after birth. The lower limit of acceptable **blood pressure** (BP) that will ensure adequate CBF is unknown and may vary with age. Likewise, excessive BP elevation may exceed the limits of autoregulation at different pressures at different ages.

C. **Cerebral perfusion pressure.** Since CBF is not easily determined, **cerebral perfusion pressure** (CPP) is often used to estimate global cerebral circulation (CPP = MAP− ICP); however, regional ischemia can exist with normal global cerebral perfusion. As with CBF, acceptable limits for young children are not known and probably vary with age. It is helpful to be familiar with normal BP values for different ages (Table 15-1.).

D. **Intracranial pressure.** Elevation of ICP may not be apparent on clinical examination. Pupillary dilatation, increasing BP, and bradycardia do not always develop in association with intracranial hypertension [9,18]; however, when they occur, they are usually late and dangerous signs [44]. Papilledema may not be present in children who die as a

Table 15-1. Vital signs of children

Age	Weight (kg)	Blood pressure (mean systolic) (mmHg)	Heart rate (per min)	Respiratory rate (per min)
Premature	< 2.5	50	120–160	35–80
Term neonate	> 2.5	60	120–170	35–60
1 yr	10	90	100–130	20–40
6 yr	20	100	80–120	20–25
12 yr	40	115	60–110	18–20

result of intracranial hypertension. An abnormal level of consciousness, especially when associated with abnormal motor responses to painful stimuli, is frequently associated with elevated ICP [9]. An increase in ICP occurring soon after head injury in children is not often from intracranial hematoma (as in adults), but is more likely to be secondary to diffuse brain swelling caused by a hyperemic response to injury [10].

1. **Techniques used to monitor ICP** in adults have also been useful in children. Unfortunately, in children, ventricular catheters may be difficult to insert into the small ventricles further compressed by brain swelling. Subarachnoid bolts are commonly used to monitor ICP in children but are difficult to stabilize in infants less than 1 year old because of the thin calvaria. Epidural transducers, placed surgically in older children, or secured noninvasively to the anterior fontanelle in neonates, have also been used to assess ICP [62].

2. **Normal values** for ICP are generally accepted as less than 15 mmHg. Occurrence of plateau waves (frequent pressure waves despite a normal baseline ICP) in children who have intracranial disorders should be considered hazardous [9]. Before the fontanelles have closed, significant increases in head circumference can occur, and ICP may remain in the normal range on intermittent measurements.

II. Anesthetic management

A. **Preoperative evaluation** for neurosurgical patients is similar to that performed for all pediatric patients with special attention to birth history, developmental age, and associated medical problems. A typical evaluation emphasizes the following:

1. **History**

a. **Birth history and neonatal course**, particularly any history of prematurity. Anesthesia for premature and term neonates requires familiarity with fetal, transitional, and normal neonatal physiology, as well as pharmacokinetic and pharmacodynamic differences from older patients. A complete discussion is beyond the scope of this chapter, although several texts are available [3,60]. Postoperative care in these infants demands heightened vigilance with particular attention to the potential for respiratory complications [37,40,64]. Prematurity is associated with a number of congenital malformations, genetic syndromes, and intra-uterine insults and can itself be the cause of persistent medical problems. Table 15-2 highlights some of the more common concerns.

  b. Developmental versus chronologic age (Tables 15-3 and 15-4).

  (1) First trimester. Neurologic development begins very early in the embryonic period. The tubular structure destined to become the brain and spinal cord is fully formed by the end of the fourth week of gestation. During the fifth and sixth weeks, the basic form of the cerebral hemispheres and ven-

Table 15-2. Concerns for the premature and ex-premature infant

Diagnosis/condition	Consequences/comments
Intraventricular hemorrhage (similar consequences with hypoxic ischemic encephalopathy)	Hydrocephalus Ventriculoperitoneal shunt Cerebral palsy Seizures Developmental delay
Neonatal meningitis	Severe morbidity as above
Hyaline membrane disease	Bronchopulmonary dysplasia Bronchospasm Infection (pneumonia/bronchitis) Cor pulmonale Subglottic stenosis
Necrotizing enterocolitis	Short-gut syndrome Total parenteral nutrition Hepatitis Vitamin deficiencies
Retinopathy of prematurity (previously retrolentofibroplasia)	Impaired vision/blindness
Apnea and bradycardia	May be exacerbated by anesthesia [37, 40, 64]
Patent ductus arteriosus	Congestive heart failure Hypoxemia
Sudden infant death syndrome	More frequent in premature infants
Physiologic anemia	Nadir lower and earlier in prematures than term infants

Table 15-3. Significant primary neonatal reflexes [24,48,54]

Reflex	Age at appearance	Age at disappearance (mon)
Moro	28 wks' gestation	4
Palmar grasp	28 wks' gestation	4
Plantar grasp	Present at birth	9–10
Tonic neck	44 wks' postconceptual age	7
Ankle clonus (< 10 beats)	Normal in neonate without other neurologic abnormalities	1–2

tricular system appears at the rostral end. Elements of the peripheral nervous system, including sensory and sympathetic ganglia, are developing simultaneously. Insults interfering with these first-trimester events usually result in major structural deformities (e.g., meningomyelocele, encephalocele, holotelencephaly) that are immediately apparent at birth. The presence of major deformities, particularly those affecting both the cerebrum and the midline facial structures, should alert one to the probability of multiple congenital malformations involving additional organ systems. **Meningomyelocele** and **encephalocele** are generally associated only with other CNS anomalies (e.g., Arnold-Chiari malformation, polymicrogyria). Even when cord development progresses normally, positional changes in the caudal extent of the cord have clinical relevance for conduction anesthesia. In utero, the spinal cord initially extends the entire length of the vertebral canal; however, because the bony column grows more rapidly than the spinal cord itself, the caudal end of the cord gradually comes to lie at higher vertebral levels. At birth, the cord extends to the bottom of the third lumbar vertebra. Continued differential growth rates result in the final adult position at the L1–L2 interspace.

(2) Second and third trimesters

    (a) Neuronal multiplication and **migration** occur predominantly in the second and third trimesters with forebrain development preceding similar events in the cerebellum [59,65]. Immature neurons multiply in subependymal germinal matrixes along the neuraxis and migrate to their ultimate locations. Failure of these processes results in some forms of microcephaly and cortical malformations (e.g., schizencephaly, lissencephaly, pachygyria, and neuronal heterotopias) that may go unnoticed until the infant fails to achieve the usual

Table 15-4. Normal neurobehavioral development [24,48,54]

Age	Motor	Language	Interactive
28 wk	"Athetoid" Decreased tone Extension UE and LE	—	Briefly awakens with stimulation
32 wk	Extension UE Flexion LE	—	Spontaneous wakefulness
37 wk	Coordinated oral feeding without tiring	—	Cries when awake
Term	Flexion UE and LE	—	Distinct periods of attention
1 mon	Lifts chin when prone	Alerts to sound	Follows object or face 90-degree arc
2 mon	Lifts head when prone	Listens to voice	Responsive smile
3 mon	Lifts head/chest when prone	Coos	Clumsy reach toward familiar object or person
4 mon	Sits with support Grasps object	Orients toward voice	Laughs out loud
5–6 mon	Rolls supine to prone; hand-to-hand transfer	Babbles	Recognizes stranger; prefers mother
9–10 mon	Pulls to stand	Nonspecific "mama/dada"	Plays peek-a-boo and pat-a-cake
1 yr	Cruises; walks with support	Few words	Responds to name when called
15 mon	Walks well; neat pincer grasp	Follows simple commands	Gives hugs; indicates desires by pointing
18 mon	Runs stiffly	Identifies one or more body parts	Feeds self with spoon
2 yr	Walks up and down stairs	Calls self by name	Listens to story with pictures

UE = upper extremity; LE = lower extremity.

postnatal developmental milestones [27]. Hemorrhage into the periventricular germinal matrix is also a frequent cause of morbidity in premature infants.

(b) Brain mass increases early in life with 80% of adult weight being achieved by 2 years of age [39, 47]. Maximal growth rate occurs during the late fetal period and early infancy. It is largely due to proliferation of axons and dendrites and their supporting elements (glia, blood vessels, and myelin) with little increase in the number of individual neurons [13]. The appearance of synaptic connections accompanies the elaboration of axons and dendrites. This period of rapid growth is vulnerable to a variety of insults including hypoxia, ischemia, acidosis, and hemorrhage. The resulting major neurologic abnormalities (e.g., cerebral palsy) are thought to be due to interference with normal cellular differentiation and organization.

(c) **Myelination** begins during the sixth month of gestation and continues throughout adult life. Accomplishment of various motor and cognitive skills coincides with myelination of the corresponding neuronal pathways. Myelination is adversely affected by various metabolic and genetic defects (e.g., leukodystrophies) predominantly unrelated to fetal and perinatal events.

The **manifestation of significant neurologic impairment** may be subtle during infancy. Consequently, familiarity with normal neurobehavioral development is important for accurate assessment of a child scheduled for anesthesia and surgery. Both failure to achieve developmental milestones and persistence of primitive reflexes beyond their expected time of disappearance are significant findings on neurologic examination. Tables 15-3 and 15-4 provide reference for normal neurobehavioral development.

c. **Associated medical problems** (particularly those more common in children such as croup, asthma, or seizures), which may influence the choice of anesthetic agent.

d. **Use of medications** (e.g., anticonvulsants, corticosteroids, antihypertensives) that may require a change in dose or route of administration, or may affect the metabolism of other drugs used in the perioperative period.

e. **Previous drug reactions, allergies, or asthma** (especially if contrast agents are to be used for neuroradiologic studies).

f. **Family history** of adverse reaction to anesthetics, sudden infant death syndrome, metabolic disease, coagulopathy, sickle cell disease.

2. **Physical examination**

a. **Weight.** To guide drug administration, intraoperative fluid management, and estimation of allowable blood loss.

b. **Vital signs.** Normal values vary with age. Average awake, normal values are illustrated in Table 15-1.

c. **Temperature** exhibits diurnal variation with a nadir in the morning and zenith in the evening. This pattern is maintained even with illness. Children normally exhibit temperature elevation in hot weather, after exercise, and (important to the neurosurgical population) with **dehydration**. Some individuals normally exhibit temperatures slightly higher than average, and toddlers frequently have a rectal temperature of 37.7°C (99.8°F). In children with chronic illnesses, higher normal temperatures are occasionally seen. Average temperatures at rest are:

Oral: 35.8°C (96.5°F) to 37.2°C (99.0°F)
Rectal: up to 1.0°F higher than oral
Axillary: up to 1.0°F lower than oral

d. **Head and neck.** Adenotonsillar hypertrophy, macroglossia, dentition (present, absent, loose), anticipated ease of intubation.

e. **Respiratory system.** Evidence of upper respiratory infection (nasal crusting or rhinnitis), wheezing, cough, pneumonia.

f. **Cardiovascular system.** Congenital heart disease, especially right-to-left shunts that predispose the patient to paradoxical air emboli.

g. **Gastrointestinal system.** Nausea or vomiting, delayed gastric emptying, or increased gastric acidity may result from increased ICP.

h. **Neurologic assessment**

(1) Presence of **intracranial hypertension** (signs may be subtle; see sec. **I.D**). Headache is an infrequent complaint in young children; irritability, however, may represent its equivalent.

(2) **Level of consciousness** (airway protection, ability to cooperate with induction of anesthesia).

(3) **Respiratory pattern** (regularity, apnea).

(4) **Motor function** (strength, tone, denervation)

(a) **Strength** (ability to cough and breathe adequately, presence of adequate gag and swallowing mechanisms for airway protection).

(b) **Tone** (spasticity or hypotonia) may alter response to muscle relaxants or confuse assessment of their effectiveness. Contractures may cause difficulty with positioning for surgery.

(c) **Denervation** (spinal shock, autonomic instability, altered response to succinylcholine).

(5) **Deep tendon reflexes,** coordination, gait.

(6) **Pupillary responsiveness** and equality (detection of benign congenital anisocoria).

(7) **Cranial nerves.** Abnormality or asymmetry of function

may indicate increased ICP. **An abducens nerve (VI) palsy** often occurs in children with increased ICP, particularly in those with shunt obstruction. **Ophthalmoplegia** (setting sun sign) is also frequently apparent in infants with elevated ICP.

 i. **Hydration** may be altered as a result of prolonged vomiting, poor appetite, diabetes insipidus, inappropriate antidiuretic hormone secretion, fluid restriction, and osmotic diuretics or contrast agents. In the case of multiple trauma with closed head injury, occult bleeding must also be considered. Unlike adults, infants can demonstrate a significant drop in hematocrit as a result of intracranial bleeding alone. Furthermore, significant losses can occur from scalp lacerations. One should remember that skin turgor, moistness of mucous membranes, and urine output are more reliable signs of volume status in children than are BP and pulse rate. BP will be maintained until compensatory mechanisms have been exhausted, after which a precipitous decline will occur.

3. Laboratory data

 a. **Hematocrit** is useful both as a baseline and as a screening for disease states. It is the only test required for all children prior to anesthesia for neurosurgical procedures.

 b. **Additional studies** may include chest radiograph, electrocardiogram, urinalysis, urine electrolytes and osmolality, serum chemistries, sickle cell preparation, arterial or capillary blood gases, and anticonvulsant drug levels. An assessment of endocrine function is obtained in children with pituitary tumors. **Evaluation of clotting parameters is particularly important** in preparation for major intracranial or spinal surgery. The consequences of unexpected intraoperative or even moderate postoperative bleeding into the CNS may be devastating.

 c. **Neuroradiologic studies** may include skull radiograph, **computed tomography** (CT) scan, **magnetic resonance image** (MRI), and angiogram.

 d. Blood is sent for **type and crossmatch** for all major procedures. For infants weighing less than 5 kg, it is sometimes helpful to request that a unit of blood be split into two smaller aliquots. The reserved aliquot is maintained under usual storage conditions until subsequent transfusion is required, thereby limiting patient exposure to a minimal number of blood donors.

4. Permission for anesthesia is obtained from the parent or legal guardian for all but the emancipated minor. Good rapport with the parent and patient will facilitate a smooth induction.

5. NPO orders. No solid food or milk products for at least six to eight hours before induction. Clear liquids are withheld for varying lengths of time depending on age:

      a. **Neonate.** Offer clear liquids two hours before induction; then NPO.

      b. **1 to 6 months.** Offer clear liquids four hours before induction; then NPO.

      c. **6 to 36 months.** Offer clear liquids six hours before induction; then NPO.

      d. **Over 3 years.** Offer clear liquids eight hours before induction; then NPO.

Currently, preoperative fasting guidelines are undergoing re-evaluation, at least in the healthy pediatric outpatient population [55]; however, in neurosurgical patients who are likely to have delayed gastric emptying, it remains prudent to adhere to the aforementioned recommendations.

B. Premedication

    1. **Atropine** is not given on the ward as the vagolytic effect is usually gone by the time of induction, the antisialagogue effect is annoying and usually unnecessary, and it may be administered during induction if needed.

    2. **Narcotics** are avoided if intracranial hypertension, CNS depression, or hypotonia is suspected due to the adverse effects of potential respiratory depression and airway obstruction in these settings.

    3. **Sedatives** are avoided if intracranial hypertension, CNS depression, or hypotonia is suspected due to the adverse effects of potential respiratory depression and airway obstruction in these settings. Diazepam (0.1–0.5 mg/kg) or midazolam (0.3–0.5 mg/kg) may be given orally with a sip of water to anxious and alert patients who are 10 months or older; however, they should then be closely observed. Much smaller doses may be given intravenously to facilitate separation from parents.

    4. **Corticosteroids** are continued in the perioperative period. If recently discontinued after chronic use, adrenal suppression is assumed and supplemental steroids are given preoperatively or at induction and continued throughout the perioperative period.

    5. **Anticonvulsants** are continued in the perioperative period. Intravenous administration will be necessary if oral intake is restricted perioperatively. When the usual drug is unavailable in a parenteral form, it can frequently be given rectally. Fortunately, the half-life of most commonly used anticonvulsants is long, so that a missed dose intraoperatively can be made up later. Some anticonvulsants alter the metabolism of other medications.

    6. **Histamine-blocking agents** and **gastrointestinal motility agents** may be useful in the setting of elevated ICP and other medical conditions associated with delayed gastric emptying; however, **extrapyramidal side effects** may occur.

    7. **Rectal hypnotics.** The ability to promise no perioperative injections often greatly improves cooperation in children. **Methohexi-**

tal (25–30 mg/kg as a 10% solution in sterile water) is a safe and effective drug.

a. Advantages and contraindications

(1) Particularly useful in patients between 1 and 5 years of age who may be uncooperative. Sleep is induced within 10 minutes and persists for 30 minutes to an hour if the child is not disturbed. A second full or partial dose may be given if the first fails.

(2) Often administered to healthy children in their parents' presence but should only be given by an anesthesiologist in an area where resuscitation equipment is available.

(3) Does not require preoperative bowel preparation; however, the buttocks must be held together to prevent expulsion of the drug.

(4) Probably lowers ICP in the same manner as intravenous barbiturates if airway obstruction is prevented.

(5) Lower dose may calm a child sufficiently to allow placement of an intravenous catheter, or a smooth inhalation induction.

(6) May be given intramuscularly, 8 to 10 mg/kg, as a 5% solution in sterile water.

(7) Best avoided in patients who have complex psychomotor, temporal, or mixed seizure disorders as it can induce convulsions in the presence of these conditions. Rectal thiopental in the same dose is then preferable.

C. Monitoring

1. Standard monitoring includes BP, electrocardiogram, stethoscope, neuromuscular blockade, temperature, oxygen saturation by **pulse oximetry** (SpO_2) and **end-tidal carbon dioxide** ($EtCO_2$). Precordial Doppler, ICP, electroencephalogram, and **somatosensory evoked potentials** (SSEPs) are used when indicated as in adults. The small size of the patient may actually be an indication for a more aggressive, if necessarily invasive, approach since changes occur more rapidly and are often more difficult to detect accurately. Many monitors have limitations peculiar to children, including:

a. Stethoscope. Precordial or esophageal. Precordial is preferable for detection of a mainstem intubation.

b. Blood pressure. Appropriately sized cuff (should cover about two-thirds of the upper arm) with measurement by palpation, oscillation, or Doppler device; direct intra-arterial pressure monitoring is indicated for most intracranial procedures.

c. Pulse oximetry allows for noninvasive measurement of oxygen saturation. It is particularly useful in children by limiting repeat blood sampling, serving as an early detection device for **hypoxia** from any cause, and permitting titration of oxygen to avoid hyperoxia in infants less than 44 weeks post conceptual age. Any pulsatile vascular bed can be monitored, but digits (or palm/sole in premature infants) are usual sites.

d. Expired gas monitors. In small children, small tidal volumes, rapid respiratory rates, large fresh gas flows, and high sampling rates all contribute to the potential for **underestimation** of end-tidal gas concentrations. Displayed values frequently reflect a mixture of inspired and expired gas more than end-tidal values in the smallest patients. Increased dead space volume introduced by sensors is also a consideration in spontaneously breathing infants, although controlled ventilation is usually used during neurosurgical procedures. Endotracheal tube adapters with sampling ports are available, as are small sampling catheters for insertion into the endotracheal tube. These devices, coupled with manipulation of gas flow and respiratory parameters, usually provide useful data in most children. In-line, infrared carbon dioxide analyzers may be more accurate for use in very small patients than devices that aspirate gas samples. They weigh more, however, and care must be taken to ensure that they do not lead to an accidental extubation. Continuous capnography is essential for monitoring $EtCO_2$ when a significant risk of air embolism exists. Intermittent sampling by shared mass spectroscopy is insufficient under these circumstances.

e. Evoked potentials are monitored in children for similar indications as in adults. Additionally, however, SSEPs are particularly useful during surgery for spinal fusion, which is frequently done in the pediatric population for the treatment of scoliosis. Because SSEPs monitor only dorsal column function, they may **occasionally miss potential compromise** of the anterior spinal cord. Communication between the anesthesiologist and neurophysiologist is important to interpret changes that may be due to anesthetic agents.

2. Technical problems. Catheters are easier to insert following induction of anesthesia in children.

a. Arterial catheters. Catheters (22 or 24 gauge) can be placed percutaneously (or by cutdown) in the radial or dorsalis pedis artery, even in infants weighing less than 1000 gm. In the first days of life, an umbilical artery can be cannulated, providing, in addition to an intra-aortic catheter for monitoring and blood sampling, a portal for drug and fluid administration. It is important to position these catheters away from the renal arteries (either below T10 or above the diaphragm) to minimize the risk of renal infarction. Proper position should be confirmed radiographically.

b. Central venous catheters may be inserted through the umbilical vein in the first days of life. Portal vein thrombosis is an associated risk. Commercially available kits provide small catheters and wires (as small as 2.5 French for neonates) for percutaneous venous cannulation. Any vein used for access to the central circulation in adults can be used in children; however, there are a few special considerations:

(1) It may be helpful to cannulate the vein with a short plastic catheter and subsequently use that catheter as an introducer for the longer central line. This not only makes passage of the long catheter easier, it allows for repositioning without fear of shearing the catheter with a needle. In the event the central circulation cannot be entered, the initial catheter can be used for peripheral venous access.

(2) The basilic vein is often difficult to cannulate in children under five years of age; however, because of its safety, it should probably be attempted if visible or palpable.

(3) **Caution** is advised in cannulating the internal jugular vein, particularly in small children with intracranial pathology, because of the risk of occlusion of the relatively small vessel and resultant obstruction to cerebral venous drainage. In small infants, lateral positioning of the head alone is sufficient to markedly retard venous outflow [14,22]. The external jugular vein should be attempted first if visible.

(4) Cannulation of the femoral vein is easy and reliable at any age; however, special care must be exercised in small infants since an undeveloped hip capsule makes percutaneous entry into the joint more likely with the potential complication of septic necrosis.

   c. Urinary catheters. Infant feeding tubes are useful if Foley catheters are too large, although leaking may occur around them. Urine volume is more accurately estimated when collected into large syringes rather than drainage bags.

D. Special problems

1. Inaccessibility is frequently encountered during neurosurgical procedures and is more pronounced with pediatric patients. All tubes, catheters, and devices must be **securely fastened,** preferably with liquid adhesive prior to taping. Vascular catheters can be further protected by hard plastic "tents" placed over limbs to prevent pressure from surgical drapes and personnel. Slight displacement of the endotracheal tube (whether from motion of the tube or change in head position) can cause either extubation or bronchial intubation in small children. The small diameter of pediatric endotracheal tubes makes them especially vulnerable to kinking. Disconnection of vascular catheters under the drapes can rapidly result in hypovolemia, hypotension, or air embolism. When possible, a small, well-lit tunnel is created to provide a view of the patient, the airway, and the catheters.

2. **Positioning.** Children are at great risk if all pressure points are not protected during positioning. The consequences of surgical personnel leaning on the patient may be serious. Mechanical devices (such as a metal triangle or Mayo stand) may be secured to the operating table and placed between the surgeon and the patient. **Care** must be taken to avoid stretch or pressure on peripheral nerves (e.g., a limb extending over the edge of the table) and compression of vital areas (e.g., pressure on the eyes with incorrect positioning on a headrest). **Eyes** should be further protected with lubricant and taped closed. Once properly positioned, complete immobility must be ensured.

   a. **Sitting.** Fortunately, the sitting position is rarely used for children less than 3 years of age. When it is required, essential monitoring includes a capnograph and a precordial Doppler to assist in the early detection of air emboli. A right atrial catheter can be helpful if massive air embolism occurs. Because of a greater risk of paradoxical air emboli, this position is avoided in children with a known intracardiac shunt. The 20% incidence of probe patent foramen ovale has led some to question whether the sitting position should be used at all [1]. Early detection and prevention of entrainment of large volumes of air are essential.

   b. **Prone.** For the prone position, care must be taken to ensure free abdominal and chest wall motion to avoid both impairment of respiration and increased intra-abdominal pressure leading to an increase in venous pressure and, therefore, increased bleeding. The child is usually supported by padding under the chest and pelvis; pressure on the genitalia is avoided. Inevitably, some equipment must be disconnected while the patient is positioned; **constant attention should be directed toward the heart tones** audible with the esophageal stethoscope, and periods of monitoring "blackout" should be minimal.

3. **Temperature control**

   a. **Hypothermia** is a common problem during anesthesia for pediatric neurosurgery. Children have a greater surface area–to-weight ratio, less insulating fat, and higher metabolic rates than adults. They, therefore, produce more heat that potentially can be lost. CNS abnormalities may predispose children to autonomic dysfunction and temperature instability. Pediatric operations are also often performed in rooms with ambient temperature controlled for the comfort of the operating room personnel.

   Although mild hypothermia decreases brain energy requirements and may be beneficial in paralyzed patients, its deleterious effects become important during the recovery period. Shivering will increase ICP and oxygen consumption. Metabolic acidosis may depress cardiac output, and arrhythmias commonly occur when the body temperature falls below 30°C. If the patient is to remain paralyzed and sedated, then mild hypothermia is permissible. If extubation is anticipated, efforts must be made to maintain near normal body temperature, since it is difficult to rewarm a patient in the operating room once the temperature has fallen.

b. Normothermia

(1) Aids in maintaining normothermia in children include the following:

(a) Warm the room before induction and maintain the warm environment at least until surgical preparation is completed.

(b) Limit time of body exposure, especially to cleansing solutions.

(c) Provide **overhead warmers** for infants (servo-controlled to body temperature to avoid overheating) and heating lamps for older children. Lamps should be at least 36 in. away from the skin to avoid burns.

(d) Provide a **heated water mattress,** especially for children less than 10 kg (about 1 year of age).

(e) Place **covers** over uninvolved areas of the body.

(f) Heat and humidify inspired gases. Measuring inspired gas temperature will help to avoid airway burns. Alternatively, heat/moisture exchangers may be used, but these can occlude with airway secretions.

(g) Warm all intravenous solutions and blood products.

4. **Anesthesia circuits.** All systems applicable to the general practice of pediatric anesthesia can be used for neurosurgical procedures. Mechanical ventilation is desirable for procedures that require careful, stable control of $PaCO_2$. All systems should provide a method of humidifying inspired gases. Unnecessary dead space should be eliminated. For children over 3 years of age, the standard semi-closed reabsorber circuit is used. The resistance created by one-way valves may be excessive for younger children unless ventilation is controlled. If spontaneous ventilation is desired for neonates and small children, a Mapleson D or Bain circuit is frequently used, with fresh gas flows of at least twice the minute ventilation to prevent rebreathing (a normal minute ventilation in the neonate is approximately 100 ml/kg). It should be remembered that $EtCO_2$ will be underestimated under these circumstances (see sec. **II.C.1.d).**

5. **Fluid and electrolyte replacement.** Various formulas are used to

estimate maintenance fluid requirements. An easily remembered one for calculating hourly fluid requirement is the following:

4 ml/kg/hour	0 to 10 kg
2 ml/kg/hour	10 to 20 kg
1 ml/kg/hour	>20 kg

Example: 25-kg child:

4 ml/kg/hour × 1st 10 kg	40 ml/hour
2 ml/kg/hour × 2nd 10 kg (10–20 kg)	20 ml/hour
1 ml/kg/hour × 5 kg (20–25 kg)	5 ml/hour
Total hourly requirement	65 ml/hour

In cases where blood loss is not a major concern, the estimated deficit is replaced, if necessary, with crystalloid solution slowly during the case. If blood loss is likely, half the estimated deficit is replaced over the first hour, and one-fourth of the deficit is replaced over each of the subsequent two hours. The choice of electrolyte solution is similar to that for adults except, perhaps, that very small infants receive supplementation with glucose-containing solutions to avoid hypoglycemia. When large quantities of glucose-containing solutions are given, however, hyperglycemia usually occurs. Elevated serum glucose may be detrimental to ischemic brain because it provides more substrate for anaerobic metabolism and results in more severe lactic acidosis [56]. Serum glucose usually remains within acceptable limits during surgery when deficit, third space, and allowable blood loss are replaced with a glucose-free, salt solution (e.g., normal saline or lactated Ringer's solution). If glucose administration is indicated, a rate equal to one-half the calculated hourly maintenance requirement is usually adequate. Hypotonic solutions are best avoided, and normal saline (with an osmolality of 308 mosm/L) may be preferable to lactated Ringer's solution (with an osmolality of 273 mosm/L) when brain edema is a concern.

6. **Blood loss and replacement.** Blood loss is often difficult to estimate accurately. Much of the blood lost is absorbed onto the drapes, and irrigation solutions confuse sponge weights and suction measurements. Nevertheless, it is important to attempt to **estimate losses.** Accuracy can be improved if the surgeon communicates the volume of blood lost as it occurs and if all suctioned blood is collected in calibrated bottles (such as empty 250-ml intravenous fluid bottles). Serial measurement of the hematocrit will reflect blood loss during replacement with crystalloid solution.

   a. **Crossmatched blood.** Preoperatively, an adequate amount of crossmatched blood should be available, and clotting studies should be normal. It is important to be sure that all neonates have received **prophylactic vitamin K₁,** (1 mg IM), to prevent hemorrhagic disease of the newborn. Preoperative dehydration may cause a false elevation in hematocrit so that blood requirements may actually be greater than initially anticipated.

b. **Adequate and timely blood replacement is imperative.** Whereas an adult must lose approximately 500 ml to suffer a 10% loss of blood volume, the comparable amount in a neonate may be less than 25 ml. The hematocrit at which blood transfusion is indicated has become less rigidly defined as the risks associated with transfusion have increased. Transfusion can probably be avoided if a postoperative hematocrit in the 20s is anticipated for children older than 3 months of age; however, in accepting a low hematocrit, one must ensure an otherwise healthy patient with a preponderance of hemoglobin A, cardiovascular and respiratory stability, and no anticipated postoperative blood loss. In infants under 3 months of age, a postoperative hematocrit of 30 or greater is desirable as apnea may be more likely in the severely anemic infant and hematopoiesis may not yet be occurring. When blood transfusion is required, sufficient blood should be given from one donor to raise the hematocrit to the mid-40s in an effort to avoid repeat transfusions with blood from additional donors. Each 10 cc of packed red cells transfused per kilogram of body weight will raise the hematocrit approximately 4%. In small patients, packed cells can be administered more rapidly and accurately if they are drawn into a 60-cc syringe and then warmed. Calcium, 10 mg/kg, is useful when hypotension accompanies rapid administration of blood or blood components containing citrate as an anticoagulant. Because of the risk of communicable disease, fresh-frozen plasma should be used only when a coagulopathy exists. If simple dilution or volume expansion is needed, 5% albumin is an effective choice.

c. **Procedure.** When **extensive blood loss** is anticipated, blood is administered on a milliliter-for-milliliter basis from the start of the procedure. Intravenous access, with catheters of adequate caliber and number, must be secured preoperatively, even if surgical cutdown is required. Great care is necessary to **prevent air bubbles** from entering lines as unsuspected right-to-left intracardiac shunts may be present (especially in neonates).

d. **Blood volume** is estimated as 90 ml/kg in premature infants, 85 ml/kg in full-term infants, 80 ml/kg in children, and 70 ml/kg in adolescents. Acceptable blood loss can be estimated by multiplying the percentage of tolerable hematocrit loss (based on a lower limit of 25) by the blood volume. **Example:**

1. Beginning hematocrit = 40
   Lowest acceptable hematocrit = 25
   Weight = 20 kg
   Estimated blood volume = 20 kg × 80 ml/kg = 1600 ml
2. Estimated acceptable blood loss = $\dfrac{40 - 25}{40}$ × 1600 = 600 ml

If the amount of actual blood loss is less than half the acceptable blood loss, replacement is with crystalloid solution. If the loss is greater than this but less than the acceptable blood loss, 5% albumin is then used. Losses greater than the calculated acceptable blood loss are replaced with packed red cells. In cases of massive replacement (more than the child's blood volume), the administration of fresh-frozen plasma (10 ml/kg) and platelets (0.1–0.2 units/kg) may be necessary to correct coagulopathies. In special circumstances when cryoprecipitate is required, 1 unit per 5 to 10 kg will bring fibrinogen and factor VIII levels into the normal range.

7. **Drug dosing.** All medications should be titrated to effect, although familiarity with average mg/kg requirements is helpful. For emergency situations, doses for children can be estimated as a percentage of the average adult dose. **Dose estimates:**

Age	Weight (kg)	Fraction of adult dose
Neonate	3	$\frac{1}{10}$
1 year	10	$\frac{1}{4}$
7 years	25	$\frac{1}{2}$
12 years	40	$\frac{3}{4}$

E. Induction

In general, all patients who have major medical problems, whether adults or children, should have an **intravenous cannula securely in place before the induction of anesthesia.** Because of the high metabolic rates in children, a critical situation can develop rapidly. Attempts to insert an intravenous catheter under emergency conditions during or after induction can be difficult. Pediatricians routinely place catheters in children of all ages without the child's cooperation; when necessary, anesthesiologists should do the same. The procedure is greatly simplified if local anesthesia is used at the insertion site prior to placing the catheter. The sicker the child, the easier the procedure.

Once an intravenous catheter is in place, induction can proceed as with adults. In the presence of intracranial hypertension, voluntary hyperventilation with oxygen in the cooperative child, and the use of mannitol, 0.5 to 1.0 mg/kg, can improve intracranial compliance.

1. **Emergency surgery.** Intubation is often performed in neonates while they are awake to ensure an adequate airway; however, awake intubation in the neonate has been associated with significant increases in BP and ICP [31, 42, 50] and may be a contributing factor in the pathogenesis of intraventricular hemorrhage in premature babies. In neonates with elevated ICP and a normal airway, an intravenous induction with cricoid pressure may be preferred. By approximately 1 month of age, the infant is sufficiently vigorous to make awake intubation difficult unless he or she is gravely ill. Older infants and children with a full stomach also receive a rapid-sequence induction using a barbiturate, muscle relaxant, and cricoid pressure. **Atropine** (0.01–0.02 mg/kg) is frequently given prior to induction to prevent a vagal response to laryngoscopy. Because of the delayed gastric emptying associated with intracranial hypertension, gastric contents are emptied via a large-bore suction catheter prior to awake intubation or following rapid-sequence intubation and throughout surgery.

2. **Elective surgery**
   a. **Neonates.** Awake intubation or intravenous induction as described in sec. **II.E.1.** Inhalation induction (as described for older children below) may also be used.
   b. **Children under 5 years of age.** Children between 1 and 5 years of age usually resist separation from their parents. Furthermore, they may be frightened by an anesthesia mask and smell of inhalation anesthetics. Rectal barbiturates or oral benzodiazepines (see sec. **II.B**) are particularly useful. Once consciousness is blunted, an intravenous catheter can be placed using local anesthesia or an inhalation induction can be performed, as described below.
   c. **Children over 5 years of age.** Older children will usually cooperate with an inhalation induction when offered as an alternative to a needle. Of the volatile agents, **halothane** provides the smoothest induction. Hyperventilation prior to the introduction of halothane appears to blunt the increase in ICP caused by this cerebral vasodilator in adults, but the effect of this maneuver in children is unknown. It would certainly appear safe, however, to combine the use of low concentrations of halothane with muscle relaxants and controlled hyperventilation. Deep levels of anesthesia necessary to accomplish intubation using inhalation drugs alone will reduce BP and simultaneously elevate ICP, thereby decreasing CPP.

3. **Barbiturates. Thiopental,** 4 to 6 mg/kg, or **methohexital,** 1 to 2 mg/kg, given intravenously, are ultrashort-acting hypnotics that

have ICP-lowering properties and may be used for induction. Other barbiturates (pentobarbital and phenobarbital) take longer to equilibrate with the CNS and have more prolonged effects. They are, therefore, not generally used for surgical anesthesia but may have a role in sedation for neuroradiologic procedures or in the intensive care unit.

4. **Narcotics.** Infants, especially those less than 3 months of age, have an unpredictable response to narcotics. Because of the potential for respiratory depression, they are avoided as premedicants; however, in the controlled operating room setting, they can be titrated cautiously once ventilation is assured. Typical doses are 1 to 3 μg/kg of **fentanyl** or 0.1 to 0.2 mg/kg of **morphine,** with subsequent doses of approximately 1 to 2 μg/kg/hour of fentanyl or 0.05 mg/kg/hour of morphine. Sufentanil and alfentanil are also potentially useful in infants and children. Infants less than 3 months of age who receive narcotics should be monitored in the postoperative period to ensure adequate respiration.

5. **Propofol** is a recently approved intravenous anesthetic finding wide application both in induction and maintenance of anesthesia. Because it allows for rapid recovery, it is especially useful for short procedures in both inpatient and outpatient populations. Propofol has been found to reduce both CBF and $CMRO_2$ but decreases MAP somewhat more than thiopental [7]; however, recent data suggest that it can be used safely for sedation in intensive care unit patients with both normal and compromised intracranial compliance [63]. Experience with propofol in pediatric anesthesia is limited, particularly in small children. In unpremedicated children, 2.5 to 3.0 mg/kg has been found to be an effective induction dose [28]. It may also prove to be particularly useful as a sedative for neuroradiologic procedures [61] and for brief outpatient procedures in pediatric oncology patients [4].

F. **Intubation**

1. A **small air leak** should be audible around the endotracheal tube when an airway pressure of approximately 25 cm H_2O is applied. If no leak is audible, the tube is probably too large and may increase the risk of postoperative croup or lead to ischemia of the subglottic region, which can ultimately result in subglottic stenosis.

2. A rough guide to the choice of endotracheal tube size is as follows:

Age	Size (mm I.D.)
< 28 weeks' gestation (about 1000 gm)	2.5
28 to 38 weeks' gestation (1000–3000 gm)	3.0
Term neonate	3.5
9 months to 1 year	4.0
2 years and older: calculate mm I.D. by the following formula:	

$$\text{Endotracheal tube size} = \frac{16 + \text{age (years)}}{4}$$

3. **Cuffed endotracheal tubes** are generally used only in children who require size 6.0 mm or greater (i.e., over 8 years of age by the formula given here).
4. **Straight laryngoscope blades** are easier to use in children under 5 years of age.
5. Endotracheal tubes must be **securely fastened** with liquid adhesive and tape, since slight motion can cause displacement. If oral tubes are used, they should be placed on the side of the mouth that will be turned upward so that saliva will not loosen the tape.
6. **Nasal tubes** are easier to secure.
7. To prevent gastric dilatation, an oral airway can be inserted to allow for the venting of gases that leak around the endotracheal tube. Alternatively, the gastric tube used for aspiration of stomach contents at induction may be left in place and open throughout the case.
8. **Relaxants**
   a. **Depolarizing drugs. Succinylcholine** is frequently used to facilitate intubation because of its rapid onset and brief duration; however, it may induce a hyperkalemic response in patients who have been at prolonged bedrest with ongoing disuse muscular atrophy, or, in those who have stroke, encephalitis, muscular dystrophies, tetanus, spinal cord dysfunction, severe head injuries, burns, or massive trauma. The hyperkalemic response has not been reported with isolated intracranial hypertension, but caution is advised if motor dysfunction is present. Interestingly, meningomyelocele does not appear to increase the risk of hyperkalemia following succinylcholine [17]. Succinylcholine can also cause myoglobinemia and myoglobinuria, and can initiate malignant hyperthermia in susceptible children. It has also been shown to elevate ICP due to an increase in $CMRO_2$ resulting from muscle spindle afferents; however, this response is less significant following barbiturate induction and pretreatment with nondepolarizing relaxants. The dose for intubation is 1.0 to 1.5 mg/kg IV or 3 to 4 mg/kg IM. It is helpful to pretreat children with **atropine,** 0.01 to 0.02 mg/kg, to prevent dysrhythmias due to the vagomimetic properties of succinylcholine.
   b. **Nondepolarizing drugs. Pancuronium** (0.1–0.15 mg/kg) is particularly useful in children since cardiac output is better maintained when the heart rate is high. Increasing the dose will effect a more rapid onset so that pancuronium may be used, even under emergency conditions, if succinylcholine is contraindicated. Curare or atracurium, 0.5 mg/kg, provides intubating conditions in a few minutes, but are generally avoided because of their histamine-releasing properties (unless hypotension is desired or

ICP is not elevated). **Metacurine,** 0.25 mg/kg, or **vecuronium,** 0.1 mg/kg, provides cardiac stability and is used when tachycardia is not desirable. A more rapid onset of muscular blockade can be achieved by increasing the intubating dose by 50 to 100%. One must, however, expect a **prolonged duration of paralysis,** particularly in small infants. Additional drug should be given in increments of one-fourth to one-third the intubating dose. A neuromuscular blockade monitor is helpful in guiding drug administration.

9. **Lidocaine.** 1.0 to 1.5 mg/kg IV given a few minutes before laryngoscopy and intubation may help blunt the ICP-increasing effects of these procedures in patients who have poor intracranial compliance [26]. Additional thiopental or fentanyl may be equally effective for this purpose.

G. **Extubation.** The **neurologic exam** is the most useful means of assessing a neurosurgical patient in the postoperative period. It is, therefore, desirable to have an awake and responsive patient at the completion of surgery. Effort must also be directed toward control of hypertension, coughing, and struggling as the patient emerges from anesthesia. Adequate narcotic analgesia, with or without intravenous lidocaine, and maintenance of muscle relaxation until just prior to extubation, will all help to realize these goals. Early discontinuation of any inhalational agent is also helpful. Antihypertensive agents are usually unnecessary for emergence in children when analgesia is adequate.

H. **Anesthetic techniques**

1. **Local anesthesia** alone is usually insufficient for children undergoing neurosurgical procedures but may be helpful as an adjuvant to minimize the depth of general anesthesia required. It may permit insertion of a ventricular catheter for CSF drainage prior to induction when ICP is markedly elevated. Local anesthetic solutions are also frequently used as "carriers" for epinephrine when vasoconstriction is necessary to limit blood loss with incision of highly vascular structures such as the scalp. An easy method to administer a safe dose of both local anesthetic and epinephrine is to use 0.5 ml/kg of 0.5% lidocaine (or bupivacaine) with 1 : 200,000 epinephrine. This limits the local anesthetic to 2.5 mg/kg and the epinephrine to 2.5 μg/kg. Local anesthesia may also be supplemented with intravenous sedation in adolescents to facilitate brief, usually radiologic, procedures involving little stimulation.

2. **General anesthesia. Ventilation** is controlled in all infants. All halogenated inhalation anesthetics are cerebral vasodilators and should be used in low concentrations and coupled with hyperventilation when ICP is elevated until the dura is opened. Isoflurane has

some theoretic advantages for neurosurgical patients in that it provides cardiovascular stability while provoking the smallest increase in CBF and greatest decrease in $CMRO_2$. When used with hyperventilation, effects on ICP are usually minimal. Halothane, however, generally offers a smoother mask induction, and in children, the ability to induce anesthesia without breath holding, coughing, and laryngospasm (thereby avoiding the adverse effects on ICP) far outweighs the potential advantages of isoflurane. Once induction and intubation are complete, isoflurane may be substituted for halothane. Enflurane offers no advantage over these agents and may be epileptogenic, especially when combined with hyperventilation. Additionally, enflurane may lead to an increase in CSF production, thereby increasing ICP in a manner unresponsive to hyperventilation [32].

All of the intravenous anesthetics used in adults produce similar effects in children. Numerous cases of sudden and severe increases in ICP have been reported after administration of ketamine, especially in infants and children with hydrocephalus. Most other intravenous sedatives reduce CBF and metabolism when ventilation is controlled. A **balanced technique** using nitrous oxide, oxygen, barbiturates, muscle relaxants, narcotics, and sedatives can be used for all age groups.

I. **Postoperative care.** Repeated neurologic examination is the most important factor in assessing postoperative recovery. Deterioration in neurologic function is often a sign of intracranial bleeding. Therefore, it is usually desirable to have the child as fully **alert** as possible immediately following surgery. Neuromuscular blockade can be pharmacologically reversed with neostigmine (0.06–0.08 mg/kg) and atropine or glycopyrulate. ICP can be assessed most effectively in the unconscious or paralyzed patient by continuous monitoring.

CT scans are extremely valuable in evaluating increasing ICP or deteriorating neurologic status to determine the presence of surgically correctable causes. Cranial ultrasound techniques may be useful if the fontanelles are open. Careful assessment of fluid and electrolyte status is necessary, particularly after operations in the region of the pituitary gland. Close observation in an intensive care unit familiar with the care of children is essential to the early detection and treatment, if not prevention, of postoperative complications. Screaming and combativeness can elevate ICP and increase bleeding. The **judicious use of narcotics** may be helpful for control of pain and agitation; however, arterial blood gases should be monitored closely to avoid carbon dioxide retention. Postoperative vomiting will also increase ICP. **Droperidol** is a useful antiemetic, and, in doses of 10 to 20 μg/kg, does not produce noticeable sedation.

III. Special procedures. With an understanding of the special problems presented by children, the anesthesiologist can offer the same standard of care to patients of all ages. Special requirements for each procedure should be considered. The following is a brief discussion of the more **common operations and diagnostic studies** that require anesthesia and their relevant concerns.

A. Neurosurgical disorders

   1. Tumors. Most craniotomies in children are for tumors. **Brain tumors** are the most common solid tumor in childhood and are second only to leukemia as the leading cancer. Contrary to the situation in adults, most pediatric brain tumors are **infratentorial** and are still occasionally approached surgically with the patient in a sitting position (see sec. **II.D.2**). Intracranial hypertension is always a possibility. Because of the small posterior fossa compartment, patients are frequently symptomatic with brainstem compression. Intraoperatively, further compression or surgical trauma can result in dysrhythmias or BP instability [2]. The surgeon should be immediately informed of any such occurrence as it will usually abate with cessation of direct surgical stimulation. Delayed awakening, altered airway reflexes, vocal cord paralysis, and abnormal respiratory patterns may become apparent on emergence. In the postoperative period, the child is closely monitored in an intensive care unit for bleeding, seizures, level of consciousness, and electrolyte abnormalities.

   a. Craniopharyngioma is usually a benign tumor presenting in childhood. Associated morbidity is related to its proximity to the pituitary gland and optic chiasm. Preoperative evaluation should assess thyroid and adrenal function, as well as fluid and electrolyte status. Resection is often via a transphenoidal approach but may entail frontal craniotomy. Accurate monitoring of fluid intake and output is essential as diabetes inspidus is a potential perioperative problem. Initial treatment is replacement of free water; intranasal or intravenous DDAVP is used when replacement is inadequate.

   2. Vascular anomalies include **arteriovenous malformations** (AVM) and aneurysms. It is unusual for elevated ICP to be present except where CSF drainage is obstructed due to the abnormal vessels themselves, or due to a prior bleed. Premedication is, therefore, both safe and desirable in older infants and children. Aneurysms are rare in children. AVMs most frequently present in infancy as high-output congestive heart failure (CHF). Seizures and intraparenchymal hemorrhage are more usual in older children. The vein of Galen aneurysm is actually the result of increased flow, usually due to a deeper AVM that drains into the vein of Galen or one of its tributaries [38]. This lesion, which represents about 1% of

AVMs in children, is almost uniformly fatal in the neonate whether medically or surgically managed. If presentation is later in life, mortality drops significantly and is about 25% if surgical repair is undertaken after 1 year of age. Cardiac death is most frequent. CHF, usually present preoperatively, can also occur acutely during surgery as systemic vascular resistance abruptly increases with clipping of the aneurysm. Infarction may result from poor coronary perfusion (low diastolic pressure). Uncontrolled hemorrhage is also responsible for both preoperative and surgical deaths. The long-term outlook for survivors is poor with significant neurologic impairment the rule. The anesthetic regimen should minimize cardiovascular depression (CHF) and maintain a reduced, but stable BP (minimize transmural pressure gradients to prevent rupture), while providing adequate cerebral and coronary perfusion, all in a setting of markedly changing systemic vascular resistance. Venous air embolism is also a concern. Smaller AVMs, especially those that are surgically inaccessible, may be treated with stereotactic radiosurgery.

3. **Trauma.** Accidents are the most frequent cause of death in children. The majority of these fatalities are caused by **head injury.** Initial evaluation and managment is focused on airway (trauma, bleeding, reflexes), breathing (rate, tidal volume, pattern), and circulation (rhythm, BP, perfusion). Unlike adults, infants can demonstrate a significant drop in BP (and hematocrit) as a result of intracranial bleeding alone. Of course, the possibility of intrathoracic and intra-abdominal bleeding should not be ignored. A Glasgow coma score below 6 is associated with high mortality in children [8,10,36]. Because of incomplete ossification, cervical spine fractures may not always be detected on standard neck films in small children. If a CT is not available, a fracture should be considered, and axial traction to immobilize the neck should be provided by an assistant during tracheal intubation and positioning of the patient. The cribriform plate is easily fractured with trauma, making placement of nasal tubes inadvisable in a child with midfacial injury or nasal discharge or bleeding. The response to head injury in children is more frequently global brain swelling rather than hematoma formation as in adults [8,10]. With early aggressive management to control ICP and maintain CPP, the prognosis for children suffering head injury is better than that for adults with similar presentations [11,36].

4. **Craniofacial deformities. Craniosynostosis** is the premature closure, usually in utero, of one or more cranial sutures. Most commonly, only one suture is involved and the problem is essentially cosmetic. Elevated ICP is prevented by expansion of the skull at the unfused suture sites. Multiple synostoses are more commonly

associated with increased ICP, and, if not corrected, can lead to retardation and optic atrophy. Multiple synostoses are frequently seen in combination with facial anomalies (such as Apert's and Crouzon's syndromes).

   a. **Brain growth,** which is the normal stimulus for expansion and shaping of the head, occurs very rapidly in infancy. Brain size doubles in the first 6 months of life and reaches 80% of the adult weight by 2 years of age. Surgical intervention is usually recommended at 4 to 6 weeks of age to achieve the greatest cosmetic benefit [19]. Correction of extensive craniofacial malformations is staged to allow for differing rates of growth between the skull and facial bones. The sutures are opened early and facial correction delayed for several years.

   b. **Intraoperative concerns** are numerous. Large blood loss is frequent in all but single-suture repairs, and the minimal requirement for available blood should equal the patient's blood volume. Occasionally blood loss can be massive if a sinus is accidentally opened. Air emboli can occur even in the supine position, particularly in infants with large heads and large bony excisions. Occasionally, it is helpful to shrink the brain with diuretics, osmotic agents, or CSF drainage. The oculocardiac reflex may result from traction on the eye muscles or globe during surgery. Additionally, the potential for an abnormal airway must be considered. When the surgical procedure involves the facial structures, it is helpful to secure the endotracheal tube by suturing it to the nasal septum or by wiring to the teeth. Despite these maneuvers, one must remain watchful for changes in position of the endotracheal tube with changes in head position. Aspiration of blood and debris can be minimized during intraoral procedures by packing the pharynx with sponges. Pneumothoraxes may develop when rib grafts are used as part of the repair. The possibility of airway edema and obstruction must be carefully considered prior to any decision to extubate at the completion of surgery.

   c. **Monitoring** for all cases, with the exception of a single-suture repair, should include an arterial line. Since air emboli are possible, a capnograph and precordial Doppler are useful. Placement of a right atrial catheter may also be considered [29,30]. A postoperative chest radiograph is obtained when rib grafts have been used in reconstruction.

5. **Dysraphism.** Failure of closure of the neural tube during the fourth week of gestation results in a spectrum of defects ranging from anencephaly to spina bifida occulta. Neurologic deficits accompany most defects involving neural tissue; however, the size of the sac is not indicative of the amount of neural tissue involved. Whether dysraphism occurs in the spine (myelocele or meningomy-

elocele), or in the head (encephalocele or encephalomeningocele), repairs are usually undertaken at an early age because of the risk of infection. Preservation of viable nervous tissue is also a goal.

Hydrocephalus usually coexists in infants with meningomyelocele and paralysis below the lesion. This is most often due to an associated aqueductal stenosis or Arnold-Chiari malformation (a downward displacement of cerebellar and brainstem structures into a deformity of the upper cerival spine). Extremes of neck extension can cause brainstem compression, as can occur with tumors of the posterior fossa. Positioning for intubation is complicated by the presence of exposed neural tissue, which must remain free of pressure. If supine, the infant is elevated onto rolls at the shoulders and pelvis. The meningomyelocele can be protected with a sterile "doughnut." The left lateral position may also be used. Neuromuscular blockade is avoided (or carefully monitored) if the surgeon plans direct stimulation to identify viable neural tissue. Although blood loss is usually only moderate, extensive undermining of skin to facilitate closure of larger defects may make transfusion necessary. Autonomic control below the level of the lesion is abnormal and effort must be directed toward conserving body heat.

Encephaloceles most commonly occur in the occipital area. When large amounts of brain tissue within the defect appear viable, a dural graft preserves function and prevents bradycardia associated with returning the brain to the intracranial compartment under tension. Additional anesthetic considerations are similar to those for meningomyelocele repair. Prognosis for neurologic development depends on the amount of herniated brain tissue and the presence of hydrocephalus. Frontal encephaloceles, although much less common, are often associated with midline facial defects.

6. **Hydrocephalus.** Most hydrocephalus in neonates is due to obstruction of the CSF circulation either within the ventricular system (noncommunicating hydrocephalus) or at the sites of reabsorption of CSF (communicating hydrocephalus). Obstruction can result from congenital malformations, or from scar tissue or fibrin deposits following intraventricular hemorrhage or infection. CSF is usually shunted from the lateral ventricle to the peritoneal cavity. Occasionally, the distal end is placed in the right atrium. In this setting, care must be taken to ensure accurate positioning and to avoid intravascular air. Ventriculoperitoneal shunts are preferable because of their lower rate of complications and less frequent need for revisions with growth.

The child with hydrocephalus usually has intracranial hypertension, and its presence affects the anesthetic plan. If shunt revision is to be performed, ICP may be reduced preoperatively by withdrawing CSF from the shunt reservoir when only the distal end of the catheter is obstructed. The sudden removal of large volumes of CSF from the ventricles may, however, result in upward displacement of the brainstem, producing signs similar to herniation. Replacement of fluid (CSF or saline) can be an effective temporizing measure.

B. Neuroradiologic procedures entail special risks. They are usually performed in an environment not designed for pediatric anesthesia and located far from support facilities. When contrast agents are used, the danger of allergic reactions exists, and an osmotic diuresis occurs, which may complicate fluid management. Frequently, the patient must be monitored via closed-circuit television while radiation is in use. Whenever possible (see limitations sec. **2**), **monitoring** should be similar to that in the operating room and be visible, along with the patient, from outside the room. It is **essential that the anesthesiologist be certain all necessary supplies and equipment are available and functioning.**

1. **CT scan** requires that the patient be immobilized. Sedation (oral, rectal, intramuscular, or intravenous) and occasionally general anesthesia may be necessary for uncooperative patients; however, young children are usually well controlled with rectal barbiturates. Neonates and small babies can sometimes be scanned while they sleep immediately after feeding, but they often benefit from oral or rectal **chloral hydrate,** 50 to 75 mg/kg, to ensure that they remain still.

2. **MRI** uses a strong magnetic field and radiofrequency pulses to generate an image. Scanning is a relatively slow process and therefore requires that the patient be immobilized longer than for CT scanning. In addition, image quality is degraded by the presence of ferrous material or deflection of the radiofrequency pulses. Objects made of ferrous metals can become airborne missiles in the presence of the magnet and may result in injury. Consequently, anesthesia and monitoring equipment must be constructed entirely of nonferrous metal or placed far away from the magnet. Through modifications with long cords, SpO_2 and Doppler BP monitoring are possible. Modification of the anesthesia machine, and lengthening of the anesthesia circuit, allow safe general anesthesia when necessary [51]; however, intravenous sedation provides satisfactory conditions for scanning in many patients. MRI itself is attractive for pediatric neuroradiologic diagnosis since it does not use ionizing radiation, and provides excellent resolution in the posterior fossa and brainstem. Additionally, intravenous contrast agents are often unnecessary. Although brief exposure to the magnetic field appears to be safe, the effect of long-term exposure, and therefore the risk to medical personnel, are unknown [12].

3. **Arteriography.** The intraarterial injection of contrast material produces pain and causes children to respond by moving. **General**

anesthesia is usually required. In the presence of elevated ICP, ventilation is controlled to produce hypocapnia. Cerebral vasoconstriction induced by hyperventilation slows transit time and diverts contrast agents from normal (vasoconstricting) to abnormal (poorly responsive) areas of the brain and may improve the resolution of the angiogram. The anesthesiologist should be familiar with **dose limitations** and **potential side effects** of the particular agent being used. Approximately 5 to 8% of radiologic procedures using contrast agents are complicated by systemic reactions [21]. **Resuscitation drugs and equipment** must be available at all times. Prophylaxis with steroids and antihistamines has been beneficial in patients with a history of allergies and those with a prior reaction to contrast agents [23]. Contrast agents have also been associated with nephrotoxicity. **Adequate hydration** is necessary to minimize this risk, particularly in patients with preexisting renal dysfunction.

4. **Pneumoencephalography** is rarely performed since the advent of CT scanning. If intracranial hypertension is suspected, the study is performed through a ventriculostomy and not via the lumbar subarachnoid space. Extreme changes in position during the procedure require that all tubes and lines be firmly anchored. The patient is closely monitored and is promptly returned to the supine position at any sign of distress. If air is used as the contrast medium, the administration of **nitrous oxide** as part of the anesthetic can cause expansion of the intracranial gas bubble and tension pneumocephalus. This problem may be eliminated by using either oxygen or nitrous oxide as the contrast agent [6]. In comparison with air, the more rapid absorption of nitrous oxide from the ventricles appears to reduce postcontrast headache, but large volumes must be used and the study must be completed quickly before absorption occurs. Rapid or excessive injection of any gas as contrast agent can precipitate an acute increase in ICP. Moderate hyperventilation (to reduce ICP) and light anesthesia (to support blood pressure during changes in body position), coupled with muscle relaxation, are indicated. Any injected gas may embolize intravascularly if the patient has a ventriculoatrial shunt.

5. **Myelography and polytomography.** Like pneumoencephalography, these procedures often involve a frequent change in the patient's position. All tubes and lines must be well secured and any sign of distress recognized immediately to initiate therapy. **Metrizamide,** a water-soluble contrast agent, can produce seizures if allowed to enter the intracranial compartment in high concentrations. The patient's head should remain slightly **elevated** to avoid intracranial ascent.

6. **Radiation therapy** usually involves a series of treatments given daily for several weeks. Tolerance to anesthetic drugs can develop.

Children are often managed as outpatients, and, consequently, **rapid recovery from anesthesia is a priority.** Occasionally, treatment is several times a day. The procedure itself requires that the anesthesiologist observe the patient from outside the room, usually via **closed-circuit television.** The patient and all monitors should be readily visible. Although each treatment is of short duration, accurate focusing of the radiation demands that the patient be motionless. As with CT and MRI scans, rectal barbiturates, or ketamine (2–4 mg/kg IM, if ICP is not elevated) with or without midazolam, may be used. **Propofol** may be an excellent drug in this setting [61], particularly if the child has an indwelling central line to avoid pain on injection; however, to date, there is little experience with this agent in small children. Techniques for general inhalational anesthesia by mask [20] and laryngeal airway have also been described.

References

1. Albin, M. The paradox of paradoxical air embolism. *Anesthesiology* 61:222, 1984.
2. Allan, D., Kim, H. S., and Cox, J. M. The anesthetic management of posterior fossa exploration in infants. *Can. Anaesth. Soc. J.* 17:227, 1970.
3. Avery, G. B. *Neonatology: Pathophysiology and Management of the Newborn* (3rd ed.). Philadelphia: Lippincott, 1987.
4. Barst, S., et al. Anesthesia for pediatric cancer patients: ketamine, etomidate or propofol? *Anesthesiology* 73,3A:A1114, 1990.
5. Bell, W. E., and McCormick, W. F. *Increased Intracranial Pressure in Children.* Philadelphia: Saunders, 1978.
6. Betts, E. K. A simplified technique of air encephalography. *Anesth. Analg.* 56:469, 1977.
7. Biebuyck, J. F. Propofol: A new intravenous anesthetic. *Anesthesiology* 71:260, 1989.
8. Bruce, D. A. Special Considerations in the Pediatric Age Group. In P. R. Cooper (ed.), *Head Injury.* Baltimore: Williams & Wilkins, 1980.
9. Bruce, D. A., Berman, W. A., and Schut, L. Cerebrospinal fluid pressure monitoring in children: physiology, pathology and clinical usefulness. *Adv. Pediatr.* 24:233, 1977.
10. Bruce, D. A., et al. Diffuse cerebral swelling following head injuries in children: the syndrome of "malignant brain edema." *J. Neurosurg.* 54:170, 1981.
11. Bruce, D. A., et al. Outcome following severe head injury in children. *J. Neurosurg.* 48:679, 1978.
12. Budinger, T. F. Nuclear magnetic resonance (NMR) in vivo studies: known thresholds for health effects. *J. Comput. Assist. Tomogr.* 5:800, 1981.
13. Conel, J. L. *The Postnatal Development of the Human Cerebral Cortex* (Vols. I–VI). Cambridge: Harvard University Press, 1939–1960.
14. Cowan, F., and Thoresen, M. Changes in superior sagittal sinus blood velocities due to postural alterations and pressure on the head of the newborn infant. *Pediatrics* 75:1038, 1985.
15. Cross, K. W., et al. An estimation of intracranial blood flow in the newborn infant. *J. Physiol.* 289:329, 1979.
16. Cutler, R. W. P., and Spertell, R. B. Cerebrospinal fluid: A selective review. *Ann. Neurol.* 11:1, 1982.
17. Dierdoff, S. F., et al. Failure of succinylcholine to alter plasma potassium in children with myelomeningocele. *Anesthesiology* 64:272, 1986.

18. DiRocco, C., et al. Continuous intraventricular cerebrospinal fluid pressure recording in hydrocephalic children during wakefulness and sleep. *J. Neurosurg.* 42:683, 1975.

19. DiRocco, C. Iannelli, A., and Velardi, F. Early diagnosis and surgical indication in craniosynostosis. *Childs Brain* 6:175, 1980.

20. Glauber, D. T., and Audenaert, S. M. Anesthesia for children undergoing craniospinal radiation. *Anesthesiology* 67:801, 1987.

21. Goldberg, M. Systemic reactions to intravascular contrast media. *Anesthesiology* 60:46, 1984.

22. Goldberg, R. N., et al. The effect of head position on intracranial pressure in the neonate. *Crit. Care Med.* 11:428, 1983.

23. Greenberger, P. A., Patterson, R., and Tapio, C. M. Prophylaxis against repeat radiocontrast media reactions in 857 cases. *Arch. Intern. Med.* 145:2197, 1985.

24. Greene, M. G. (ed.). *The Harriet Lane Handbook: A Manual for Pediatric House Officers* (12th ed.). Chicago: Year Book, 1990.

25. Grubb, R. L., et al. The effects of changes in $PaCO_2$ on cerebral blood volume, blood flow and vascular mean transit time. *Stroke* 5:630, 1974.

26. Hamill, J. F., et al. Lidocaine before endotracheal intubation: Intravenous or laryngotracheal? *Anesthesiology* 55:578, 1981.

27. Hanaway, J., Lee, S. I., and Netsky, M. Pachygyria: Relation of findings to modern embryologic concepts. *Neurology* 18:791, 1968.

28. Hannallah, R., et al. Induction dose of propofol in unpremedicated children. *Anesth. Analg.* 70:S143, 1990.

29. Harris, M. H., et al. Venous air embolis and cardiac arrest during craniectomy in a supine infant. *Anesthesiology* 65:547, 1986.

30. Harris, M. H., et al. Venous air embolism during craniectomy in supine infants. *Anesthesiology* 67:816, 1987.

31. Hinkle, A. J. Awake neonatal laryngoscopy: pre-oxygenation alone versus continuous oxygenation. *Anesthesiology* 59:A437, 1983.

32. Jones, R. M. Clinical comparison of inhalation anesthetic agents. *Br. J. Anaesth.* 56:57S, 1984.

33. Kennedy, C., and Sokoloff, L. An adaptation of the nitrous oxide method to the study of the cerebral circulation in children; normal values for cerebral blood flow and cerebral metabolic rate in childhood. *J. Clin. Invest.* 36:1130, 1957.

34. Kety, S. S., and Schmidt, C. F. Nitrous oxide method for the quantitative determination of cerebral blood flow in man: theory, procedure and normal values. *J. Clin. Invest.* 27:476, 1948.

35. Kety, S. S., and Schmidt, C. F. The effects of altered arterial tensions of carbon dioxide and oxygen on cerebral blood flow and cerebral oxygen consumption of normal young men. *J. Clin. Invest.* 27:484, 1948.

36. Kraus, J. F., Fife, D., and Conroy, C. Pediatric brain injuries: the nature, clinical course and early outcomes in a defined United States' population. *Pediatrics* 79:501, 1987.

37. Kurth, C. D., et al. Postoperative apnea in preterm infants. *Anesthesiology* 66:483, 1987.

38. Lasjaunias, P., et al. The role of dural anomalies in vein of Galen aneurysms: report of six cases and review of literature. *A.J.N.R.* 8:185, 1987.

39. Lemire, R. J., et al. *Normal and Abnormal Development of the Human Nervous System.* Hagerstown, MD: Harper & Row, 1975.

40. Liu, L. M. P., et al. Life threatening apnea in infants recovering from anesthesia. *Anesthesiology* 59:506, 1983.

41. Lofgren, J., and Zwetnow, N. N. Cranial and spinal components of the cerebrospinal fluid pressure-volume curve. *Acta Neurol. Scand.* 49:575, 1973.

42. Marshall, T. A., et al. Physiologic changes associated with endotracheal intubation in preterm infants. *Crit. Care Med.* 12:501, 1984.

43. McComb, J. G. Recent research into the nature of cerebrospinal fluid formation and absorption. *J. Neurosurg.* 59:359, 1983.
44. McDowall, D. G. Monitoring the brain. *Anesthesiology* 45:117, 1976.
45. Mehta, S., et al. Energy metabolism of brain in human protein calorie malnutrition. *Pediatr. Res.* 11:290, 1977.
46. Milhorat, T. H. Hydrocephalus. In T. H. Milhorat (ed.), *Pediatric Neurosurgery*. Philadelphia: Davis, 1978. Pp. 91–135.
47. Minkowski, A., et al. Development of the Nervous System in Early Life. In F. Falkner (ed.), *Human Development*. Baltimore: Saunders, 1966.
48. Nelson, W. E. (ed.). *Textbook of Pediatrics* (13th ed.). Philadelphia: Saunders, 1987.
49. Rahilly, P. M. Effects of 2% carbon dioxide, 0.5% carbon dioxide and 100% oxygen on cranial blood flow of the human neonate. *Arch. Dis. Child.* 55:265, 1980.
50. Raju, T. K. N., et al. Intracranial pressure during intubation and anesthesia in infants. *J. Pediatr.* 96:860, 1980.
51. Rao, C. C., McNiece, W. L., and Emhardt, J. Modification of an anesthesia machine for use during magnetic resonance imaging. *Anesthesiology* 68:640, 1988.
52. Reivich, M. Arterial PCO_2 and cerebral hemodynamics. *Am. J. Physiol.* 206:25, 1964.
53. Rogers, M. C., Nugent, S. K., and Traystman, R. J. Control of cerebral circulation in the neonate and infant. *Crit. Care. Med.* 8:570, 1980.
54. Saint-Anne Dargassies, S. Neurologic Maturation of the Premature Infant of 28–41 Weeks' Gestational Age. In F. Falkner (ed.), *Human Development*. Philadelphia: Saunders, 1966. Pp. 306–325.
55. Schreiner, M. S., Triebwasser, A., and Keon, T. P. Oral fluids compared to preoperative fasting in pediatric outpatients. *Anesthesiology* 72:593, 1990.
56. Seiber, F. E., et al. Glucose: A reevaluation of its intraoperative use. *Anesthesiology* 67:72, 1987.
57. Settergren, G., Lindblad, B. S., and Persson, B. Cerebral blood flow and exchange of oxygen, glucose, ketone bodies, lactate, pyruvate and amino acids in infants. *Acta Paediatr. Scand.* 65:343, 1976.
58. Shapiro, H. M. Intracranial hypertension: Therapeutic and anesthetic considerations. *Anesthesiology* 43:445, 1975.
59. Sidman, R. L., and Rakic, P. Neuronal migration with special reference to developing human brain: a review. *Brain Res.* 62:1, 1973.
60. Smith, C. A., and Nelson, N. M. *The Physiology of the Newborn Infant* (4th ed.). Springfield: IL: Thomas, 1976.
61. Vangerven, M., et al. Total intravenous anesthesia with propofol and without intubation for magnetic resonance imaging (MRI) in pediatric patients. *Anesthesiology* 73,3A:A1239, 1990.
62. Vidyasagar, D., and Raju, T. N. K. A simple noninvasive technique of measuring intracranial pressure in the newborn. *Pediatrics* 59:957, 1977.
63. Weinstabl, C., et al. Impact of propofol on intracranial dynamics in head trauma ICU patients. *Anesthesiology* 73,3A:A1217, 1990.
64. Welborn, L. G., et al. Post anesthetic apnea and periodic breathing in infants. *Anesthesiology* 65:658, 1986.
65. Yakovlev, P. I., and Lecours, A. R. The Myelogenetic Cycles of Regional Maturation of the Brain. In A. Minkowski (ed.), *Regional Development of the Brain in Early Life*. Philadelphia: Davis, 1967.
66. Younkin, D. P., et al. Noninvasive method of estimating human newborn regional cerebral blood flow. *J. Cereb. Blood Flow Metab.* 2:415, 1982.

16

Pediatric Neurogenic Airway and Swallowing Disorders

LEE D. ROWE

This chapter presents a neuroanatomic approach to the evaluation and management of neurogenic airway and swallowing disorders in children. An understanding of pediatric neurogenic abnormalities of the aerodigestive tract also provides guidelines for successful treatment of acquired adult neurogenic airway dysfunction. Anesthetic techniques, perioperative problems, and surgical approaches to supranuclear, nuclear, and infranuclear lesions of the ninth and tenth cranial nerves are analyzed.

I. **Functional anatomy.** Neuronal control of the pharynx and larynx is divided into three elements: supranuclear, nuclear, and infranuclear (Fig. 16-1).

A. **Supranuclear.** Corticobulbar motor fibers originate in area 4 on the rostral side of the sylvian (lateral) fissure, enter the corona radiata, and pass into the internal capsule. Neurons emerge from the cerebral peduncle, forming the pyramidal tracts, and descend through the pons. Decussating and uncrossed fibers terminate in the nucleus ambiguus.

B. **Nuclear**

1. The nucleus ambiguus is the primary source of pharyngeal and laryngeal motor supply. The orientation of adductor and abductor nuclei (which innervate the intrinsic and extrinsic laryngeal muscles) is dorsoventral. **Adductor neurons,** which innervate the lateral cricoarytenoid, cricothyroid (the sole extrinsic laryngeal muscle), interarytenoid, and external thyroarytenoid muscles, are loosely arranged in the dorsal portion of the medulla. **Abductor neurons** innervate the posterior cricoarytenoid muscle (the *only* laryngeal abductor) and form the more compact ventral division [12].

2. The retrofacial nucleus, rostral to the nucleus ambiguus, is a second source of abductor neurons to the posterior cricoarytenoid muscle and of adductor neurons to the lateral cricoarytenoid muscle.

3. Nuclei controlling deglutition are located within the nucleus ambiguus.

C. **Infranuclear**

1. Efferent axons from laryngeal motor nuclei emerge in the rostral first and second rootlets of the vagus nerve. These neurons cross the posterior cranial fossa and enter the superior (jugular) ganglion at the level of the jugular foramen. Below the jugular foramen, axons

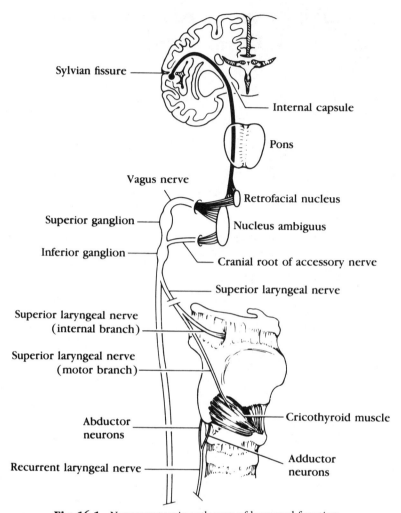

Fig. 16-1. Neuroanatomic pathways of laryngeal function.

are joined by the cranial (bulbar) spinal accessory nerve, which is proximal to the inferior (nodose) ganglion. This ganglion contains sensory cell bodies of the internal branch of the superior laryngeal nerve, which innervates the entire larynx above the level of the true vocal cords. The external branch of the superior laryngeal nerve carries efferent motor output to the cricothyroid muscle, the chief tensor of the vocal cord.

2. The recurrent laryngeal nerve carries the remaining vagal innervation to the larynx. Abductor and adductor neurons separate into two distinct groups, approximately 1 to 2 cm above their entrance into the larynx. Additional afferent sensory fibers, carrying stretch

and mucosal receptor information from the true vocal cords and subglottic space, terminate in the nodose ganglion. Secondary neurons ascend to the nucleus solitarius.

3. The pharyngeal plexus, which is separate from the superior laryngeal and recurrent laryngeal nerves, carries motor input to the superior, middle, and inferior pharyngeal constrictor muscles and to striated muscles of the upper esophagus. Pharyngoesophageal sensory output is primarily carried to the nucleus solitarius in the glossopharyngeal and vagus nerves.

II. Physiology
A. Respiration

1. The primitive role of the larynx is to function as a sphincter separating the tracheobronchial tree from ingested material and secretions. Phylogenetically, abductor fibers have appeared only recently and are fewer in number ($4 : 1$ ratio of adductor to abductor neurons). With gradual evolutionary conversion to additional respiratory and phonatory roles, the abductor nuclei have received increasing input from the reticular formation neurons and coordinate inspiration through neuronal interconnections with the posterior cricoarytenoid muscle, diaphragm, intercostal muscles, and accessory neck muscles [5].

2. Respiration requires a complex interaction of the adductor and abductor laryngeal nuclei and reticular formation neurons [4]. During inspiration the vocal cords abduct (Fig. 16-2A). Neuronal output to the posterior cricoarytenoid muscle is increased through the recurrent laryngeal nerve; adductor activity is inhibited. During expiration, slight adduction maintains a physiologic positive end-expiratory pressure.

3. Phonation requires tensing of the cricothyroid muscle, increased adductor activity, and approximation of the vocal cords in the median position (Fig. 16-2B).

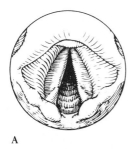 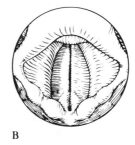

A   B

Fig. 16-2. Endoscopic view of the endolarynx. *A.* Inspiration: abduction of the true vocal cords. The posterior cricoarytenoid muscle is the sole abductor of the true vocal cords. *B.* Phonation: midline approximation of the true vocal cords.

4. Voluntary coughing and reflex clearance of foreign material from the airway are mediated by the nucleus ambiguus.

B. Swallowing

1. Deglutition is initiated by a voluntary oral phase that moves a bolus of food to the base of the tongue and oropharynx. The palate elevates and the lateral wall narrows, stimulating the involuntary pharyngeal phase. Respiration ceases and the larynx rises under the base of the tongue. The constrictor muscle fibers contract sequentially in a rostral-to-caudal direction, and the tonically contracted (15–40 cmH$_2$O resting pressure) cricopharyngeal muscle relaxes.

2. Food enters the proximal esophagus and is carried by gravity and striated muscle activity in a 100-cm pressure zone to the gastroesophageal junction in three to seven seconds. Normal swallowing function depends, therefore, on adequate mobility of the tongue, sequential relaxation of the cricopharyngeal muscle, and separation of ingested food from the tracheobronchial tree.

III. Etiology and clinical findings

A. Supranuclear lesions

1. Isolated supranuclear anomalies are difficult to recognize in the neonate because lower nuclear pharyngeal and laryngeal reflexes remain intact and speech has not yet been acquired. As a result, supranuclear lesions produce minimal airway, swallowing, or speech dysfunction unless associated with cerebral agenesis, hydrocephalus, or severe encephalitis (Table 16-1).

2. Clinical features include persistent abnormal reflexes such as snout, jaw jerk, Moro, and Babinski. Delayed acquisition of speech and disorders of the basal ganglia, including rigidity and hyperkinesia, may be present. Cough and swallowing reflexes are intact. Characteristic signs of spastic dysarthrophonia and slurring of articulation often occur in older children and adolescents (Table 16-2).

Table 16-1. Supranuclear lesions

Congenital	Acquired
Hydrocephalus	Hydrocephalus
Cerebral agenesis	Tuberculosis
Kernicterus	Meningoencephalitis
Cerebral palsy	Birth trauma
Charcot-Marie-Tooth syndrome	Cryptococcosis
Toxoplasmosis	
Neurosyphilis	
Intraventricular hemorrhage	
Intra-axial neoplasms	

Table 16-2. Supranuclear lesions: clinical findings

Persistent jaw jerk, snout, Moro, or Babinski reflexes
Delayed speech acquisition
Basal ganglia disorders: rigidity and hyperkinesis
Intact cough and swallowing reflexes

B. Nuclear lesions

1. Nuclear lesions produce striking aerodigestive tract impairment in neonates and infants including dysphagia, aspiration, and upper airway obstruction. Concomitant cranial neuropathies and congenital anomalies are frequently encountered (Table 16-3).
2. The Arnold-Chiari malformation, a congenital anomaly of the lower brainstem and inferior cerebellum associated with caudal displacement of the medulla, cerebellar tonsils, and fourth ventricle into the upper vertebral canal, is the most common cause of nuclear pharyngolaryngeal dysfunction. Hydrocephalus is severe, and meningomyelocele is almost always present.
3. Neurogenic airway and swallowing dysfunction probably results from increased intracranial pressure (ICP), which causes intracranial stretching of the vagus, traction on vagal rootlets, and ischemia or hemorrhage from medullary compression. These conditions frequently develop after removal of the accompanying meningomyelocele or after obstruction of a ventriculoperitoneal shunt previously placed to correct the hydrocephalus. Bilateral impairment of the phylogenetically newer abductor neurons results in paralysis of the vocal cords in the median or paramedian position (Fig. 16-3A). Paradoxically, the cry is normal with high-pitched inspiratory stridor exacerbated by agitation. Persistent adductor neuronal activity probably permits normal phonation (Table 16-4) [6, 7,15].

Table 16-3. Nuclear lesions

Congenital	Acquired
Brainstem neoplasms	Trauma
Arteriovenous malformations	Polioencephalitis
Dandy-Walker snydrome	Diphtheria
Arnold-Chiari malformation	Rabies
Syringobulbia	Brainstem hemorrhage
Nuclear dysplasia or agenesis	Guillain-Barré syndrome
Riley-Day syndrome	Tetanus
Klippel-Feil syndrome	

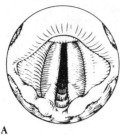 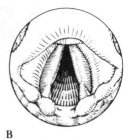

A   B

Fig. 16-3. Endoscopic view of the endolarynx in an infant with bilateral vocal cord paralysis secondary to the Arnold-Chiari malformation. *A.* Inspiration: bilateral abductor vocal cord paralysis with the true vocal cords in the paramedian position. *B.* Phonation: bilateral abductor *and* adductor vocal cord paralysis with both vocal cords in the intermediate position. Failure to achieve closure of the vocal cords during swallowing results in life-threatening aspiration.

4. With additional nuclear adductor neuronal involvement, the vocal cords assume a more abducted or intermediate position (Fig. 16-3B). The cry becomes weak and the stridor decreases. However, severe dysphagia and life-threatening aspiration also develop. Children who have the Arnold-Chiari malformation who exhibit these signs should be examined for evidence of increasing ischemia of the brainstem.

5. Bilateral abductor vocal cord paralysis may, in rare circumstances, be inherited as a genetic defect. In addition, dysphagia and aspiration can occur because of either an isolated congenital crico-

Table 16-4. Nuclear lesions: clinical findings

Bilateral vocal cord paralysis	Unilateral vocal cord paralysis
Abductor neurons	Weak or hoarse cry
Normal cry	Minimal stridor or aspiration
Inspiratory stridor	Frequent associated cranial
Minimal aspiration	neuropathies
Vocal cords in paramedian position	Swallowing function: feeding difficulties
Abductor and adductor neurons	
Weak cry	
Minimal inspiratory stridor	
Significant aspiration	
Vocal cords in intermediate position	
Swallowing function	
Feeding difficulties with	
cricopharyngeal achalasia	
Associated cranial neuropathies and	
congenital anomalies	

pharyngeal achalasia or pharyngoesophageal dyskinesia. Discoordination of pharyngeal and palatal mobility with failure of cricopharyngeus relaxation results in excessive oropharyngeal secretions, nasal reflux, recurrent aspiration, and bronchopneumonia [24].

6. Isolated unilateral nuclear vocal cord paralysis is rare but does occur more commonly in association with other brainstem nuclear dysplasia or agenesis. Clinically, the cry is weak or hoarse with minimal stridor and aspiration (Table 16-4).

C. Infranuclear lesions

1. Congenital infranuclear lesions of the vagus nerve in the neonate are primarily caused by congenital heart disease, mediastinal neoplasms, vascular anomalies, or tracheoesophageal fistulas. Frequently, these disorders are associated with unilateral vocal cord paralysis secondary to recurrent laryngeal nerve involvement (Table 16-5).

2. The cry is weak and one vocal cord is in either the median or the paramedian position (Fig. 16-4A). Aspiration and swallowing difficulties may be significant clinical problems, depending on the degree of compensatory glottic closure by the opposite vocal cord (Table 16-6; Fig. 16-4B).

3. Acquired infranuclear lesions of the vagus nerve, on the other hand, frequently involve both vocal cords and affect the recurrent laryngeal nerve, superior laryngeal nerve, and pharyngeal plexus (see Table 16-5). Infants who have polyneuritis, demyelinating disorders, and botulism exhibit a weak or absent cry, vocal cords in an intermediate position, no stridor, recurrent aspiration, and difficulty in swallowing [22]. Neonates who sustain significant cervical trauma during forceps delivery may demonstrate transient unilateral or bilateral vocal cord paralysis [3]. Prolonged intubation of the larynx

Table 16-5. Infranuclear lesions

Congenital	Acquired
Congenital heart disease	Trauma
Tracheoesophageal fistula	Botulism
Mediastinal neoplasms	Polyneuritis
Aortic arch anomalies	Demyelinization disorders
	Idiopathic
	Meningitis
	Mediastinitis
	Diphtheria
	Parapharyngeal neoplasms

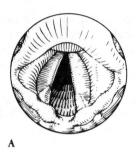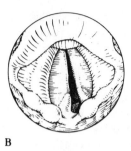

A   B

Fig. 16-4. Right vocal cord paralysis secondary to recurrent laryngeal nerve paralysis. *A.* Inspiration: right vocal cord in paramedian position fails to abduct. *B.* Phonation: the left true vocal cord crosses the midline to approximate the opposite cord incompletely resulting in a weak, breathy cry. Failure to effect glottic closure completely during swallowing may lead to aspiration.

and trachea may also be associated with recurrent laryngeal nerve injury.

IV. **Diagnosis.** Neurogenic laryngeal and swallowing abnormalities are unrecognized in the neonatal period unless associated with significant airway obstruction, aspiration, or other congenital anomalies [11]. Respiratory failure secondary to perinatal anesthetics, hypoxia, or central nervous system damage because of maternal incompatibility or diabetes mellitus must be excluded. In addition, hyaline membrane disease and congenital obstructive lesions of the aerodigestive tract must be ruled out. The congenital lesions include laryngomalacia (the most common cause of congenital laryngeal stridor), subglottic stenosis, and subglottic hemangiomas.

A. In the neonatal period and early infancy, **direct laryngoscopic examination** of the larynx and pharynx provides information concern-

Table 16-6. Infranuclear lesions: clinical findings

Unilateral vocal cord paralysis	Bilateral vocal cord paralysis

Recurrent laryngeal nerve
  Weak cry
  Minimal aspiration
  Normal swallowing
  Vocal cord in paramedian position
	Recurrent laryngeal nerve, superior
	    laryngeal nerve
	  Severe dysphagia
	  Aspiration
	  Recurrent bronchopneumonia

Recurrent laryngeal nerve, superior
    laryngeal nerve, pharyngeal plexus
  Weak or absent cry
  Recurrent aspiration
  Vocal cord in intermediate position
  Swallowing function variably
    impaired	

ing vocal cord mobility and the presence or absence of congenital laryngeal and pharyngeal lesions [8].

B. Careful examination of the cranial nerves and assessment of the quality of respiration provide clues for sites of possible airway obstruction.

1. Stridor represents partial obstruction of the respiratory tract from either external compression of, or partial occlusion within, the air channels. Occurring during inspiration, expiration, or both, the source of the compression may vary from the external nares to the distal bronchioles. The character and intensity of the noise depend on the site and degree of obstruction and the air flow, velocity, and pressure gradient across the point of obstruction. In the evaluation of an infant who has neurogenic airway and swallowing disorders, several signs are useful in localizing the site of obstruction [17].

a. Normally, inspiration and expiration require approximately equal periods of time. The phase of respiration in which stridor occurs is more likely to be inspiratory in the presence of upper respiratory obstruction.

b. When there is obstruction at the level of the true vocal cords, the stridor is usually high pitched in character.

c. Stridor during expiration is associated with tracheal and bronchial obstruction. The expiratory phase of respiration is prolonged and the tone of the stridor is lower.

d. Stridor can occur during both inspiration and expiration when there is tracheal obstruction.

2. The quality of the cry remains normal in the majority of infants who have airway obstruction but no laryngeal lesion. A weak or absent cry at birth suggests neurogenic impairment of the vocal cords. Paradoxically, infants who have Arnold-Chiari malformation and bilateral abductor paralysis of the vocal cords may have marked impairment of the airway but a normal cry [18, 20].

3. With compression of the trachea by either supraglottic tumors or vascular rings, **hyperextension of the neck** is frequently observed. This finding is rare in neurogenic vocal cord disorders, subglottic stenosis, and endotracheal lesions.

4. Recurrent pneumonitis is frequently associated with tracheobronchial obstruction, tracheoesophageal fistulas, bilateral abductor, *and* adductor neuronal impairment, bilateral recurrent laryngeal and superior laryngeal nerve disorders, and a tracheobronchial foreign body.

C. Radiographic techniques

1. Chest films during inspiration and expiration are necessary to rule out foreign bodies in the tracheobronchial tree, neoplasms, or cardiac or great vessel anomalies in the mediastinum. Fluoroscopy of the chest during respiration provides additional information when a lucent foreign body of the main bronchus is suspected.

Obstructive emphysema will produce a mediastinal shift away from the site of obstruction; atelectasis secondary to complete occlusion of the main bronchus will shift the mediastinum toward the involved side.

2. Nuclear and infranuclear lesions affecting swallowing are most effectively evaluated by rapid **cineradiography** of palatopharyngeal and esophageal motility. Tracheoesophageal fistulas with associated bronchopneumonia and failure to thrive may mimic infranuclear lesions of the vagus nerve and require a **barium swallow** (Fig. 16-5). Occasionally, the diagnosis requires careful endoscopy of the esophagus and tracheobronchial tree under general anesthesia. Cineesophagography is also necessary to rule out isolated cricopharyngeal achalasia.

3. **Plain films of the skull and cervical spine** are obtained in patients in whom congenital nuclear lesions are suspected. The Klippel-Feil syndrome includes a characteristic malformation of the atlanto-occipital joint and vertebrae. Bulging of the lower occipital region is diagnostic of the Dandy-Walker syndrome.

4. Confirmation of the Arnold-Chiari malformation requires **posterior fossa pneumoencephalography or computed tomography (CT)** with metrizamide. CT is also useful in assessing the size of the ventricles before and after insertion of a shunt.

5. **Magnetic resonance imaging (MRI)** may provide more accurate brainstem detail than CT.

6. Sleep disorders may be associated with supralaryngeal airway collapse secondary to skeletal muscle hypotonicity. The most obvious manifestation of this upper airway obstruction is snoring. Pediatric patients who snore may have a potentially lethal condition, obstructive sleep apnea, and should be carefully evaluated with a physical examination of the upper airway with a fiberoptic nasopharyngoscope and possibly a polysomnogram. There appears to be at least two groups of children described in the literature [9]: with specifically surgically correctible lesions such as adenotonsillar hypertrophy and those who eventually need tracheotomy because of collapse of upper airway musculature during sleep. In this latter group of children, it is necessary to hypothesize an additional defect in the central nervous system regulation and respiration during sleep. Numerous other potential obstructors of the upper airway in children such as facial dysmorphia, including the Pierre Robin syndrome, micrognathia, retrognathia, Treacher Collins syndrome, and trisomy 21. It is obvious that those with neuromuscular disorders such as the Arnold-Chiari malformation, syringobulbia, cerebral palsy, and myotonic dystrophy may have associated obstructive sleep apnea [19, 21].

D. To fully evaluate the degree of sleep-associated obstructive airway

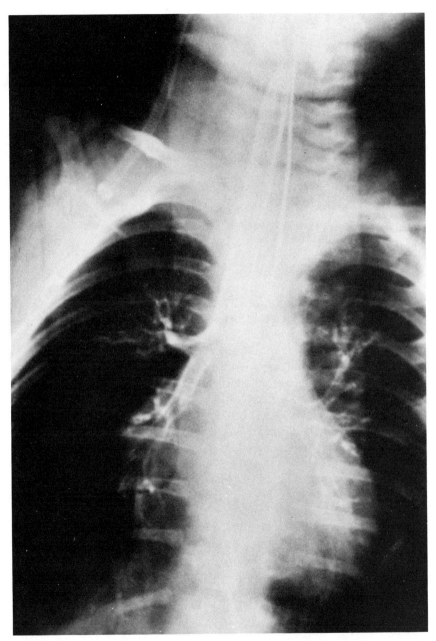

Fig. 16-5. Barium swallow in an infant with bilateral abductor and adductor vocal cord paralysis. A characteristic tracheobronchogram results from nuclear neurogenic dysfunction in an infant with the Arnold-Chiari malformation. There is no filling of the esophagus, and a feeding nasogastric tube can be seen.

dysfunction, a polysomnogram is essential. The monitoring consists of simultaneous recording of numerous physiologic variables. Cardiopulmonary measures recorded are naso-oral airflow, determined by measuring end-tidal carbon dioxide with an infrared CO_2 analyzer. Concomitant respiratory efforts are evaluated by mercury-filled capillary strain gauges mounted on the chest wall and abdomen. Oxygen saturation is measured by a pulse oximeter [13]. EKG and EEG activity is measured. This measures the broad categorization of the various states of sleep and permits a distinction among three types of apnea: obstructive, central, and mixed. Upper airway obstruction is the cessation of nasal and oral airflow for more than 10 seconds in the presence of persistent chest wall and abdominal movement. Central apnea is the simultaneous sensation of both airflow and thoracic breathing movements, and mixed apnea is a central apnea of 10 seconds or longer followed by obstructive apnea [10]. Reporting parameters include the apnea index or the number of apneas per hour (six or more apneas per hour are defined as obstructive sleep apnea), the percent of oxygen desaturation, the duration and site of the desaturation in a histogram form, the types of arrhythmias noted, and the position of the patient in relationship to the apneas.

V. Neuroanesthesia: general principles. Early diagnosis and treatment of pediatric neurogenic and swallowing abnormalities require direct laryngoscopy initially and additional bronchoscopy and esophagoscopy under general anesthesia. Of primary concern is maintaining an adequate airway and avoiding aspiration in patients who have vocal cord paralysis and impaired cough and gag reflexes [23].

A. Anesthesia is induced with an inhalation anesthetic (halothane or isoflurane) and 100% oxygen by mask while the child breathes spontaneously. The operating table is in the Trendelenburg position [1, 2].

    1. Suction is immediately available. Muscle relaxants are not used to preserve pharyngolaryngeal muscle tone and spontaneous respiration, permitting either direct laryngoscopy or intubation. Ventilation may be assisted or controlled to prevent hypoventilation, accumulation of CO_2, and ventricular arrhythmias [16].

    2. The surgeon is prepared to perform either bronchoscopy or an **emergency tracheotomy** if the airway becomes obstructed.

    3. When the depth of anesthesia is adequate, direct laryngoscopy is performed to evaluate intrinsic laryngeal muscle function during quiet respiration and to rule out congenital laryngeal anomalies such as laryngomalacia or webs. Care is taken not to insert the tip of the laryngoscope into the glottic folds and provoke laryngospasm.

    4. Bronchoscopy may be accomplished under general anesthesia without the use of an endotracheal tube. After achieving adequate anesthesia by mask, a pediatric ventilating bronchoscope of appropriate size is inserted with the aid of a Jackson pediatric laryngoscope. This plane of anesthesia should be maintained at the conclusion of bronchoscopy to facilitate direct laryngoscopy without danger of laryngospasm.

It is important to note that during bronchoscopy, the suctioning of secretions and saline introduced into the tracheobronchial tree should be limited to brief periods of time to prevent altered ventilation-perfusion relationships and hypoxia. A mean decrease in arterial O_2 of 12 mmHg has been observed secondary to loss of effective tidal volume during overzealous suctioning and bronchial lavage.

5. When **esophagoscopy** is planned, an endotracheal tube is inserted initially. After completion of endoscopic inspection of the esophagus, the endotracheal tube is removed while the child is still deeply asleep, and the bronchoscope is inserted into the trachea. The function of the vocal cords during quiet respiration may be assessed by direct laryngoscopy after removal of the bronchoscope if a plane of anesthesia sufficient to prevent laryngospasm is maintained.

B. The **endotracheal tube** is removed from infants and children who have neurogenic airway disorders while they are still deeply asleep to prevent laryngospasm, coughing, and straining, which may increase ICP if there is decreased intracranial compliance. Patients are transported and nursed in the lateral decubitus position until fully awake. This places the pharynx in a dependent position and avoids potential aspiration.

VI. **Treatment.** Surgical management of neurogenic disorders of the aerodigestive tract is directed toward alleviation of laryngeal airway obstruction, recurrent aspiration, and dysphagia because these conditions, when coupled with the effect of concomitant hypoxia and poor nutrition on developing brainstem nuclei, may cause periodic apnea, sudden infant death syndrome (SIDS), and impaired intellectual development (Table 16-7).

Table 16-7. Treatment of neurogenic disorders of the aerodigestive tract

Swallowing	Respiration
Upright position	Tracheotomy
Nasogastric tube	Brainstem decompression
Hyperalimentation	Arytenoidectomy
Gavage	Laryngeal reinnervation
Gastrostomy	Ventriculoperitoneal shunt
Cricopharyngeal myotomy	Laryngeal closure
	Teflon injection or collagen
	Tonsillectomy and/or adenoidectomy

A. Supranuclear lesions (see Table 16-1)

    1. Neonates and infants who have congenital supranuclear lesions rarely require surgical intervention unless the lesions are secondary to hydrocephalus or intra-axial neoplasms. Airway and swallowing reflexes remain intact although there is intellectual and functional impairment.

    2. Extensive speech therapy, physiotherapy, and feeding assistance may ultimately be necessary for many of these patients.

B. Nuclear lesions (see Table 16-3)

    1. Infants who have the **Arnold-Chiari malformation who develop hydrocephalus without vocal cord impairment** are candidates for ventriculoperitoneal shunt. Close observation is necessary because the subsequent development of inspiratory stridor may be an indication of shunt obstruction and increasing ICP, meningitis, or high pressure in the cervical subarachnoid space (with normal ICP). Obstruction of the shunt necessitates immediate revision.

    2. Infants who have the **Arnold-Chiari malformation who develop hydrocephalus with bilateral abductor vocal cord paralysis** and airway obstruction require immediate intubation and insertion of a shunt. Airway obstruction and vocal cord immobility resolve within two weeks of shunt placement in more than 50% of patients.

        a. Persistent stridor, aspiration, and cyanosis during feeding are indicative of bilateral abductor vocal cord paralysis. Treatment includes decompression of the posterior fossa and cervical canal to the level of the cerebellar tonsils.

        b. Infants who exhibit unremitting bilateral abductor vocal cord paralysis will require a permanent tracheotomy to improve respiratory function, prevent airway obstruction and aspiration, and permit increased oral feedings. Tracheotomy may not relieve episodes of central apnea, hypoxia, or cyanosis, so the patient will require apnea monitoring during sleep.

    3. Bilateral abductor paralysis of the vocal cords, in association with additional adductor neuronal impairment or bilateral superior and recurrent laryngeal nerve paralysis, causes life-threatening aspiration and bronchopneumonia and mandates closure of the larynx.

        a. The larynx may be closed by suturing the vocal cords through a laryngofissure approach. A tracheotomy is mandatory.

        b. The larynx may be separated from the trachea by closure of the subglottic space and first tracheal ring with creation of a permanent tracheostoma.

    4. Nuclear swallowing dysfunction is initially treated with semirecumbent positioning, gavage or nasogastric feeding, and frequent nasopharyngeal suctioning.

        a. Cricopharyngeal myotomy through a transverse lower left cervical incision is indicated for those children who have isolated cricopharyngeal achalasia but no gastroesophageal reflux.

b. Gastrostomy is reserved for those infants who have severe feeding difficulties and failure to thrive.

c. Parenteral hyperalimentation with carbohydrates, proteins, essential fatty acids, and phospholipids may prevent brain damage from malnutrition.

C. Infranuclear lesions (see Table 16-5)

1. Isolated unilateral paralysis of the left recurrent laryngeal nerve is the most common type of congenital or acquired infranuclear lesion. When no underlying surgically treatable lesion is identified, these patients are evaluated periodically by direct laryngoscopy. Persistent positioning of the true vocal cord in the paramedian position results in a weak, breathy voice.

This vocal cord malposition is subsequently treated in early adulthood by injection of Teflon or collagen lateral to the paralyzed vocal cord. The involved cord is mobilized medially and vocal quality is improved by providing an accessible vibratory point for the nonparalyzed cord. This technique is not feasible in neonates or infants because of the extremely small size of the airway, need for general anesthesia, and rapid laryngeal growth. The procedure is done with local anesthesia so the patient can phonate, permitting a judgment as to when an adequate amount of Teflon has been injected. In addition to topical 4% lidocaine, bilateral superior laryngeal nerve blocks are performed by injecting two milliliters of 1% lidocaine with a 22-gauge needle 1 cm anterior to the superior corner of the thyroid cartilage in a line drawn midway between the hyoid bone and thyroid cartilage. The ECG is monitored throughout the procedure.

2. Bilateral paralysis of the recurrent laryngeal nerve is commonly treated with a tracheotomy and valved Tucker tracheostomy tube. Although used in adults, arytenoidectomy, through either an external or a transoral approach, is not recommended in children because of the aggravation of aspiration and the resultant poor vocal quality.

3. Functional reinnervation of the larynx in adults who have **bilateral abductor paralysis of the vocal cords** has been successful. Neurotization of the posterior cricoarytenoid muscle, the only laryngeal abductor, is achieved through the implantation of a neuromuscular pedicle of the ansa cervicalis nerve and a block of the associated omohyoid muscle. The value of this technique in children is currently unknown, however. Patients who do not have intact posterior cricoarytenoid muscle fibers capable of accepting implanted motor endplates are not candidates for this surgery. Congenitally denervated abductor muscle fibers or fibers traumatically denervated for more than 18 months will probably not be successfully reinnervated. These unique neurogenic airway problems will require a permanent tracheotomy.

D. Infants and children with sleep disorders and associated apnea are treated on an individual basis. Patients exhibiting only tonsilloadenoidal hyperplasia may benefit from a tonsillectomy and adenoidectomy. Infants with the Pierre Robin syndrome, micrognathia, or retrognathia may benefit from sliding osteotomies and reposition of the mandible. Macroglossia may be treated with a tongue plasty and excision of excess lymphoid tissue at the base of the tongue. Patients exhibiting obstructive sleep apnea due to primary collapse of the pharynx and hypotonicity will require a tracheotomy. Central sleep apnea is best managed by a tracheotomy. Mixed central and obstructive sleep apnea may require both correction of the upper airway obstruction as well as a tracheotomy [10]. At present the value of using continuous positive pressure therapy as a technique of correction of sleep apnea in children has not been fully evaluated. However, its success in adults has been well demonstrated.

References

1. Brown, E. S. Anesthesia in pediatric otolaryngology. *Otolaryngol. Clin. North Am.* 10:113, 1977.
2. Burtner, D. D., and Goodman, M. Anesthetic and operative management of potential upper airway obstruction. *Arch. Otolaryngol.* 104:657, 1978.
3. Fearon, B. Respiratory distress in the newborn. *Otolaryngol. Clin. North Am.* 3:185, 1970.
4. Haddad, G. G., and Mellins, R. B. The role of airway receptors in the control of respiration in infants: A review. *J. Pediatr.* 91:281, 1977.
5. Hart, C. W. Functional and neurological problems of the larynx. *Otolaryngol. Clin. North Am.* 3:609, 1970.
6. Holinger, L. D., Holinger, P. C., and Holinger, L. D. Etiology of bilateral abductor vocal cord paralysis. *Ann. Otol. Rhinol. Laryngol.* 85:428, 1976.
7. Holinger, P. C., Holinger, L. D., Reicher, T. J., et al. Respiratory obstruction and apnea in infants with bilateral abductor vocal cord paralysis, meningomyelocoele, hydrocephalus, and Arnold-Chiari malformation. *J. Pediatr.* 92:368, 1978.
8. Holinger, P. H. Clinical aspects of congenital anomalies of the larynx, trachea, bronchi and esophagus. *J. Laryngol. Otol.* 75:1, 1961.
9. Mandel, E. M., Reynolds C. F. 3d. et al. Sleep disorders associated with the upper airway obstruction in children. *Pediatr. Clin. N. Am.* 28:897, 1981.
10. Orr, W. C., and Moran, W. B., Diagnosis and management of obstructive sleep apnea: A multidisciplinary approach *Arch Otolaryngol.* 111:583, 1985.
11. Naeye, R. L. The sudden infant death syndrome. *Arch. Pathol. Lab. Med.,* 101:165, 1977.
12. Rontal, M., and Rontal, E. Lesions of the vagus nerve: Diagnosis, treatment, and rehabilitation. *Laryngoscope* 87:72, 1977.
13. Rowe, L. D., Hansen, T. N., Nielson, D., et al. Continuous measurements of skin surface oxygen and carbon dioxide tensions in obstructive sleep apnea. *Laryngoscope* 90:1797, 1980.
14. Rowe, L. D., et al. Adaptation of function in pharyngeal constrictor muscles. *Otolaryngol. Head Neck Surg.* 92:392, 1984.

15. Rowe, L. D., and Newfield, P. Airway and swallowing disorders in the Arnold-Chiari malformation. In *Trans. Pac. Coast Otoophthalmol. Soc.* Vol. 61, 1980. Pp. 203–210.
16. Smith, R. M. Pediatric anesthesia in perspective. *Anesth. Analg.* (Cleve.) 57:634, 1978.
17. Snow, J. B., Jr. Clinical evaluation of noisy respiration in infancy. *Lancet* 2:504, 1965.
18. Snow, J. B., and Rogers, K. A. Bilateral abductor paralysis of the vocal cord secondary to Arnold-Chiari malformation and its management. *Laryngoscope* 75:316, 1965.
19. Strohl, K. P., Saunder, N. A., Feldman, N. T., et al. Obstructive sleep apnea in family members. *N. Engl. J. Med.* 299:969, 1978.
20. Venes, J. L. Multiple cranial nerve palsies in an infant with Arnold-Chiari malformation. *Dev. Med. Child Neurol.* 16:817, 1974.
21. Wealthall, S. R., Whittaker, G. E., and Greenwood, N. The relationship of apnea and stridor in spina bifida to other unexplained infant deaths. *Dev. Med. Child Neurol.* 16 (Suppl. 32): 107, 1974.
22. Wolfe, J. A., Rowe, L. D., Pasquariello, P., et al. Tracheotomy for infant botulism. *Ann. Otol. Rhinol. Laryngol.* 88:861, 1979.
23. Wolfsdorf, J. The acute care of respiratory problems in the neonate, infant, and child. *Int. Anesthesiol. Clin.* 13:73, 1975.
24. Work, W. P. Paralysis and paresis of the vocal cords. *Arch. Otolaryngol.* 34:267, 1941.

17

Neuroradiologic Procedures

BERNARD WOLFSON

WILLIAM D. HETRICK

KHURSHED J. DASTUR

Radiology has played an integral part in neurodiagnosis since the introduction of roentgenography in 1895. Although the bony skull and vertebral column provide excellent protection for the enclosed brain and spinal cord, they also make it difficult to obtain information about their contents from simple x-ray films. Contrast material has therefore been injected intravascularly and intrathecally to delineate specific portions of the brain and spinal cord. Dandy injected air into the lateral ventricles in 1918 and into the spinal subarachnoid space in 1919 (pneumoencephalogram). In 1922, Sicard and Forestier injected a radiopaque substance, iodized oil (Lipiodol), into the spinal subarachnoid space (myelogram). Moniz injected radiopaque sodium iodide directly into the carotid artery in 1927, thus performing the first cerebral angiogram. In 1973, the first computed tomographic (CT) brain scanning units were introduced to the United States. This technique provides information about intracranial contents quickly, efficiently, and noninvasively. Magnetic resonance imaging (MRI) is the latest diagnostic technique to be introduced into clinical practice. Like CT it is noninvasive. It too produces superior images but without the use of ionizing radiation.

All these techniques are used today. Most of the changes through the years have involved improvements in apparatus, technique, and contrast media to enhance the quality of the radiographs and reduce their general toxic effects.

I. General considerations

A. Evaluation. The patient requiring a diagnostic procedure should initially undergo a general evaluation. According to the nature of the disease, additional factors must be considered. The presence or absence of increased intracranial pressure (ICP) should be noted. Systemic vascular disease may suggest cerebrovascular disease and, conversely, transient ischemic attacks may suggest generalized as well as cerebral arteriosclerotic disease. Prolonged bed rest after trauma or neurologic disease may cause general debility, which may compound the depressant effect of anesthesia. A hyperkalemic response to succinlycholine has now been noted not only in patients who have burns and acute trauma but also in a variety of neurologic diseases including (but not limited to) upper and lower motor neuron lesions, multiple sclerosis, encephalitis, and some muscular dystrophies. Acute head trauma, a common reason for neuroradiologic investigation, may cause unconsciousness, which precludes taking an adequate history. In such instances, the possibility of a full stomach, cervical spine injury, and multiple organ damage must always be considered.

B. Choice of technique. Although most neurodiagnostic procedures are to some degree invasive and may involve considerable discomfort, none is so traumatic or painful as to make general anesthesia mandatory. These procedures require the patient's total immobility, but in most instances, discomfort can be mitigated and immobility produced by vocal encouragement and sedation. In some cases the patient will not or cannot adequately cooperate, a situation most commonly found in children who do not comprehend what the procedure involves. An adult may be unable to cooperate because of either fear or disease-related impairment of cerebral function (as in the case of retarded or semicomatose patients). In some instances, general anesthesia with endotracheal intubation, by providing complete airway control and avoiding hypoxia and hypercapnia, may be preferable to the less predictable effects of intravenous sedatives, especially for poor-risk patients.

In most hospitals, radiology suites have not been designed as anesthetizing locations. Anesthetic apparatus must often compete for space with x-ray machines and, in general, conditions are less than optimal. It is essential, however, not to compromise the fundamental requirements of an adequate anesthetic machine and all equipment necessary for administering a general anesthetic and for cardiopulmonary resuscitation. Suction should be available, and monitoring capabilities should be equivalent to the general operating room. Electrocardiographic (ECG) monitoring is particularly important because, in the presence of controlled ventilation, an arrhythmia may be the earliest sign of pressure on the brainstem. In addition, a defibrillator should be immediately available. This equipment should also be available when sedation is used because of the possibility that general anesthesia may be needed and, more important, because of the potential for complications from the diagnostic procedure.

II. CT. CT has become the most widely used neuroradiologic procedure. The quality and detail of the images produced by this noninvasive combination of x-ray and computer instrumentation, coupled with almost total safety, are unparalleled by older, more conventional techniques.

A. Basic considerations

1. Technical facts. A CT scan provides tomographic images of serial sections through the head. Each image is produced by computer integration of measurements of x-ray absorption obtained by scanning the periphery of the head. The differences in the radiation absorption coefficient between different normal tissues and between normal and abnormal tissues enable the computer to separate these tissues. The image of the brain structures is generated by feeding the relative absorption values (CT numbers) into a cathode ray tube, the brightness of the image being proportional to the absorption value. In addition to being displayed on the cathode ray tube, the image may be obtained on x-ray film, photographed with an instant camera, or transferred to a magnetic disc for permanent storage.

2. **Procedure.** For scanning of the brain, the patient lies on a table with his or her head inside a rotating gantry (a large square "donut" with a hole in the center, the periphery of which contains the x-ray source, detectors, and associated electronics). In old scanners, the head was encased in a water jacket to eliminate computer artifacts at the scalp level. The water jacket is no longer necessary in new scanners, and the patient's head is simply immobilized with a Velcro belt applied across the forehead. One rotation of the gantry produces one axial slice or "cut." A series of cuts is made; the usual interval is 8 mm but can be larger or smaller, depending on the particular diagnostic information sought. The duration of the procedure reflects the sophistication of the scanner. The first-generation scanners took 4 ½ minutes per cut, whereas the newest scanners take only 2 to 4 seconds per cut. A complete examination of the head usually consists of about 8 cuts. The whole procedure may be repeated after rapid intravenous infusion of contrast medium if contrast enhancement is indicated.

3. **Complications.** Since CT is noninvasive, there are no complications associated with its performance per se. However, examination in the coronal projection may occasionally require extreme degrees of head positioning, which may either compromise blood flow to the brain or obstruct the airway (by possible kinking of the endotracheal tube). Many of the CT body scanners can tilt on their axis, eliminating these extremes of positioning with their associated problems. When contrast medium is injected intravenously, its attendant complications are also possible (see sec. **VIII**).

4. **Exposure of personnel to radiation.** It has been estimated that anesthesia personnel standing behind a lead screen at the side of a patient undergoing CT scanning will receive a skin dose of 1 to 2 mrad/hr [1]. This level would make it feasible, if necessary, to participate in a full daily schedule without receiving excessive exposure to radiation.

B. **Management**

1. **Sedation.** Most adults and older children require no medication for a CT scan. Young children may respond well to intramuscular or peroral sedation. Pentobarbital, 6 mg/kg IM in children weighing up to 15 kg and 5 mg/kg IM in children weighing more than 15 kg, may be used. The maximum recommended dose is 200 mg given 20 to 30 minutes before the examination. A mixture contain-

ing meperidine hydrochloride (Demerol) 25 mg, chlorpromazine (Thorazine) 6.25 mg, and promethazine hydrochloride (Phenergan) 6.25 mg in each milliliter has also been suggested. The dose is 1 ml/10 to 12 kg IM with a maximum dose of 2 ml given 10 to 20 minutes before the procedure. This "cocktail" has been associated with respiratory depression [7]. Rectal barbiturates (e.g., methohexital, 25 mg/kg) have been used successfully for relatively short procedures (20-25 minutes). Disoriented or very nervous adults may be given sedative doses of diazepam (2.5-mg increments IV) or, more recently, midazolam in 0.5- to 1.0-mg increments IV and/or small doses of a short-acting narcotic such as fentanyl (0.025-mg increments IV); the usual precautions against respiratory depression must be observed. Special care must be taken when giving sedatives to patients who have head injury or suspected increased ICP. In these cases, it may be preferable to administer general anesthesia with controlled ventilation.

2. **General anesthesia.** General anesthesia may be indicated in situations in which sedation is either hazardous or ineffective (e.g., combativeness or cardiovascular instability). It may also be preferable when there are potential airway problems or when control of ICP is critical. As the patient's head is inaccessible during the CT scan, it is mandatory to place an endotracheal tube, no matter what the reason for using general anesthesia. The scan itself demands only that the patient remain motionless and tolerate the endotracheal tube. Thus, if spontaneous ventilation is acceptable, topical anesthesia (4% lidocaine) to the larynx may be helpful. When ICP is increased, controlled ventilation is essential. When the patient has intracranial hypertension, total flaccidity should be produced before intubation, either with succinylcholine, 1.5 mg/kg, after pretreatment with tubocurarine, 3 mg, or with a nondepolarizing relaxant such as vecuronium or atracurium in accepted intubating dosage. Monitoring of neuromuscular blockade with a peripheral nerve stimulator before intubation is helpful.

   a. **Induction of anesthesia** is performed with thiopental. Anesthesia is maintained with nitrous oxide (N_2O), oxygen, small doses of narcotics, and muscle relaxants. When an inhalation induction is necessary, the lowest concentration permitting insertion of an intravenous cannula should be used; hyperventilation should be instituted as soon as possible. Ketamine increases cerebral blood flow (CBF) and ICP and does not predictably prevent the patient from moving. It is therefore not advocated.

   b. **Control of temperature** is especially important because many of the patients are babies or small children. Scanner rooms are maintained at cool temperatures (approximately 65°F) to avoid artifacts and damage to the circuits (x-ray equipment is heat sensitive). With early scanners, it was possible to fill the water bag surrounding the head with warm water. Because the water bag is not used with the new machines, the use of standard techniques such as heating lamps and warmed intravenous solutions may be necessary.

III. MRI. MRI is a new imaging modality that does not use ionizing radiation, depending rather on magnetic fields and radiofrequency (RF) pulses for the production of its images. Its use is spreading rapidly and although it is by no means as ubiquitous as the CT scanner, there is little doubt that it will become so. Although MRI produces images similar to those obtained with CT, it has certain advantages over this technique. For example, MRI has greatly increased sensitivity in the diagnosis of diseases involving the white matter of the brain, thus making possible the in vivo diagnosis of multiple sclerosis. MRI images can be displayed in sagittal, coronal, or axial planes without reliance on reconstruction. There is no dental or bony artifact, facilitating visualization of the posterior fossa, and no absolute requirement for intravenous contrast.

Two types of magnets are in use: resistive magnets, which can be turned off but that then require several hours to re-establish a stable field, and super conductors, which cannot be turned off. As one type cannot be turned off and as it may be predicted that nothing short of imminent disaster will induce the radiologist to turn off the other, the anesthesiologist will do well to learn to cope with whatever problems may ensue in the continued presence of the magnetic field.

Ferromagnetic objects within the range of the magnet pose a considerable hazard, and they may be moved with remarkable speed. In the less dangerous but still annoying category, credit cards may be erased, as may magnetic storage material, and damage may be done to some wristwatches. Laryngoscopes may be difficult to use within range of the magnet. It has been shown, however, that it is not the laryngoscope but the battery that is the source of magnetic attraction. This problem may be resolved with the use of plastic or paper-coated batteries. Patients who have implanted metal must be viewed with caution. A magnetic clip on an intracranial aneurysm may contraindicate this form of examination lest it be moved. Demand pacemakers may be inhibited by induced currents in the leads. A patient who has a total hip prosthesis may be scanned until or unless he or she complains of heat at the site of the prosthesis.

When the anesthesiologist is uncertain of the ferromagnetic properties of any given object, he or she may gauge this by approaching the magnet gradually while controlling the object by hand. The magnetic pull can then be estimated directly.

The machine itself is typically six feet in length, but with a very small internal diameter. This renders the patient extremely inaccessible, and, in addition, is potentially claustrophobic. The nature of the MRI scanner produces two sets of problems for the anesthesiologist. The powerful magnet precludes the use of ferromagnetic substances in anesthesia equipment, and the intermittent RF signals used during imaging interfere with many pieces of monitoring equipment.

Like CT, MRI is basically atraumatic, but, also as with CT, sedation or anesthesia may be required. MRI, however, presents greater difficulties than CT. On the positive side, as there is no radiation, the anesthesiologist may be present within the imaging room after divestment of credit cards, watches, ect. Although there is still relatively little available in the literature, guidelines are beginning to appear.

A. Monitoring. Heart tones may be monitored with a nonmetal chest piece or an esophageal stethoscope. In either event, this is made more difficult by the MRI-generated noise [12].

Blood pressure can be measured using ordinary cuffs and long pressure tubing without metal connections [9]. An ordinary blood pressure dial can be used if it is kept away from the magnet. Alternatively, the use of an automated blood pressure device ("Dynamap"), again without metal connectors, has been described. Heart rate and regularity can be observed with a vascular Doppler. The probe may be placed over the radial or the dorsalis pedis artery. Reports of the effects of a pulse oximeter on image degradation have varied, so that the anesthesiologist should test this for each specific scanner. The use of a long probe lead, enabling the oximeter to be distanced from the magnet, may be helpful, or it may be necessary to turn off the oximeter during actual imaging [3]. In either event, valuable information may be obtained either on a continuous or intermittent basis.

Respiratory monitoring may be difficult, especially during sedation without endotracheal intubation. Suggested techniques include monitoring respiratory sounds via a precordial stethoscope, which may be difficult because of the scanner-induced noise. Capnography may be used with the sampling tube taped beside the mouth or nostril. Long tubing and high-power suction should be used. Although the value of the CO_2 reading may not reflect the actual end-tidal CO_2, the changes give an indication of respiratory rate. Apnea alarm mattresses and a pneumatic bellows have also been used. The latter is linked to a pressure-sensitive piezo-electric crystal outside the magnet room. Some scanners utilize a pneumatic bellows connected via the machine's computer to an outside monitor.

ECG monitoring is also a problem. Any wires within the unit will interfere with the image. Some MRI units have a wireless ECG that gives good tracings in the absence of an RF signal from the unit. During the RF pulses, there may be some distortion of the ECG tracing. Telemetric ECG systems have also been described [9]. More sophisticated intra-arterial pressure monitoring has also been described with the transducers within the MRI chamber coupled to a monitor located outside the magnet room [2].

B. Anesthetic management. Where sedative techniques are considered applicable, these are utilized at the discretion of the anesthesiologist. Rectal methohexital has proved useful in small children, and, presumably, techniques such as those described for CT scanning could be used. Monitoring, particularly respiratory monitoring as described above, is of great importance and any problem or suspicion of problem mandates immediate removal from the scanner.

Where general anesthesia is deemed necessary endotracheal intubation is essential, and the same considerations apply as for CT. Anesthesia is commonly induced in an adjoining room, and the patient is brought into the scanning room after stabilization. The lack of vertical space within the unit makes a prebent (RAE) tube very helpful. Some form of Mapleson D device with very long delivery tubing and either a wall source of gases or a remotely placed anesthetic machine are commonly used. There must also be long breathing tubing between the patient and the bag so that this is outside the scanner and available to the anesthesiologist. If an anesthetic machine is used in the scanning room, the cylinders should be of aluminum to avoid interference with the MRI signal. Anesthesia is maintained with intravenous drugs, thiopental, narcotics, and muscle relaxants if ventilation is to be controlled. Spontaneous respiration is one of the best forms of monitoring available but may be difficult to maintain. A ventilator (225/SIMVr ventilator, "MRI compatible," Monaghan Medical Corp., Plattsburg, NY) has been specifically designed with MRI in mind and has been used successfully [11]. It is usually situated at the foot of the magnet. It is powered by high-pressure oxygen delivered either by a wall source or from large cylinders outside the imaging suite. This is of particular value for poor-risk patients, especially when combined with some of the sophisticated monitoring described previously.

IV. Angiography. CT has reduced the use of angiography in neurodiagnosis. Unlike pneumoencephalography, however, angiography is still used fairly frequently to delineate the vasculature of either the brain or the spinal cord. Technical advances in recent years include the use of catheter techniques for selective angiography and of contrast media that are less toxic and cause less discomfort. The introduction of catheters through the femoral and axillary arteries has virtually replaced the direct puncture of the common carotid artery. In addition to eliminating the hazards of puncturing the common carotid artery, the use of catheters allows the selective study of the posterior circulation. The injection of contrast into the internal carotid artery eliminates facial discomfort in the distribution of the external carotid artery, which was one of the main subjective complaints associated with common carotid injection. Patients may still, however, experience a burning sensation behind the eye or a flash of light. The use of newer low ionic (Hexabrix) and nonionic contrast material, iopamidol and iohexol (Omnipaque), has even further reduced this discomfort.

Accompanying the reduction in discomfort has been a reduction in the number of patients requiring general anesthesia. The anesthesiologist may be asked, however, to administer sedative medications and to monitor the patient's vital signs and neurologic function. It is therefore important to understand the risks and problems associated with angiographic techniques.

A. Spinal cord angiography. Angiography of the spinal cord, pioneered by Djindjian in France, virtually always involves selective studies and subtraction techniques. Many of the patients have damage to the cord already. The possibility of further spinal cord damage induced by the injection of contrast is a significant hazard. Although the examination may be prolonged and therefore uncomfortable, it is usually performed without general anesthesia so the patient's neurologic status can be assessed after each injection of contrast medium. Paroxysmal contractions of the lower limbs (which may occur when dye is injected into the anterior spinal artery) respond to the direct injection of diazepam, 5 mg, through the angiography catheter.

B. Complications. Arterial puncture and catheterization may produce arterial spasm, hematoma, or embolization of arteriosclerotic plaques or thrombi forming at the tip of the catheter. Injection into the wall of the vessel may cause either subintimal dissection or occlusion of the vessel. The contrast media, all of which are iodine-containing salts, produce vasodilatation that in turn causes burning discomfort in the area supplied by the vessels injected. The degree of vasodilatation is affected by the osmolality of the contrast medium. Solutions of low osmolality are becoming available. Those currently in common use, such as meglumine iothalamate (Conray), are highly ionized with resultant high osmolality.

Serious neurologic complications from contrast media include dizziness, convulsions, unconsciousness, hemiplegia, blindness, and aphasia. These effects are related to the hyperosmolality of the contrast medium, which may temporarily impair the blood-brain barrier and allow the medium access to brain cells. The damage may also be caused by hypoxic microvascular damage. The concentration of the agent appears to be the critical factor.

Premonitory signs such as slurring of speech or confusion should suggest the need for termination of the procedure. For more serious problems (e.g., hemiplegia, aphasia, or blindness) that do not resolve swiftly after discontinuation of the procedure, a number of therapies have been recommended, including the use of steroids and low molecular weight dextran and the elevation of systemic blood pressure by vasopressors to restore blood flow to the areas that have presumably become ischemic.

Allergic reactions to contrast media include itching nose, sneezing, and conjunctival swelling; mild cardiovascular changes such as bradycardia or tachycardia; and marked hypotension and arrhythmias (see sec. **VIII**). Respiratory problems include bronchospasm, laryngeal edema, and respiratory arrest. Pulmonary edema, congestive heart failure, and even cardiac arrest may occur.

C. Anesthetic management

1. Sedation. Sedation has a number of advantages over general anesthesia for angiography. These advantages may be lost, however, if the patient becomes confused or unconscious from the drugs administered. For this reason the drugs should be selected with care and given in small incremental intravenous doses. The use of a short-acting narcotic such as fentanyl may ameliorate some of the discomfort and provide some mood elevation, but care should be taken to avoid respiratory depression. The addition of diazepam in incremental doses may also be valuable but the achievement of hypnosis may be quite unpredictable with this combination. Early experience with midazolam suggests that it may have some advantages over diazepam but dosage must be discrete. The patient's level of consciousness should therefore be ascertained regularly. The phenothiazines, although effective sedatives, should not be used in these cases because of their ability to lower the convulsive threshold. Droperidol rarely produces unconsciousness in modest doses and, when combined with a narcotic, may be valuable; its ability to produce Parkinson-like central nervous system symptoms should be kept in mind.

2. General anesthesia. General anesthesia for angiography is more comfortable for the patient and ensures complete immobility during x-ray exposures. Some European radiologists believe that general anesthesia is essential where subtraction techniques* are used, but in the United States, general anesthesia is rarely requested to improve the radiologic technique. General anesthesia may be necessary, however, for uncooperative patients and for young children.

In planning the anesthetic technique, some factors should be considered. If hyperventilation is used to produce a moderate reduction in arterial carbon dioxide tension ($[PaCO_2]$ 30–35 mmHg), a greater concentration of the contrast medium will be

---

* A radiologic process in which the shadows of the bony skeleton are "subtracted" from the final x-ray picture, leaving the vascular shadows intact. It requires obtaining a series of identical films before and after the injection of dye.

produced by constricting cerebral vessels and showing cerebral circulation. This improvement in the clarity of the film is of particular value in children whose fast cerebral circulation times make it difficult to obtain good angiograms. Rapid-filming techniques have made hyperventilation a refinement rather than a necessity, however. Hyperventilation has also been shown to improve the quality of angiograms in patients who have brain tumors because it provokes intracerebral steal. In contrast, the cerebral vasodilatation induced by the inhalation drugs may produce the opposite effect. If these drugs are necessary, hyperventilation should be established before their introduction and continued during the study. However, a technique using thiopental, muscle relaxant, N_2O/O_2, and controlled ventilation, with or without additional narcotics, is usually satisfactory.

V. Myelography. It is uncommon for the anesthesiologist to be involved in myelography, except for studies in children who may not cooperate during the spinal puncture and required positioning. Since the patient is prone, almost any anesthetic technique that ensures protection of the airway may be used. The traditional contrast agents were oily solutions. Newer water-soluble agents give better definition in the myelogram and do not lead to arachnoiditis. The introduction of these water-soluble agents has produced greater involvement on the part of the anesthesiologist, however, because of the absorption of the agent from the cerebrospinal fluid (CSF) and the potential for allergic response. For example, pharmacokinetic studies of metrizamide, the first agent to become widely used, revealed appearance of the agent in the blood within approximately 15 minutes and a peak at about two hours. After the use of metrizamide, headache occurred in 21 to 62% of patients, and nausea in 13 to 39%. Most reactions occurred six hours after the injection of material into the lumbar sac, reflecting a mean time for peak intracranial concentration. Metrizamide also caused mental changes including confusion, disorientation, nightmares, hallucinations, hyperacusis, lightheadedness, depression, dysphasia, and anxiety, as well as convulsions presumably from cortical irritation. Seizures were more likely to occur with concomitant use of drugs that lower the epileptogenic threshold (e.g., phenothiazines, monoamine oxidase [MAO] inhibitors, and alcohol) and in patients who had a seizure disorder.

The newer nonionic contrast media (iohexol and iopamidol) have greatly reduced the incidence of these side effects and virtually eliminated metrizamide from practice. Nevertheless, if general anesthesia is required during myelography with these agents, the use of ketamine should probably be avoided because of its associated electroencephalogram (EEG) changes. Similarly, good hydration before and after the study, as recommended for metrizamide myelography, should be maintained. The semierect position after the examination is also important to limit the rostral spread of the contrast agent, thus reducing the possibility of cortical effects.

VI. Pneumoencephalography. This diagnostic procedure is now seldom performed in centers possessing CT scanners. For this reason, only an abbreviated description of anesthetic management will be given, and readers are referred to larger texts for greater detail [14]. In the conscious patient, pneumoencephalography may cause headache and nausea, as well as many cardiovascular complications. The least common but most serious complications are air embolus or brainstem herniation. Intravenous sedation using diazepam in 2.5-mg increments or perhaps midazolam in 1-mg increments plus a narcotic such as fentanyl in 0.025-mg increments may be used to mitigate the headache, with the addition of droperidol in 2.5-mg increments for nausea. Cardiovascular side effects should be treated symptomatically with appropriate drugs. If general anesthesia is preferred, nitrous oxide should be avoided as it will diffuse into the air in the ventricles. A technique involving thiopental, muscle relaxants, and controlled ventilation, with or without the addition of small doses of narcotic, is usually satisfactory. Due care must be given to control the endotracheal tube during the numerous positional changes and cardiovascular complications.

VII. Therapeutic embolization. The expertise obtained by the radiologist during selective angiography has now been applied to producing selective occlusion of extracranial and intracranial vessels to obliterate feeding arteries of arterial venous malformations, to close carotid-cavernous sinus fistulas, or to decrease the vascularity of tumors. Embolization may be either an adjunct to or a substitute for surgery. Occlusion may be produced by particulate emboli (e.g., absorbable gelatin sponge [Gelfoam]), by polymerizing agents (glue), or by detachable balloons.

   A. Complications. Each technique is associated with problems: vessels may be occluded inadvertently; arterial hemorrhage may occur after injury to the vessel wall by a balloon. In addition, as selective angiography is part of each technique, the possibility of a reaction to the contrast medium is always present.

   B. Management

   1. Sedation. It is essential that the diagnosis of neurologic complications be made immediately. The procedures are therefore preferably performed without general anesthesia. Because the procedures are potentially hazardous and may be prolonged, uncomfortable, and, at some stages, even painful, the involvement of the anesthesiologist is essential to ensure adequate monitoring, cooperation, and comfort. Modest doses of neuroleptic drugs (droperidol, 0.1 mg/kg; fentanyl, 0.002 mg/kg) may be used, either alone or as an adjunct to the use of hypnotic suggestion to produce the necessary conditions. Constant monitoring is essential with particular attention to level of consciousness, motor strength, respiratory and cardiac rhythms, and blood pressure. If signs suggestive of cerebral ischemia appear (e.g., hemiplegia, slurred speech, altered level of consciousness, or aphasia), the procedure should be discontinued immediately. Other measures to promote CBF include the use of low molecular weight dextran and maintenance of blood pressure in the high normal range, using pressors if necessary, in an effort to maintain cerebral perfusion.

2. **General anesthesia.** General anesthesia is required for infants and children. It is important to prevent movement during the procedure, but consciousness should be restored as soon as possible so that a neurologic evaluation may be carried out. The most practical method of achieving these aims involves the use of N_2O/O_2, a muscle relaxant, and controlled ventilation. Whether thiopental or an inhalation drug is used for induction will depend on the availability of suitable veins and the cooperation of the patient. Normocapnia or modest hypocapnia should be maintained; hypocapnia is necessary when inhalation drugs are used. Sudden changes in vital signs should be correlated with the radiologist's activity. The presence of hypertension and bradycardia should raise concern about a possible intracranial hemorrhage.

VIII. Adverse reactions to contrast media. Reactions to intravascularly administered contrast media vary from pruritus, mild rashes, and vasomotor phenomena (flushing, burning) on injection to anaphylactic reactions including dyspnea, wheezing, syncope, and cardiovascular collapse. Although these reactions are immediate in onset and mimic IgE-mediated allergic responses, they most likely result from the nonimmunologic release of histamine and other vasoactive mediators from mast cells and basophils [8]. Pulmonary function studies have shown reduction in the peak flow rate and FEV_1 after contrast administration in normal patients. This effect is more pronounced in patients who have a history of allergies. The mildest of these reactions require little, if any, treatment other than reassurance, whereas the most severe of these reactions are truly life-threatening and necessitate immediate treatment.

A. **Basic considerations**

1. **Incidence.** In a prospective study reported by the Committee on Contrast Media of the International Society of Radiology in 1975 [10], there was a 2.33% incidence of nonfatal reactions and 4 fatal reactions in 27,628 vascular studies. As many as 500 deaths occur in the United States each year [5]. Repeat studies in patients who have had a previous untoward response were associated with a threefold increase in reactions as compared to the general population.

2. **Predictive tests.** There are no generally accepted predictive tests. Intradermal testing is unreliable [13] and has been virtually aban-

doned. The use of small intravenous doses of contrast before the procedure is not a sure method of detection and has been associated with some deaths.

B. Management

1. Prophylaxis. Patients who have either allergies or a history of reaction to intravascularly administered contrast media should be evaluated by an allergist and medicated with corticosteriods and antihistamines for 36 to 48 hours before the proposed injection of contrast [15]. A suggested regimen consists of prednisone, 25 mg q.i.d., and either hydroxyzine, 25 mg, or diphenhydramine (Benadryl), 50 mg q.i.d., starting two days before injection of contrast and continued for 24 hours after the investigation [6]. In addition, diazepam, 10 mg, is given intramuscularly 30 minutes before the patient comes to the x-ray department; diphenhydramine, 50 mg, is given intravenously immediately before the examination. More recently, ephedrine sulfate, 25 mg orally one hour prior, has been added to the prednisone, diphenhydramine regime with a reported further reduction in reaction rate [4]. In this same report, the results suggested that an H_2 blocker (cimetidine) might actually worsen rather than improve results. It is essential to be prepared for all degrees of resuscitation.

2. Treatment. Rashes or mild vasomotor reactions require little except reassurance and intravenous diphenhydramine. A severe anaphylactic reaction, including respiratory distress from bronchospasm or laryngeal edema, severe hypotension, or syncope, may be treated with epinephrine 1 : 1000 subcutaneously or intravenously in doses of 0.3 to 0.5 ml in an adult. Bronchospasm may respond to aminophylline, terbutaline (0.25 mg subcutaneously), or nebulized isoproterenol. Intravenous fluids and pressors will be necessary to treat hypotension. Arrhythmias should be controlled with antiarrhythmic drugs, cardioversion, or both. Corticosteroids may be required in pharmacologic doses. Endotracheal intubation with positive pressure ventilation may be necessary, as well as cardipulmonary resuscitation if cardiac arrest occurs.

References

1. Aidinis, S. J., Zimmerman, R. A., Shapiro, H. M., et al. Anesthesia for brain computer tomography. *Anesthesiology* 44:420, 1976.
2. Barnett, G. H., Ropper, A. H., and Johnson, K. A. Physiological support and monitoring of critically ill patients during magnetic resonance imaging. *J. Neurosurg.* 68:246, 1988.
3. Goudsouzian, N. Monitoring for MRI. APSF Newsletter, December 1987.
4. Greenberger, P. A., Patterson, R., and Tapio, C. M. Prophylaxis against repeated radiocontrast media reactions in 857 Cases. *Arch. Intern. Med.* 145:2197, 1985.
5. Lieberman, P., Siegle, R. L., and Taylor, W. W. Anaphylactoid reactions to iodinated contrast material. *J. Allergy Clin. Immunol.* 62:174, 1980.

6. Miller, W. L., Doppman, J. L., and Kaplan, A. P. Renal arteriography following systemic reaction to contrast material. *J. Allergy Clin. Immunol.* 56:291, 1975.
7. Mitchell, A. A., Louik, C., Lacouture, P., et al. Risks to children from computed tomographic scan premedication. *J.A.M.A.* 247:2385, 1982.
8. Olin, T. Adverse reactions to intravascularly administered contrast media. *Acta Radiol. (Diagn.) (Stockh.)* 27:257, 1986.
9. Roth, J. L., Nugent, M., Gray, J. E., et al. Patient monitoring during magnetic resonance imaging. *Anesthesiology* 62:80, 1985.
10. Shehadi, W. H. Adverse reactions to intravascularly administered contrast media: A comprehensive study based on a prospective survey. *Am. J. Roentgenol. Radium Ther. Nucl. Med.* 124:145, 1975.
11. Smith, D. S., Askey, P., Young, M. L., et al. Anesthetic management of acutely ill patients during magnetic resonance imaging. *Anesthesiology* 65:710, 1986.
12. Weston, G., Strunin, L., and Amundson, G. M. Imaging for anaesthetists: A review of the methods and anaesthetic implications of diagnostic imaging techniques. *Can. Anaesth. Soc. J.* 32:552, 1985.
13. Witten, D., Hirsch, F. D., and Hartman, G. W. Acute reactions to urographic contrast medium. Incidence, clinical characteristics, and relationship to history of hypersensitivity states. *Am. J. Roentgenol.* 119:832, 1973.
14. Wolfson, B., and Hetrick, W. D. Anesthesia for Neuroradiologic Procedures. In J. E. Cottrell and H. Turndorf (Eds.), *Anesthesia and Neurosurgery.* St. Louis: Mosby, 1986. Pp. 105–107.
15. Zweiman, B., Mishkin, M. M., and Hildreth, E. A. An approach to the performance of contrast studies in contrast material-reactive persons. *Ann. Intern. Med.* 83:159, 1975.

Index

Index